Neural Mechanisms
of Behavior in
the Pigeon

Neural Mechanisms of Behavior in the Pigeon

Edited by

A. M. Granda
and
J. H. Maxwell

University of Delaware
Newark, Delaware

Plenum Press · New York and London

Library of Congress Cataloging in Publication Data

Main entry under title:

Neural mechanisms of behavior in the pigeon.

Includes bibliographies and index.
1. Vision — Congresses. 2. Neuropsychology — Congresses. 3. Nervous system — Congresses. 4. Pigeons — Behavior — Congresses. 5. Pigeons — Congresses. I. Granda, A. M. II. Maxwell, J. H.
QP474.N46   598.6'5   78-24064
ISBN 0-306-40096-0

© 1979 Plenum Press, New York
A Division of Plenum Publishing Corporation
227 West 17th Street, New York, N.Y. 10011

Printed in the United States of America

To

ARNOLD LEROY LIPPERT

who, as Dean of the Graduate School at the University of Delaware, provided encouragement, funds and steady support for the creation of an Institute for Neuroscience and Behavior, and for this Conference; this dedication is made on the occasion of his retirement

and

LORRIN ANDREWS RIGGS

who trained several of us gathered here, on the eve of his retirement from Brown University; this dedication is made for his deep interest in things visual, and for the tools to appreciate the endless fascination of eye and brain.

Contributors

PATRICIA M. BLOUGH
Department of Psychology
Brown University
Providence, Rhode Island

R. L. BOORD
School of Life and Health Sciences
  and Institute for Neuroscience
  and Behavior
University of Delaware
Newark, Delaware

J. K. BOWMAKER
MRC Vision Unit
Centre for Research on Perception
  and Cognition
University of Sussex
Falmer, Brighton, East Sussex,
  England
Present address: Department of
  Zoology and Comparative
  Physiology
Queen Mary College
London, England

W. J. CROSSLAND
Department of Anatomy
Wayne State University School of
  Medicine
Detroit, Michigan

JUAN D. DELIUS
Psychologisches Institut
Ruhr-Universität
Bochum, West Germany

JACKY EMMERTON
Psychologisches Institut
Ruhr-Universität
Bochum, West Germany

KATHERINE V. FITE
Department of Psychology
University of Massachusetts
Amherst, Massachusetts

H. GIOANNI
Laboratoire de Psychophysiologie
  Sensorielle
Université Pierre et Marie Curie
Paris, France

VIRGIL A. GRAF
Department of Psychology
Dartmouth College
Hanover, New Hampshire

A. M. GRANDA
Institute for Neuroscience and
  Behavior
University of Delaware
Newark, Delaware

O. HARDY
Laboratoire de Psychophysiologie
  Sensorielle
Université Pierre et Marie Curie
Paris, France

D. JASSIK-GERSCHENFELD
Laboratoire de Psychophysiologie
  Sensorielle
Université Pierre et Marie Curie
Paris, France

H. J. KARTEN
Departments of Psychiatry and
  Behavioral Science and
  Anatomical Sciences
Health Sciences Center-School of
  Medicine
State University of New York
Stony Brook, New York

WILLIAM T. KEETON
Section of Neurobiology and
  Behavior
Cornell University
Ithaca, New York

MELVIN L. KREITHEN
Division of Biological Sciences
Langmuir Laboratory
Cornell University
Ithaca, New York

MEL LOCKHART
Department of Psychology
Lafayette College
Easton, Pennsylvania
Present address: Jules Stein Eye
  Institute
University of California at Los
  Angeles
Los Angeles, California

GRAHAM R. MARTIN
Laboratory of Experimental
  Psychology
University of Sussex
Falmer, Brighton, Sussex, England
and Department of Extramural
  Studies
University of Birmingham
Birmingham, England

J. H. MAXWELL
Institute for Neuroscience and
  Behavior
University of Delaware
Newark, Delaware

D. MICELI
Laboratoire de Psychophysiologie
  Sensorielle
Université Pierre et Marie Curie
Paris, France

PATRICK MULVANNY
Department of Psychology
University of Maryland
College Park, Maryland
Present address: Department of
  Psychology
Ursinus College
Collegeville, Pennsylvania

W. R. A. MUNTZ
Laboratory of Experimental
  Psychology
University of Sussex
Falmer, Brighton, Sussex, England

J. PEYRICHOUX
Laboratoire de Psychophysiologie
  Sensorielle
Université Pierre et Marie Curie
Paris, France

J. REPÉRANT
Laboratoire de Psychophysiologie
    Sensorielle
Université Pierre et Marie Curie
Paris, France

A. M. REVZIN
Neuropharmacology Research Unit
Aviation Toxicology Laboratory
Civil Aeromedical Institute
Federal Aviation Administration
Oklahoma City, Oklahoma

JACQUES SERVIÈRE
Laboratoire de Psychophysiologie
    Sensorielle
Université de Paris VI
Paris, France

J. TEULON
Laboratoire de Psychophysiologie
    Sensorielle
Université Pierre et Marie Curie
Paris, France

JOSH WALLMAN
Biology Department, City College
City University of New York
New York, New York

ANTHONY A. WRIGHT
The University of Texas Health
    Science Center at Houston
Graduate School of Biomedical
    Sciences
Houston, Texas

STEPHEN YAZULLA
Department of Biology
State University of New York
Stony Brook, New York

Preface

This book contains the proceedings of an International Conference held at the University of Delaware in June 1977. A group composed of anatomists, ethologists, natural historians, physiologists, psychologists, and zoologists gathered to synthesize a broad range of phenomena related to the neural bases of overt behavior in a single animal, the pigeon. The topics ranged from extremely complex behaviors to the microanatomies of particular tissues. The emphasis was on vision and visually mediated behaviors as befits an animal so dependent on the sense of sight for its information on external conditions.

The beginning papers assembled here are given over to the description and analysis of large behavioral complexes. The subtleties of the pigeon navigational system are described along with several of the novel, often redundant, sensory cues that are integrated into a navigational "map." Behavioral results describing visual acuity and the detection of both polarized and short-wavelength light are discussed in relation to regional specializations in the retina, the red and yellow visual fields. There are papers that describe imaginative behavioral experiments involving color, pattern, and time perception in order to illustrate the high levels of information processing and sensory discrimination attainable by pigeons.

Subsequent papers look more closely at neural complexes governing vision. The functional properties of color processing, motion detection, directional and orientational selectivity, and center–surround receptive field relationships are found to differ for two major visual pathways to the telencephalon, the tectofugal and thalamofugal systems. Subdivisions within each pathway have their own functional characteristics defined in part by single cell recordings in the thalamus and Wulst.

Later papers increase the resolution of the analysis by looking at the tissues themselves. Much of that analysis is in the retina, for anatomical evidence suggests it plays a critical role in the early processing of visual information. It may be that some functional characteristics, e.g., directional selectivity seen in particular cells in central brain structures, have their origin in the interaction of retinal cells.

The complex and often controversial question of color processing in pigeon is addressed from several points of view. In particular, the brightly colored retinal oil droplets and the functional significance of their absorbances and distributions are pursued by several authors.

Finally, detailed anatomical views of the major visual networks are presented, along with the integration of that anatomy into an understanding of single behaviors. There is also a description of the vestibular apparatus, for that system provides the spatial platform upon which vision operates.

In the broadest sense then, the papers are arranged in an order of increased resolution of the governing thesis: the neural bases of behavior in the pigeon.

As editors, we thank the contributors for their fine papers. We believe them to be in large measure state-of-knowledge reports on the various subjects discussed. We thank the Institute for Neuroscience and the Graduate School of the University of Delaware for hosting and supporting the Conference. We are grateful to the publishing staff at Plenum Publishing Corporation for dealing with our desires in an understanding and helpful way. We are also deeply indebted to Carolina Groot, for her skillful help in assembling manuscripts, editing copy, and doing those valuable tasks that result in successful publication.

A.M. Granda
J.H. Maxwell

Newark, Delaware

Contents

1

A Brief Introduction to the Taxonomy and Ecology of the Columbiformes (Pigeons and Doves)

GRAHAM R. MARTIN

INTRODUCTION

With one exception, all of the authors in this volume, *Neural Mechanisms of Behavior in the Pigeon*, report experiments concerned with only one species of pigeon, *Columba livia*. It is from this species that the many varieties of domestic pigeon have been bred. A number of authors in this volume mention the relationships among behavior, sensory capacities, sensory physiology, anatomy, and ecology of the species. It is important for the exploration of these relationships that a comparative approach be adopted. This requires that the species under investigation be viewed within the context of its relationships with species of different avian orders, as well as with species of the families and genera of its own order. With possession of such knowledge, the principles of phylogenetic relatedness and ecological convergence may be employed to illuminate the structural and functional questions posed by the investigation of the neural mechanisms of behavior in the pigeon.

Below is a brief résumé of the order Columbiformes. Topics dealt

GRAHAM R. MARTIN • Department of Extramural Studies, University of Birmingham, Birmingham, B15 2TT, England.

with include the taxonomy, distribution, and ecology of these species, with a more detailed summary of the genus *Columba* (the typical pigeons) and emphasis on *Columba livia*. Much that is written here may be found in Goodwin (1967); that text is recommended for detailed references concerning all aspects of the order Columbiformes. More recent articles which update some of the information contained in Goodwin (1967) include Frith (1972, 1977) and Davies (1970).

Class: Aves
Order: Columbiformes
Family: Columbidae
Genus: *Columba*
Species: *Columba livia* (the rock pigeon)

COLUMBIFORMES

The pigeons are a large and successful order of birds comprising approximately 305 species, with many subspecies. They are found in all continents except Antarctica, and they populate the islands of the Pacific and Indian Oceans. (The majority of species are arboreal, living, nesting, and roosting among trees.) However, from the tropics to the temperate regions, they are found in most habitats, and there are both cliff-nesting and ground-nesting species.

Pigeons vary greatly in both size and plumage color. The smallest pigeons are about 150 mm in overall length, while the largest can reach 850 mm. Color varies from the dull and cryptic plumage of *Columba livia* to the vivid colors of the green pigeons (genus *Treron*) found throughout most of the Old World tropics. The diet of pigeons is chiefly either fruits or seeds, but invertebrates are also taken by species specializing in both of these diets.

Although authorities differ, the majority of taxonomists place all pigeons within a single family, the Columbidae, which is usually divided into four subfamilies. These subfamilies are divided into 40 genera (Goodwin, 1967). The three genera *Columba* (the typical pigeons), *Streptopelia* (the turtledoves), and *Aplopelia* (the lemon dove) are considered to form a closely related group containing a total of 67 species. It is probably with species of these genera that cross-species comparisons of physiology, anatomy, and behavior, based on the principle of phylogenetic relatedness, should begin. Goodwin (1967) suggests that the cliff- and cave-dwelling species of these orders, which inhabit rather barren, open country or mountainous districts, have evolved from arboreal forms, and this may be particularly important when considering questions concerning the behavioral biology and sensory ecology of pigeons. A number of species of the northern temperate regions are either migratory or at least travel long distances when weather conditions cut off food supplies. Cross-species comparisons between the sedentary and nonsedentary species may be important in investigations of the sensory systems and related mechanisms associated with homing and migration.

Three main feeding habits are distinguished within the Columbiformes, and these may provide a useful basis for interspecies comparisons based on the principle of ecological convergence. The feeding habits generally recognized are (1) species that normally seek food above ground in trees, shrubs, or vines; (2) species that normally seek food both in trees and on the ground; and (3) species that normally seek food on the ground. The first group is found mainly in the tropics and subtropics, and includes the fruit pigeons and some of the more arboreal species of the genus *Columba*. Species in this category eat such foods as fruits, buds, flowers, and leaves. Many species supplement their diet with invertebrates.

Of particular interest to the behavioral biologists are the display and other social behaviors of the pigeons. These have received considerable study, and the paper of Frith (1977) is the most recent example of a study of this kind where comparisons of display are employed as a means of determining the taxonomic relationships between species.

GENUS *COLUMBA* (TYPICAL PIGEONS)

The genus *Columba* contains approximately 51 species and includes the rock pigeon (*Columba livia*) from which the various varieties (Homer, White Carneaux, etc.) studied by anatomists, physiologists, and behavioral biologists have been produced. Species of this genus show considerable adaptive radiation and vary greatly in both size and plumage color. Typically, they are strong fliers which perch, nest, and roost in trees and on cliffs. They are found throughout the world wherever pigeons exist at all. Some are ground feeders, others feed partly or entirely in trees and shrubs, and Goodwin (1967) suggests that some of the American species appear to fill, or partly fill, the "fruit pigeon niche" in the New World. Hence there is ample scope for cross-species comparisons of species adapted to different ecological niches within this one genus.

COLUMBA LIVIA (ROCK PIGEON)

Five or possibly six subspecies of *Columba livia* are recognized, excluding the domestic or feral pigeon. The nominate subspecies, *Col-*

umba 1. livia, is found in the Faeroes, Shetland, the Hebrides, north-west Scotland, Ireland, the Iberian Peninsula, North West Africa, and the northern shores of the Mediterranean. Other races are found throughout North Africa, the Middle East, and most of the Indian subcontinent. These birds require cliffs, gorges, and caves with sheltered ledges for nesting and roosting, and open country for feeding. *Columba livia* is thought to have evolved in arid or semiarid, nearly treeless regions, and has spread into many of the areas it now occupies subsequent to man's agricultural activities which created suitable feeding grounds for it. It is primarily a seed eater, taking seeds of many kinds; however, it is not exclusively granivorous and takes small snails, molluscs, and some berries.

Along cliffs, it flies close to the face, and this is interpreted as an adaptation to reduce predation by raptorial birds, as is also the "tightness" of small flying flocks.

FERAL PIGEONS

Feral pigeons populate all major cities of the world and are derived from domestic pigeons which have strayed, become lost, or been abandoned by their owners. In many towns, the birds probably stem from dovecote populations bred originally for food. Eight different truly feral varieties, classified according to plumage color, are recognized. Feral pigeons are found from the tropics to north of the Arctic Circle, suggesting a high degree of adaptability. In towns, the sites chosen for roosting and nesting can be considered as manmade equivalents of caves, holes, and cliff ledges.

REFERENCES

Davies, S.: Patterns of inheritance in the bowing display and associated behavior of some *Streptopelia* doves. *Behaviour* **36**:187–214 (1970).
Frith, H. J.: Nesting of the black-banded pigeon and the Australian rock pigeons. *Emu* **72**:13–16 (1972).
Frith, H. J.: Some display postures of Australian pigeons. *Ibis* **119**:167–182 (1977).
Goodwin, D.: *Pigeons and Doves of the World.* British Museum (Nat. Hist.), London, 1967.

2

Pigeon Navigation

WILLIAM T. KEETON

INTRODUCTION

This chapter gives an up-to-date overview of the main thrusts of current research into the mechanism which enables pigeons to find their way home from hundreds of miles away through unfamiliar territory. For a more detailed (although now somewhat dated) review of pigeon homing, the reader is referred to Keeton (1974a). For a review of the related subject of migratory orientation in birds, see Emlen (1975).

THE SUN COMPASS

During the 1950s, Gustav Kramer and his students firmly established that birds can derive compass information from the sun. First, Kramer showed that starlings can be trained to a particular compass direction in a circular cage, with the sun as the only orientational cue (Kramer, 1950, 1951, 1952). Because the sun's azimuth changes throughout the day, from east in the morning to south at noon to west in the afternoon, use of the sun as a compass requires time compensation at an average rate of 15 deg per hour. That starlings can indeed perform such time compensation by coupling their "internal clock" (i.e., circadian rhythm) with their observation of the sun's azimuth was confirmed by Kramer (1952) and by Hoffmann (1954, 1960), again using

WILLIAM T. KEETON • Section of Neurobiology and Behavior, Cornell University, Ithaca, New York 14853. This research was supported by National Science Foundation Grant GB-18905 A02.

circular-cage experiments. Their findings were extended to pigeons by Schmidt-Koenig (1958), who showed that pigeons whose internal clocks have been phase-shifted 6 hr (a quarter of a day) make a 90-deg (a quarter of a circle) error in locating the training direction in a circular cage. Schmidt-Koenig (1958, 1960) then showed that clock shifts have the same effect on the initial departure bearings of pigeons released at distant test sites; birds clock-shifted 6 hr fast depart roughly 90 deg counterclockwise from control birds on normal time, and birds clock-shifted 6 hr slow depart roughly 90 deg clockwise from normal. Numerous other investigators have confirmed Schmidt-Koenig's results (Fig. 1), and clock shifting has become a valuable tool in studying many aspects of pigeon navigation.

Even at release sites less than a mile from their home loft, clock-shifted pigeons depart with deflected bearings (Fig. 1, West), showing no apparent response to the landmarks that should be familiar to them from their daily exercise flights around the loft (Graue, 1963; Alexander, 1975; Keeton, 1974a). In short, the sun compass appears to be a preferred orientational cue for pigeons even when alternative cues are readily available. It seems likely, therefore, that pigeons use their recently discovered ability to detect polarized light (Kreithen and Keeton, 1974a; Delius et al., 1976) as a means of continuing to use the sun compass on partially overcast days when the sun's disk is hidden from view; however, the appropriate field experiments to test this possibility have not yet been performed.

Important as the sun compass may be, it is clearly not sufficient for goal-directed orientation. A compass alone cannot tell an animal where it is or which direction it should choose in order to return home. Recognizing this limitation, Kramer (1953) formulated his so-called map-and-compass model of bird navigation. He suggested that when a pigeon is released at an unfamiliar site it first performs a map step, i.e., it determines its geographic position relative to home and also the theoretical home direction. Once having obtained this positional or "map" information, the bird then performs a compass step, i.e., it uses a compass (e.g., the sun compass) to locate the appropriate direction in which to fly. Kramer's model has proved to be a very powerful tool for predicting the results of many kinds of experiments.

Because the sun compass was the one element in the pigeon navigation system that had been convincingly established by the early 1960s, many investigators came to assume that it was an essential component in the system and that under totally overcast skies pigeons would be unable to orient. However, I was able to show that if pigeons have been given exercise flights around the loft on overcast and rainy

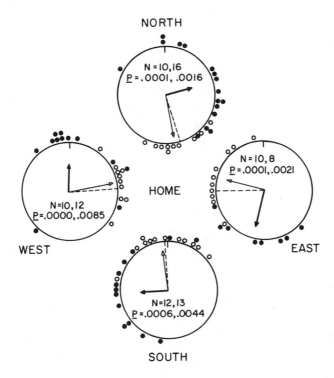

Fig. 1. Effects of 6-hr-fast clock shifts on initial bearings of pigeons released in the four cardinal compass directions from home. In each case, the controls are well oriented homeward, whereas the clock-shifted birds are oriented roughly 90 degrees to the left of the controls. Deflections of bearings by clock shifts are generally seen no matter what the distance of the release site from home; thus the release from West shown here was from a distance of only 0.9 mile, whereas the releases from North, East, and South were from 3.6, 20.8, and 30.7 miles, respectively, yet the results from all four sites are consistent. In each of the four circular diagrams shown here (and in all later figures), the home direction is indicated by a broken line and geographic north is indicated by a small line at the top of the circle. The departure bearing of each bird is shown as a small symbol on the periphery of the large circle; where an experiment utilized two different groups of birds, the bearings of the control birds are indicated by open symbols and the bearings of the experimental birds (in this case, clock-shifted) by solid black symbols. The mean vectors of the two groups are shown as arrows with open and solid heads, respectively; the lengths of the mean vectors are drawn proportional to the tightness of clumping of the bearings—i.e., the longer the vector, the better oriented (less scattered) the sample of bearings. Probabilities (P) of randomness under the Rayleigh test for circular data, together with sample sizes (N), are given inside the circular diagrams; where there are two treatments, the figures given first for P and N apply to the controls, and those given second apply to the experimentals.

days, and preferably also short training flights (3–10 miles) under such conditions, they can then orient accurately homeward when released under total overcast at distant unfamiliar test sites (Keeton, 1969). That they are not detecting the sun through the clouds even though it is not visible to us is shown by the fact that birds clock-shifted 6 hr vanish homeward just like the control birds; there is no sign of the 90-deg deflection such a clock shift would cause on sunny days (Fig. 2). It is clear, then, that when the sun compass is unavailable pigeons can still orient. Hence there must be redundancy in the birds' navigation system; there must be one or more alternative cues that can be used in lieu of the sun compass.

MAGNETIC CUES

Once I realized the existence of this redundancy, I decided to examine the possibility that magnetic cues might provide the backup information needed when the sun compass is not available. Several previous investigators had tried attaching magnets to the birds in order to distort the magnetic field around them, but they had generally reported no observable effects. My own early experiments with small bar magnets glued to the backs of pigeons likewise showed no significant effects when the birds were released at distances of 20–30 miles on sunny days (Fig. 3A). But there usually *was* an effect on totally overcast days—in most of these tests, pigeons wearing magnets vanished randomly whereas control pigeons wearing brass bars of the same size and weight oriented properly homeward (Fig. 3B) (Keeton, 1971, 1972). It appeared, then, that magnetic cues might indeed be a

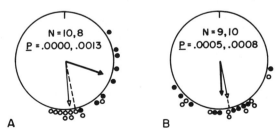

A   B

Fig. 2. Releases of clock-shifted pigeons from 41.1 miles north under sunny skies and under total overcast. A: Experienced pigeons clock-shifted 6 hr fast chose bearings deflected leftward (counterclockwise) from those of the control birds on the sunny day (19 October 1970). B: When similar pigeons were released under total overcast (12 November 1970), there was no significant difference between the mean vectors of the clock-shifted and control birds, both being well oriented homeward.

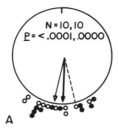 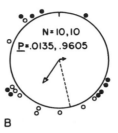

Fig. 3. Effects of bar magnets attached to experienced pigeons released at an unfamiliar site (16.6 miles north). A: On a sunny day (26 May 1969), the bearings of pigeons wearing magnets (black symbols) were as well oriented as those of control pigeons wearing brass bars (open symbols). B: On a totally overcast day (10 July 1969), the bearings of the birds wearing magnets were random but those of the control birds were oriented.

component of the pigeon navigation system, but they might be of prime importance to the birds only under conditions when the sun compass could not be used.

Suggestive as my experiments were, they did not conclusively prove that magnetic cues are actually used in orientation. Since my bar magnets had disoriented the pigeons, it was possible that the magnets had merely caused some general physiological disturbance having nothing to do with orientation per se. However, Walcott and Green (1974) soon devised a way to reorient pigeons, rather than disorient them, with imposed magnetic fields. They attached a small electro-magnetic coil to the bird's head like a cap, and another round its neck like a collar, both energized by a battery on the bird's back. When current flows through such a pair of coils, a magnetic field is induced betweed the coils, in this case pointing through the bird's head. When Walcott and Green compared the bearings of birds in whose coils the current was flowing counterclockwise with birds in whose coils the current was flowing clockwise, they found no great difference on sunny days, but on totally overcast days the group of birds with the counter-clockwise current oriented mostly toward home, whereas the other group with the clockwise current oriented mostly straight away from home (Fig. 4). (Reorientation of several species of migratory birds in circular cages surrounded by Helmholtz coils had already been reported in a series of publications by a research group at the University of Frankfurt, led first by F. Merkel and later by W. Wiltschko, e.g., Merkel and Wiltschko, 1965; Wiltschko, 1968; Wiltschko and Merkel, 1971; Wiltschko and Wiltschko, 1972.)

One of the most impressive demonstrations of animal sensitivity to very weak magnetic fields is the work of Lindauer and Martin (1968, 1972) on honeybees. They have shown that the waggle-run dance per-

WILLIAM T. KEETON

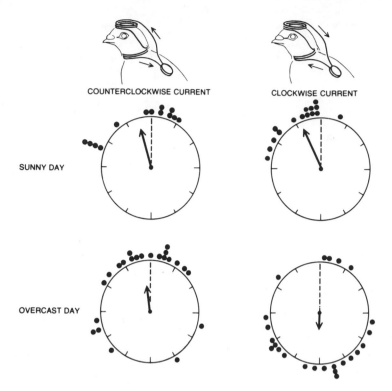

Fig. 4. Bearings of pigeons wearing current-carrying coils on their head and around their neck. On sunny days, homeward bearings are chosen by both pigeons in whose coils current is flowing counterclockwise and pigeons in whose coils current is flowing clockwise. But on totally overcast days, the bearings of the counterclockwise group are oriented homeward and the bearings of the clockwise group are oriented mostly away from home. Data from Walcott and Green (1974); figure from Keeton (1974b), used by permission of Scientific American, Inc.

formed by scout bees on the vertical comb in a darkened hive is influenced in a systematic way by the earth's magnetic field, and even by slight fluctuations of the field. Thus the bees can detect not only a magnetic field as weak as that of the earth (about 0.5 G) but also fluctuations of less than 10^{-3} G. To determine whether pigeons are equally sensitive, my colleagues and I conducted from a single test site a long series of experimental releases designed to control for as many extraneous variables as possible in order to make it easier to detect any slight effects on the birds' orientation of naturally occurring fluctuations in the earth's magnetic field. (These fluctuations are primarily caused by solar events that produce showers of high-energy particles that impinge on the ionosphere and thereby perturb the resultant field at the earth's surface.) We found that the small day-to-day differences in the bearings chosen by our pigeons were significantly correlated with the magnitude of magnetic disturbance (Keeton et al., 1974). The same relationship was found in each of 4 different years, and it was this repeatability that helped convince us that the correlation was biologically meaningful. Later experiments suggested that the correlation between bearings and magnetic fluctuations very probably reflects a true cause-and-effect relationship (Larkin and Keeton, 1976). This means that pigeons, like honeybees, are sensitive to magnetic fluctuations of less than 10^{-3} G. A similar sensitivity has been found in laughing gulls tested in circular cages (Southern, 1972) and in free-flying migrants tracked by radar over the Wisconsin Test Facility of the U.S. Navy's Project Seafarer (Larkin and Sutherland, 1977). Studies are currently in progress in my group to determine which parameter of the magnetic field—horizontal intensity, vertical intensity, or declination (or a derivative of these)—is most important to pigeons.

Exciting as it has been to be working on an apparent new sensory modality in animals, it has been somewhat disquieting that most attempts to condition pigeons to magnetic stimuli in the laboratory have failed (e.g., Kreithen and Keeton, 1974b; Beaugrand, 1976). However, Bookman (1977) has recently reported an apparently successful attempt to train pigeons to make a left-right choice of food boxes in response to two different magnetic conditions. Of special interest is his claim that the birds can choose correctly only if they first perform hovering flight within the magnetic field. Whether the hovering is essential for detection per se, or whether the birds only attend to the magnetic stimulus when in flight, is not yet known, but in either case Bookman's results may help explain why previous conditioning experiments were unsuccessful. Replication of Bookman's work under more stringently controlled conditions is urgently needed.

The mechanism of magnetic detection in pigeons remains a complete mystery. Birds have no sensory organs comparable to the ampullae of Lorenzini, which enable elasmobranch fishes to detect weak electric and magnetic fields (Kalmijn, 1973). It is possible that they possess cells containing organelles with magnetic dipoles like those in recently discovered magnetotactic bacteria (Blakemore, 1975) and that, as in the bacteria, it is the torque on the organelles that provides the transduction mechanism. Perhaps recent speculation that some organic compounds (e.g., cholesterol) may have superconductive properties at ordinary temperatures may prove to be true, and that very weak magnetic fields could therefore be detected via their effects on Josephson junction currents (Cope, 1971, 1973). Such a detection mechanism would be consistent with the evidence that suggests that the polarity of the magnetic field is unimportant to birds (Wiltschko and Wiltschko, 1972).

A theme that has appeared repeatedly in studies of the biological effects of weak magnetic fields is that animals are often responding to gravitational cues when they show the clearest reponses to magnetic stimuli (Lindauer and Martin, 1968; Wehner and Labhart, 1970; Wiltschko and Wiltschko, 1972). On the chance that magnetic and gravitational detection might somehow be linked, my colleagues and I tried to ascertain whether our pigeons' responses to natural fluctuations of the earth's magnetic field might also involve responses to gravity. Being unable to vary gravity ourselves, we decided to look for possible effects of the natural variations in gravity that accompany the monthly changes in the geometric relationships between the earth, sun, and moon (T. Larkin and Keeton, unpublished data). Somewhat to our own surprise, we did indeed find that in each of six independent field seasons there was a highly significant relationship between the birds' bearings and the day of the synodic lunar month; i.e., there was a cyclical shift in the birds' bearings from new moon to new moon (or from full moon to full moon). Periodogram analysis showed that the best frequency of the oscillations is almost exactly the period of the lunar month. Unfortunately, however, we have not yet been able to devise an experiment to test whether gravitational changes are directly causing the shifts in the birds' bearings or whether some other variable (e.g., atmospheric conditions) associated with the lunar cycle might be the cause. We conclude, nonetheless, that the possible role of gravity in bird orientation, whether as a link to magnetic cues or as a cue system in its own right, is worthy of further investigation.

STUDIES OF THE ONTOGENY OF NAVIGATIONAL BEHAVIOR

A research approach that my colleagues and I have recently found very fruitful is the manipulation of orientational cues in very young pigeons whose behavior is still sufficiently plastic so that the roles of various cues can be altered in ways that help reveal the normal pattern of integration. I shall briefly mention a few examples of our ontogenetic studies without discussing them in detail.

In the first section of this chapter, I discussed our experiments that show that experienced pigeons can orient homeward at unfamiliar release sites under conditions of total overcast (Keeton, 1969). However, we have found that this is not true of very young pigeons being released for the first homing flight of their lives; when released under

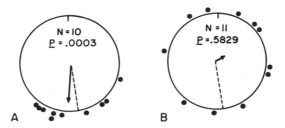

Fig. 5. Comparison of the orientation of experienced and first-flight pigeons released under total overcast at a site 16.6 miles north on 23 May 1969. The bearings of experienced pigeons were well oriented homeward (A), whereas those of the first-flight babies were random (B).

total overcast, these young first-flight pigeons depart randomly (Fig. 5) (Keeton and Gobert, 1970). They appear to require the sun compass.

Similarly, we have found that bar magnets often completely disrupt the orientation of young first-flight pigeons, even on sunny days when magnets have only minimal effect on experienced birds (Fig. 6) (Keeton, 1971, 1972). The young first-flight pigeons thus appear to require magnetic cues to orient. In short, unlike experienced pigeons, they seem to need both sun and magnetic information.

However, if young pigeons are raised without ever seeing the sun, being released for exercise at the home loft only on totally overcast days, then they can orient when given their first homing release under total overcast (Fig. 7A) (Wiltschko et al., 1976). Having never seen the sun and thus not having incorporated it into their navigation system, they have no difficulty when the solar cues required by normal first-flight youngsters are absent. That they are probably relying heavily on magnetic cues is indicated by the fact that their orientation can be systematically affected by properly aligned magnets (Fig. 7B).

We have also raised pigeons under permanently clock-shifted conditions (6 hr slow), i.e., the birds grew up with the lights going on and off 6 hr later than sunrise and sunset (Wiltschko et al., 1976). The

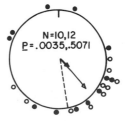

Fig. 6. Effects of bar magnets attached to first-flight pigeons released under sun 16.6 miles north on 1 October 1971. The control birds wearing brasses (open symbols) departed non-randomly, whereas the birds wearing magnets (black symbols) vanished randomly.

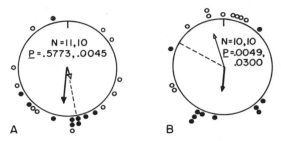

Fig. 7. Orientation under overcast of first-flight youngsters raised without view of the sun. A: When released 41.1 miles north, the experimental birds, which had never seen the sun, departed nonrandomly (black symbols), whereas the control birds (same age but with some previous exposure to the sun) departed randomly (open symbols). B: In a release from 9.6 miles southeast, no-sun youngsters wearing brasses departed in a northerly direction (open symbols), whereas no-sun youngsters wearing magnets arranged to induce a field similar to the Nup condition of Walcott and Green (1974) departed in a southerly direction (black symbols). Data from Wiltschko et al. (1976).

birds could be released for exercise flights during the afternoon, which was their physiological morning. When tested at release sites, such birds did not show the 90-deg deflection of bearings typical of normal clock-shifted pigeons; instead, they oriented toward home, like the control birds (Fig. 8A). Later, these pigeons were kept under normal time for 5–6 days and then retested. They then departed roughly 90 deg to the left of the control birds; normalization of these birds had had the same effect on them that a 6-hr-fast clock shift has on normal pigeons (Fig. 8B). In short, the permanently clock-shifted birds had learned to associate a southerly sun with early morning, a westerly sun

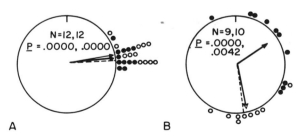

Fig. 8. Orientation of young pigeons raised under permanently clock-shifted (6 hr slow) conditions. A: Both the experimental birds (black symbols) and control birds (raised under normal time, open symbols) departed nonrandomly toward home. B: After 5–7 days of exposure to normal time, the birds raised under permanently clock-shifted conditions (black symbols) departed in a direction markedly deflected counterclockwise from the more homeward direction chosen by control birds (open symbols). From Wiltschko et al. (1976).

Cope, F. W.: Biological sensitivity to weak magnetic fields due to biological superconductive Josephson junctions? *Physiol. Chem. Phys.* **5**:173–176 (1973).

Delius, J. D., Perchard, R. J., and Emmerton, J.: Polarized light discrimination by pigeons and an electroretinographic correlate. *J. Comp. Physiol. Psychol.* **90**:560–571 (1976).

Emlen, S. T.: Migration: Orientation and navigation. In Farner, D. S., and King, J. R. (eds.): *Avian Biology*, Vol. 5. Academic Press, New York (1975). Pp. 129–219.

Graue, L. C.: The effect of phase shifts in the day-night cycle on pigeon homing at distances of less than one mile. *Ohio J. Sci.* **63**:214–217 (1963).

Hoffmann, K.: Versuche zu der in Richtungsfinden der Vögel enthaltenen Zeitschätzung. *Z. Tierpsychol.* **11**:453–475 (1954).

Hoffmann, K.: Experimental manipulation of the orientational clock in birds. *Cold Spring Harbor Symp. Quant. Biol.* **25**:379–387 (1960).

Kalmijn, A. J.: Electro-orientation in sharks and rays: Theory and experimental evidence. *Scripps Inst. Oceanogr. Contrib.* **73–39**:1–22 (1973).

Keeton, W. T.: Orientation by pigeons: Is the sun necessary? *Science* **165**:922–928 (1969).

Keeton, W. T.: Magnets interfere with pigeon homing. *Proc. Natl. Acad. Sci. USA* **68**:102–106 (1971).

Keeton, W. T.: Effects of magnets on pigeon homing. In *Animal Orientation and Navigation*. NASA SP-262. U.S. Government Printing Office, Washington, D.C. (1972). Pp. 579–594.

Keeton, W. T.: Release-site bias as a possible guide to the "map" component in pigeon homing. *J. Comp. Physiol.* **86**:1–16 (1973).

Keeton, W. T.: The orientational and navigational basis of homing in birds. *Adv. Study Behav.* **5**:47–132 (1974a).

Keeton, W. T.: The mystery of pigeon homing. *Sci. Am.* **231(6)**:96–107 (1974b).

Keeton, W. T.: Pigeon homing: No influence of outward-journey detours on initial orientation. *Monit. Zool. Ital.* (n.s.) **8**:226–234 (1974c).

Keeton, W. T., and Brown, A. I.: Homing behavior of pigeons not disturbed by application of an olfactory stimulus. *J. Comp. Physiol.* **105**:259–266 (1976).

Keeton, W. T., and Gobert, A.: Orientation by untrained pigeons requires the sun. *Proc. Natl. Acad. Sci. USA* **65**:853–856 (1970).

Keeton, W. T., Larkin, T. S., and Windsor, D. M.: Normal fluctuations in the earth's magnetic field influence pigeon orientation. *J. Comp. Physiol.* **95**:95–103 (1974).

Keeton, W. T., Kreithen, M. L., and Hermayer, K. L.: Orientation by pigeons deprived of olfaction by nasal tubes. *J. Comp. Physiol.* **114**:289–299 (1977).

Kramer, G.: Weitere Analyse der Faktoren, welche die Zugaktivität des gekäfigten Vogels orientieren. *Naturwissenschaften* **37**:377–378 (1950).

Kramer, G.: Eine neue Methode zur Erforschung der Zugorientierung und die bisher damit erzielten Ergebnisse. *Proc. 10th Int. Ornithol. Congr. Uppsala* (1951). Pp. 271–280.

Kramer, G.: Experiments on bird orientation. *Ibis* **94**:265–285 (1952).

Kramer, G.: Die Sonnenorientierung der Vögel. *Verh. Dtsch. Zool. Ges.* 1952, Pp. 72–84 (1953).

Kreithen, M. L., and Keeton, W. T.: Detection of polarized light by the homing pigeon, *Columba livia*. *J. Comp. Physiol.* **89**:83–92 (1974a).

Kreithen, M. L., and Keeton, W. T.: Attempts to condition homing pigeons to magnetic stimuli. *J. Comp. Physiol.* **91**:355–362 (1974b).

Larkin, R. P., and Sutherland, P. J.: Migrating birds react to Project Seafarer's electromagnetic field. *Science* **195**:777–779 (1977).

Larkin, T. S., and Keeton, W. T.: Bar magnets mask the effect of normal magnetic disturbances on pigeon orientation. *J. Comp. Physiol.* **110**:227–231 (1976).

Lindauer, M., and Martin, H.: Die Schwereorientierung der Bienen unter dem Einfluss des Erdmagnetfeldes. *Z. Vgl. Physiol.* **60**:219–243 (1968).

Lindauer, M., and Martin, H.: Magnetic effect on dancing bees. In *Animal Orientation and Navigation*. NASA SP-262. U.S. Government Printing Office, Washington, D.C. (1972). Pp. 559–567.

Matthews, G. V. T.: The sensory basis of bird navigation. *J. Inst. Navigat.* **4**:260–275 (1951).

Matthews, G. V. T.: Sun navigation in homing pigeons. *J. Exp. Biol.* **30**:243–267 (1953).

Matthews, G. V. T.: *Bird Navigation*. Cambridge University Press, London (1955).

Merkel, F. W., and Wiltschko, W.: Magnetismus und Richtungsfinden zugunruhiger Rotkehlchen (*Erithacus rubecula*). *Vogelwarte* **23**:71–77 (1965).

Papi, F., Fiore, L., Fiaschi, V., and Benvenuti, S.: The influence of olfactory nerve section on the homing capacity of carrier pigeons. *Monit. Zool. Ital.* (n.s.) **5**:265–267 (1971).

Papi, F., Fiore, L., Fiaschi, V., and Benvenuti, S.: Olfaction and homing in pigeons. *Monit. Zool. Ital.* (n.s.) **6**:85–95 (1972).

Papi, F., Fiore, L., Fiaschi, V., and Benvenuti, S.: An experiment for testing the hypothesis of olfactory navigation of homing pigeons. *J. Comp. Physiol.* **33**:93–102 (1973a).

Papi, F., Fiaschi, V., Benvenuti, S., and Baldaccini, N. E.: Pigeon homing: Outward journey detours influence the initial orientation. *Monit. Zool. Ital.* (n.s.) **7**:129–133 (1973b).

Schlichte, H. J., and Schmidt-Koenig, K.: Zum Heimfindevermögen der Brieftaube bei erschwerter optischer Wahrnehmung. *Naturwissenschaften* **58**:329–330 (1971).

Schmidt-Koenig, K.: Experimentelle Einflussnahme auf die 24-Stunden-Periodik bei Brieftauben und deren Auswirkungen unter besonderer Berücksichtigung des Heimfindevermögens. *Z. Tierpsychol.* **15**:301–331 (1958).

Schmidt-Koenig, K.: Internal clocks and homing. *Cold Spring Harbor Symp. Quant. Biol.* **25**:389–393 (1960).

Schmidt-Koenig, K.: Current problems in bird orientation. In Lehrman, D. S., Hinde, R. A., and Shaw, E. (eds): *Advances in the Study of Behavior*, Vol. 1. Academic Press, New York (1965). Pp. 217–278.

Schmidt-Koenig, K., and Schlichte, H. J.: Homing in pigeons with reduced vision *Proc. Natl. Acad. Sci. USA* **69**:2446–2447 (1972).

Schmidt-Koenig, K., and Walcott, C.: Flugwege und Verbleib von Brieftauben mit getrübten Haftschalen. *Naturwissenschaften* **60**:108–109 (1973).

Southern, W. T.: Influence of disturbances in the earth's magnetic field on ring-billed gull orientation. *Condor* **74**:102–105 (1972).

Walcott, C., and Green, R. P.: Orientation of homing pigeons altered by a change in the direction of an applied magnetic field. *Science* **184**:180–182 (1974).

Wehner, R., and Labhart, T.: Perception of the geomagnetic field in the fly *Drosophila melanogaster*. *Experientia* **26**:967–968 (1970).

Wiltschko, W.: Über den Einfluss statischer Magnetfelder auf die Zugorientierung der Rotkehlchen (*Erithacus rubecula*). *Z. Tierpsychol.* **25**:537–558 (1968).

Wiltschko, W., and Merkel, F. W.: Zugorientierung von Dorngrasmücken (*Sylvia communis*) im Erdmagnetfeld. *Vogelwarte* **26**:245–249 (1971).

Wiltschko, W., and Wiltschko, R.: Magnetic compass of European robins. *Science* **176**:62–64 (1972).

Wiltschko, W., Wiltschko, R., and Keeton, W.T.: Effects of a "permanent" clock-shift on the orientation of young homing pigeons. *Behav. Ecol. Sociobiol.* **1**:229–243 (1976).

Yeagley, H. L.: A preliminary study of a physical basis of bird navigation. *J. Appl. Phys.* **18**:1035–1063 (1947).

Yeagley, H. L.: A preliminary study of a physical basis of bird navigation. II. *J. Appl. Phys.* **22**:746–760 (1951).

Yodlowski, M. L., Kreithen, M. L., and Keeton, W.T.: Detection of atmospheric infrasound by homing pigeons. *Nature (London)* **265**:725–726 (1977).

3

The Sensory World of the Homing Pigeon

MELVIN L. KREITHEN

INTRODUCTION

It has become apparent that the homing pigeon lives in a sensory world quite different from our own. For the past few years, I have been testing a variety of sensory cues in the laboratory and concentrating on those that have some relevance to the problems of homing, navigation, migration, and orientation. These tests have uncovered a series of unusual sensory capabilities. The pigeon is sensitive to a surprising variety of sensory channels including polarized light, ultraviolet light, olfactory stimuli, barometric pressure changes, and very low frequency sounds (infrasounds). In this chapter, I will briefly survey a few of these sensory inputs. For more detailed descriptions of these experiments, the reader is referred to previously published accounts.

METHODS

The principal experimental method used in my laboratory has been a very simple procedure using conditioned cardiac responses. When a pigeon detects a novel stimulus, its heartbeat frequency often increases dramatically. A shock is then paired with the end of the stimulus, and

MELVIN L. KREITHEN • Division of Biological Sciences, Langmuir Laboratory, Cornell University, Ithaca, New York 14853. This research was supported by Grant BMS 75-18905 to W. T. Keeton from the National Science Foundation.

subsequent trials will result in repeated cardiac accelerations if the bird can detect the stimulus. Figure 1 shows typical cardiac responses.

The original reason for choosing cardiac conditioning was historical; it was used to repeat another experiment. As an experimental method, it has proven to be very efficient. Cardiac conditioning works—it is a fast and simple procedure requiring little training of either bird or investigator. Often a simple behavioral answer can be obtained in a matter of minutes using untrained birds. There is now a long history of successful experiments using this testing method. It has proven to be both robust and sensitive, it works well with a great variety of stimuli, and it produces threshold values equal to or better than other behavioral testing methods.

VISION

Polarized Light

The sun compass is an important element in the pigeon navigation system. Because many insects such as honeybees and ants use polarized

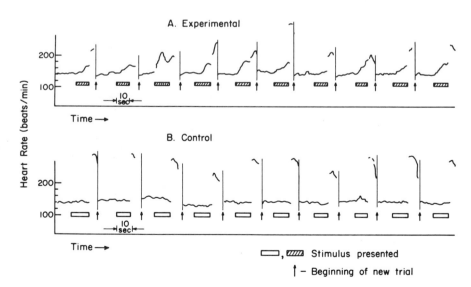

Fig. 1. Tracing of cardiac rates during an experiment. The upper trace is responses to a 20-mm H_2O pressure change. There is a random time delay of 3–8 min between each trial. The lower trace is from a control experiment with the same bird. An open vent in the chamber prevents pressure from accumulating, but the air control system works the same way as in the upper trace.

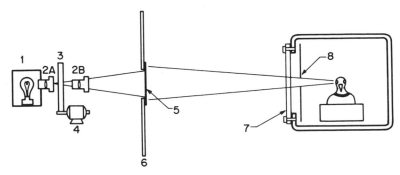

Fig. 2. Polarized light testing apparatus showing the relative positions of projector, screen, and bird. Light (1) is projected through a polarizing filter (3) on a motorized mounting (4). In the training position (2B), the lens also projects crosshairs on the nondepolarizing screen (5). When the lens is in the testing position (2A), the polarizer is out of focus and no cues except polarization remain. Opaque baffles (6 and 8) limit the beam width to reduce the possibility of unwanted reflections. Distance between chamber window (7) and screen (5) is 1.8 m.

skylight for their sun-compass orientation, it seemed worthwhile to investigate the possibility of polarized light detection in pigeons.

Several homing pigeons were successfully trained to respond to polarized light cues. Figure 2 shows the experimental configuration. This was the first evidence for polarized light detection in birds, although the last few years have produced further evidence for polarized light detection in birds and in other vertebrates such as fish and amphibians. Most remarkable is the evidence that salamanders can orient to polarized light cues using an extraocular receptor system located under the bones of the skull. Delius has shown that the pigeon can orient to overhead polarized light cues, and that the sensory mechanism is probably ocular (Kreithen and Keeton, 1974a; Delius et al. 1976; Dill, 1971; Adler and Taylor, 1973).

Ultraviolet Light

Another exciting finding in my laboratory was that pigeons can see ultraviolet light (UV). This was accomplished by further use of cardiac-conditioning methods. The birds' visual sensitivity was surprising in view of the traditional view that most vertebrate animals, like human beings, are UV blind.

Figure 3 shows the spectral sensitivity of one pigeon, obtained by behavioral testing in my laboratory, at 13 wavelengths. The pigeon apparently has the normal vertebrate maximum of sensitivity to wavelengths in the blue-green (500–600 nm) portion of the spectrum, and

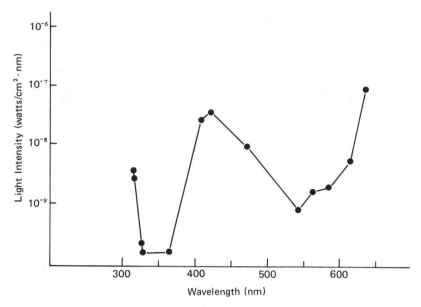

Fig. 3. Behavioral sensitivity to ultraviolet and visible light. Each circle is a behaviorally determined threshold (50%) at the wavelengths indicated. Pigeon 3075.

also has a second region of maximum spectral sensitivity in the UV (325–360 nm) range. This spectral sensitivity to UV wavelengths has recently been confirmed by Delius and Emmerton (this volume). Wright (1972) had noted earlier that UV wavelengths can interfere with the color discrimination tasks of his pigeons. Short-wavelength sensitivity has been reported even in experiments limited by the apparatus to wavelengths longer than 400 nm (Blough, 1957; Graf and Norren, 1974; Norren, 1975).

Ultraviolet light is a well-known source of information for orientation. Insects and other arthropods routinely use UV to (1) locate the sun behind clouds, (2) orient to patterns of polarized light in the sky, (3) detect hidden UV flower patterns, and (4) locate UV color patches on other insects (von Frisch, 1967; Ghiradella et al., 1972). The generalization that UV is seen and used only by invertebrate animals needs to be critically reexamined. Aside from my own results with pigeons, UV sensitivity has recently been demonstrated in such other vertebrates as hummingbirds (Huth and Burkhardt, 1972), toads (Dietz, 1972), newts (Kimeldorf and Fontanini, 1974), and lizards (Moehn, 1974). It may be that UV sensitivity is more widespread among vertebrate groups than was previously assumed.

Ultraviolet-absorbing pigments in the lens of man prevent short wavelengths from reaching the retina, but not all vertebrates have these pigments. The lenses of pigeons and other birds are very clear in the UV range, as are the cornea and ocular media (Govardovski and Zueva, 1977). Clear lenses are reported in toads (*Bufo bufo*) (Dietz, 1972), but Kennedy and Milkman (1956) reported yellow lenses in frogs (*Rana pipiens*). Fish appear to vary, some species having very clear lenses and others having yellow pigments in the optic path (Muntz, 1972).

The mechanism of UV detection is not known. There are several potential mechanisms, and experiments may help to choose which of these is being used.

Many insects including ants and bees use the polarized light of the sky for orienting and direction finding. Ultraviolet wavelengths are often used for this task since these shorter wavelengths penetrate thin cloud layers and thus are available when other cues are masked. Pigeons, like honeybees, have a well-developed sun compass and are now known to be sensitive to polarized light. I encourage future workers to determine whether pigeons can extend their proven ability to detect polarized light into the UV portion of the solar spectrum. There are many important applications of UV sensitivity in birds. Navigation, food gathering, and insect prey detection all have potential UV components. It is possible that many more vertebrates use UV vision than we previously thought.

OLFACTION

Papi and several other Italian scientists have recently obtained substantial evidence that homing pigeons use olfactory information to assist in their navigation. Their experiments range through many techniques including olfactory nerve sectioning and painting odor mixtures on the birds' bills (Papi et al., 1972; Benvenuti et al., 1973). Some experiments are quite convincing, but others may be explained by proposing other mechanisms besides olfaction (Keeton et al., 1977). Considerable effort is being expended at other laboratories to duplicate and extend these olfactory experiments.

Pigeons do have a functional olfactory system. Behavioral tests show a reasonable sensitivity to simple laboratory chemicals, but the pigeons' olfactory system is not as well developed as that of other birds such as the kiwi. Lesions to the olfactory tract often result in general behavioral and motivational deficits that may affect more than just olfactory dependent behaviors (Hutton et al., 1974).

At Cornell, several experiments are in progress to find how much navigational emphasis birds place on olfactory cues. Several birds were tested for their olfactory capabilities in an olfactory conditioning chamber which presented brief pulses of test vapors. Two procedures were then developed for altering the olfactory sensitivity of the pigeons. The first was a surgical procedure in which the olfactory nerves were cut and a 1-mm segment was removed for histology and verification. After recovery, when these birds were tested in the olfactory test chamber, they showed no olfactory responses. When these birds were further tested by releasing them from both distant and nearby sites, there was little effect on navigational performance.

The second procedure involved a reversible method for altering the birds' olfactory capability. A plastic tube was inserted into each nostril so that the birds could breathe through the tubes, but they could not smell because the olfactory epithelium was blocked. Birds fitted with tubes were tested in both laboratory and field for their olfactory and navigational capabilities. After removal of the tubes, the birds shortly regain their sense of smell. The control and experimental birds were then reversed, and over a long series of field tests each bird was evaluated against his own performance under both conditions. There were few effects of olfactory deprivation on initial flight directions and speeds. However, there was poorer homing success from long-distance releases, suggesting that decreased motivation, irritation, or other factors reduced the ability to fly long distances.

MAGNETIC FIELDS

There has been a renewed interest in the nature of biological responses to magnetic fields. I have witnessed the disoriented behavior of Cornell homing pigeons wearing magnets when released in overcast weather. Other pigeon lofts have been able to duplicate these remarkable results using appropriate training procedures. However, very few investigators have been able to produce laboratory responses to magnetic fields. I have performed over 600 hr of laboratory tests using Cornell homing pigeons under a great variety of artificial magnetic-field conditions. The birds have been placed within large coils, small coils, stationary fields, fluctuating fields, disappearing fields, and rotating fields—all to no avail (Kreithen and Keeton, 1974b). Many other workers have tried similar tests, and, with one exception (Reille, 1968), all have failed. Successful magnetic experiments have two features in common which are usually lacking in most laboratory experiments: (1) locomotion and (2) long time intervals between stimulus and response. Locomotion was one of the factors present in Bookman's (1977) food-box choice test. Long time constants and locomotion are both features of honeybee magnetic responses (Lindauer and Martin, 1968), and also of the migratory bird responses of Wiltschko and Wiltschko (1972). When the exact nature of magnetic interactions is known, the reasons for our previous failures may become clear.

BAROMETRIC PRESSURE

When cardiac conditioning was used, Cornell homing pigeons showed a remarkable sensitivity to small changes in air pressure. Positive or negative pressure changes of just a few millimeters of water could be easily detected by the pigeons (Kreithen and Keeton, 1974c). Expressed as sea level altitude changes, these pressure differentials corresponded to altitude changes of roughly 5–10 m.

There were two applications in my mind when these pressure tests began. The first grew out of the increasing evidence showing just how good migratory birds are at predicting weather changes (reviewed in Emlen, 1975). The second role of pressure detection by birds is the still-untested possibility that flying birds control their altitude in flight by using a pressure-sensitive altimeter. There is substantial radar evidence that migratory birds have good control of their altitude even when flying in darkness or within heavy cloud cover (Griffin, 1972). An animal that flies in three-dimensional space must have problems to face that may not be apparent to us since we spend most of our lives in a two-dimensional world. I would like to encourage further study of the detection of altitude changes by birds.

ATMOSPHERIC INFRASOUNDS

As a natural outgrowth of barometric pressure and weather detection studies, it was brought to our attention that there is a rich source of navigational and meteorological information available in the form of low-frequency acoustic signals (infrasounds). Reflecting our human limitations in hearing, we call airborne sounds below 10 Hz infrasounds. Infrasounds form a very loud and complex world of low-frequency sounds of which we are unaware.

Geophysicists and meteorologists, using suitable microphones, have identified many stationary and transient infrasound sources. Thunderstorms, auroras, earthquakes, ocean waves, and even mountain ranges produce coherent acoustic signals that can be detected hundreds or thousands of kilometers away (Cook, 1969; Gossard and Hooke, 1975; Procunier, 1971; Wilson, 1971). Figures 4, 5, and 6 show

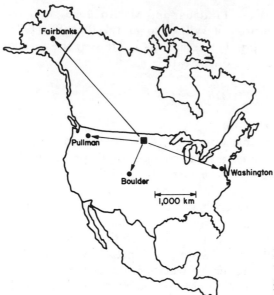

Fig. 4. Acoustic (infrasound) detection of a thunderstorm (August 4, 1969). Modified from Bowman and Bedard (1971).

several sources of infrasound, and demonstrate the scale of distances that infrasounds can travel and still be detected.

There are two features of infrasound responsible for its long-range properties. First, the sounds are usually loud; 120 dB (SPL re 0.0002 dynes/cm^2) is a common amplitude for sounds below 1 Hz. Second,

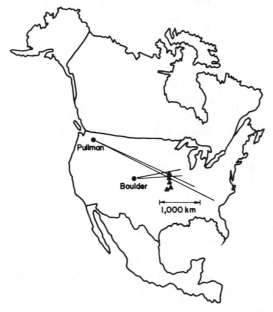

Fig. 5. Acoustic detection and tracking of a series of severe hailstorms (June 5, 1969). Modified from Bowman and Bedard (1971).

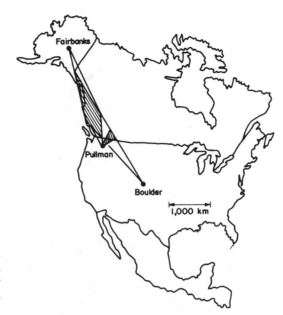

Fig. 6. Areas of continuous infra-sound production by the inter-action of suitable winds and mountains in the northwestern United States. Another steady infrasound source is located in Argentina.

sound attenuation in air is proportional to the square of frequency; hence low-frequency sounds are attenuated very little when compared to higher-frequency sounds. Sounds from the eruption of Krakatoa in 1883 were heard in Texas as distant cannon fire, and barographs recorded acoustic waves circling the earth several times (Georges and Beasley, 1977).

It has been suggested that birds use infrasounds to help locate themselves on their map or in some other way to aid the navigation process (Griffin, 1969). For this reason, I began a series of experiments on the detection of infrasounds by homing pigeons. Much to my surprise, the pigeons were capable of detecting low-frequency sounds with sufficient sensitivity to be potentially able to use this capability in the natural world.

Figure 7 shows the behaviorally determined, low-frequency hearing sensitivity of the pigeon. Each dot is a threshold (50%) at that particular frequency. Note that there are still behavioral responses as low as 0.06 Hz. To place the audiogram in perspective, the hatched area represents an estimate of some natural infrasound intensities reported in the literature. The upper curve in Fig. 7 is the low-frequency audiogram for humans (Yeowart and Evans, 1974; Whittle et al., 1972) and shows that, unlike pigeons, we cannot hear most infrasounds because our thresholds are above the intensity of these natural sounds.

The data in Fig. 7 make it reasonable to assume that pigeons can

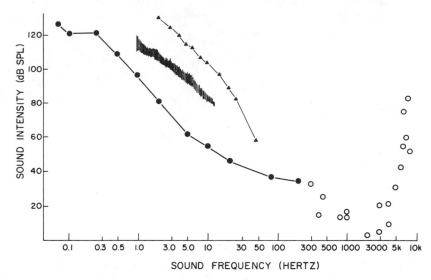

Fig. 7. Infrasound sensitivity of the pigeon. Each filled circle is a behaviorally determined threshold at that frequency. Open circles are previous audiogram data from other workers (see text). Triangles represent human thresholds. Vertical bars represent natural infrasound levels.

detect natural infrasounds, especially the loud events. A recent paper on infrasonic booms from Concorde supersonic transport planes reports intensities above the pigeon thresholds given here; therefore, our birds in Ithaca should be able to detect the trans-Atlantic passages of the SSTs (Balachandran et al., 1977).

Previous work on auditory sensitivity had implied that 200 Hz was a lower limit of hearing for birds. The data shown in Fig. 7 extend the known hearing range 11 octaves lower than previously published limits.

In an attempt to isolate the infrasound receptors, two surgical procedures were performed. The cochleas and lagenas were surgically removed from one group of pigeons and behavioral tests were performed. No auditory or infrasonic reponses could be obtained from this group (Yodlowski et al., 1977). Another group had just the columella removed. (The columella in the pigeon is a single bone, homologous to our three middle ear bones, that links the tympanic membrane to the inner ear.) The sensitivity of these birds was reduced by about 50 dB when tested at 2, 5, and 10 Hz. These data suggest but do not prove that the transducing mechanism is probably in the ear and not elsewhere in the pigeon's body. The surgically altered birds are currently being tested further.

Although these laboratory findings are exciting, they do not guarantee that pigeons can and do use natural infrasounds. There are several problems to be solved before we will know if it is possible for pigeons to use natural infrasounds. Two major obstacles are (1) confusion with pseudosounds and (2) difficulty of localization. Pseudosounds are nonpropagating pressure variations due to local winds and atmospheric turbulence. They are sometimes equal in amplitude to the long-distance infrasounds, and special filtering devices are required to separate the two types of signals. It is not yet known if the bird can perform this signal-separation task. It may be possible only if the birds fly and use spatial variations in the signals to distinguish local pseudosounds from propagated true infrasounds. This question is critical and needs to be investigated further.

Localization of sound sources is normally accomplished by recognizing some binaural differences of the incoming signals. Phase differences, time of arrival differences, or amplitude differences between the two ears are often used as cues to locate a source of sound. None of these localization methods is possible with infrasounds because of their long wavelengths. A 0.1-Hz sound has a wavelength in air of 3 km. With such long wavelengths, there are virtually no differences in the signals between the two ears. Infrasound microphone arrays used for research have several kilometers separating the microphones and therefore can use time of arrival differences in the signals. However, birds cannot use this method. In our search for alternative means of sound localization, Quine and I (unpublished data) have been investigating the possibility that Doppler shifts in infrasound frequency might provide some directional cues.

Homing pigeons fly at about 20 m/sec, or 7% of the speed of sound in air. If a pigeon flies toward and then away from a sound source, the apparent frequency can shift by as much as 14%. Quine and Konishi (1974) have shown that owls can discriminate sound frequency shifts of less than 1% (in the usual audible range). Quine is now investigating in my laboratory how much frequency shift can be detected by a pigeon in the infrasonic range. Very preliminary results show that the pigeons can discriminate as little as 5% frequency shifts at 5 Hz. This begins to make Doppler shift localization of infrasound an attractive possibility. We intend to continue these experiments.

Many gaps remain in our understanding of low-frequency hearing in pigeons. We do not yet know what is the lower limit of the hearing range; we stopped at 0.06 Hz only because we did not have an apparatus to generate lower frequencies. We need to explore the lower limits of pigeons' hearing further.

Infrasound signals arrive from all parts of the world and must present a highly complex mixture of amplitudes and frequencies. There is little doubt that pigeons can hear some of these sounds, but we do not know if they can sort them out, separate the signals from the background noise, and somehow make use of the infrasound in any meaningful way. We will attempt to answer some of these intriguing questions as work progresses.

It is difficult to imagine what the sensory world of the pigeon must be like when we cannot share its sensory capabilities.

ACKNOWLEDGMENTS. I thank my colleagues, Irene Brown, Timothy Larkin, and André Gobert for their help in conducting the releases.

REFERENCES

Adler, K., and Taylor, D. H.: Extraocular perception of polarized light by orienting salamanders. *J. Comp. Physiol.* **87**:203–212 (1973).
Balachandran, N. K., Dunn, W. L., and Rind, D. H.: Concorde sonic booms as an atmospheric probe. *Science* **197**:47–49 (1977).
Benvenuti, S., Fiaschi, V., Fiore, L., and Papi, F.: Homing performances of inexperienced and directionally trained pigeons subjected to olfactory nerve section. *J. Comp. Physiol.* **83**:81–92 (1973).
Blough, D. S.: Spectral sensitivity in the pigeon. *J. Opt. Soc. Am.* **47**:827–833 (1957).
Bookman, M.: Sensitivity of the homing pigeon to an earth-strength magnetic field. *Nature (London)* **267**:1340–1342 (1977).
Bowman, H. S., and Bedard, A. J.: Observations of infrasound and subsonic disturbances related to severe weather. *Geophys. J. R. Astron. Soc.* **26**:215–242 (1971).
Cook, R. K.: Atmospheric sound propagation. National Academy of Sciences (USA). Proceedings of the panel on remote atmospheric probing. *Proc. Natl. Acad. Sci. USA* **2**:633–669 (1969).
Delius, J., Perchard, R., and Emmerton, J.: Polarized light discrimination by pigeons and an electroretinographic correlate. *J. Comp. Physiol. Psychol.* **90(6)**:560–571 (1976).
Dietz, M.: Erdkröten können UV-Licht sehen. *Naturwissenschaften* **59(7)**:316 (1972).
Dill, P. A.: Perception of polarized light by yearling sockeye salmon (*Oncorhynchus nerka*). *J. Fish. Res. Board Can.* **38**:1319–1322 (1971).
Emlen, S. T.: Migration: Orientation and navigation. In Farner, D. S., and King, J. R. (eds.): *Avian Biology*, Vol. 5. Academic Press, New York (1975). Pp. 129–219.
Georges, T. M., and Beasley, W. H.: Refraction of infrasound by upper atmospheric winds. *J. Acoust. Soc. Am.* **61**:28–34 (1977).
Ghiradella, H., Aneshansley, D., Eisner, T., Silberglied, R., and Hinton, H.: Ultraviolet reflection of a male butterfly: Interference color caused by thin-layer elaboration of wing scales. *Science* **178**:1214–1217 (1972).
Gossard, E. E., and Hooke, W. H.: *Waves in the Atmosphere.* Elsevier, Amsterdam (1975).
Govardovski, V. I., and Zueva, L. V.: Visual pigments of chicken and pigeon. *Vision Res.* **17**:537–543 (1977).
Graf, V., and Norren, D. V.: A blue sensitive mechanism in the pigeon fovea: Lambda max 400 nM. *Vision Res.* **14**:1203–1209 (1974).

Griffin, D. R.: The physiology and geophysics of bird navigation. *Q. Rev. Biol.* **44**:255–276 (1969).

Griffin, D. R.: Nocturnal bird migration in opaque clouds. In Galler, S., Schmidt-Koenig, K., Jacobs, G., and Bellville, R. (eds.): *Animal Orientation and Navigation, A Symposium.* NASA SP 262. U.S. Government Printing Office, Washington, D. C. (1972).

Huth, H., and Burkhardt, D.: Der spektrale Sehbereich eines Violettohr-Kolibris. *Naturwissenschaften* **59**:650 (1972).

Hutton, R. S., Wenzel, B. M., Baker, T., and Homuth, M.: Two-way avoidance learning in pigeons after olfactory nerve section. *Physiol. Behav.* **13**:57–62 (1974).

Keeton, W. T., Kreithen, M., and Hermayer, K.: Orientation by pigeons deprived of olfaction by nasal tubes. *J. Comp. Physiol.* **114**:289–299 (1977).

Kennedy, D., and Milkman, R. D.: Selective light absorption by the lenses of lower vertebrates, and its influence on spectral sensitivity. *Biol. Bull.* **111**:375–386 (1956).

Kimeldorf, D. J., and Fontanini, D. F.: Avoidance of near ultraviolet radiation exposures by an amphibious vertebrate. *Environ. Physiol. Biochem.* **4**:40–44 (1974).

Kreithen, M. L., and Keeton, W. T.: Detection of polarized light by the homing pigeon, *Columba livia. J. Comp. Physiol.* **89**:83–92 (1974a).

Kreithen, M. L., and Keeton, W. T.: Attempts to condition homing pigeons to magnetic stimuli. *J. Comp. Physiol.* **91**:355–362 (1974b).

Kreithen, M. L., and Keeton, W. T.: Detection of changes in atmospheric pressure by the homing pigeon, *Columba livia. J. Comp. Physiol.* **89**:73–82 (1974c).

Lindauer, M., and Martin, H.: Die Schwereorientierung der Bienen unter dem Einfluss des Erdmagnetfelds. *Z. Vergl. Physiol.* **60**:219–243 (1968).

Moehn, L.: The effects of quality of light on agonistic behavior of iguanid and agamid lizards. *J. Herpetol.* **8**:175–183 (1974).

Muntz, W. R. A.: Inert absorbing and reflecting pigments. In Dartnall, H. (ed.): *Handbook of Sensory Physiology,* Vol. 7. Springer-Verlag, Berlin (1972).

Norren, D. V.: Two short wavelength sensitive cone systems in the pigeon, chicken, and daw. *Vision Res.* **15**:1164–1166 (1975).

Papi, F., Fiore, L., Fiaschi, V., and Benvenuti, S.: Olfaction and homing in pigeons. *Monit. Zool. Ital.* (n.s.) **6**:85–95 (1972).

Procunier, R. W.: Observations of acoustic aurora in the 1–16 Hz range. *Geophys. J. Roy. Astron. Soc.* **26**:183–189 (1971).

Quine, B., and Konishi, M.: Absolute frequency discrimination in the barn owl. *J. Comp. Physiol.* **93**:347–360 (1974).

Reille, A.: Essai de mise en évidence d'une sensibilité du pigeon au champ magnétique à l'aide d'un conditionnement nociceptif. *J. Physiol. (Paris)* **60**:85–92 (1968).

von Frisch, K.: *The Dance Language and Orientation of Bees.* Belknap Press, Cambridge (1967). 566 pp.

Whittle, L. S., Collins, S. J., and Robinson, D. W.: Audibility of low frequency sounds. *J. Sound Vib.* **21**:431–448 (1972).

Wilson, C. R.: Auroral infrasonic waves and poleward expansions of auroral substorms at Inuvik, N.W.T., Canada. *Geophys. J. Roy. Astron. Soc.* **26**:179–181 (1971).

Wiltschko, W., and Wiltschko, R.: Magnetic compass of European robins. *Science* **176**:62–64 (1972).

Wright, A.: The influence of ultraviolet radiation on pigeon's color discrimination. *J. Exp. Anal. Behav.* **17**:325–337 (1972).

Yeowart, N. S., and Evans, M. J.: Thresholds of audibility for very low frequency pure tones. *J. Acoust. Soc.* **55**:814–818 (1974).

Yodlowski, M. L., Kreithen, M. L., and Keeton, W. T.: Detection of atmospheric infrasound by homing pigeons. *Nature (London)* **265**:725–726 (1977).

4

Psychophysiological Correlates of Time Perception in the Pigeon

JACQUES SERVIÈRE

INTRODUCTION

All stimuli shorter than a certain critical duration are indistinguishable on the basis of their perceived duration, whatever their real physical length. It is impossible, for instance, to discriminate the duration of a photographic flash (shorter than 10 msec) from a lightning flash (approximately 100 μsec). The question is to determine the values of stimulus duration for which the passage from a sensation of *instantaneous* (lack of temporal thickness) to a sensation of *durable* intervenes.

Most previous studies concerned with the perception of duration have been carried out using durations in the order of seconds; however, the determination of the instantaneous-to-durable threshold (I-D threshold) has not been directly investigated. Nevertheless, Durup and Fessard (1929), in a study relating the effect of duration on brightness perception and visual acuity, mentioned the problem of the establishment of the sensation of durable. The few experimental data they obtained led them to conclude that, above 140 msec, light stimuli were perceived as being durable with certitude.

The relationship between the physical duration of very brief stimuli and their perceived duration has recently been investigated in different sensory modalities (vision, audition, touch). In experiments on the duration of a percept (Efron, 1970a,b,c) and on perceptual du-

JACQUES SERVIÈRE • Laboratoire de Psychophysiologie Sensorielle, Université de Paris VI, 75230 Paris Cédex 05, France.

35

rations (Efron, 1970d, 1973a,b), an observer was required to make simultaneous judgments regarding two events. The results indicated that for stimuli shorter than a critical duration (130 msec in vision), the "perceptual offset latency" increased as stimulus duration decreased, thus yielding a constant value for the sum of stimulus duration plus perceptual offset latency. According to Efron, the data supported the hypothesis of a "constant minimum perceptual duration" consistent with some aspects of the simultaneity data obtained by Haber and Standing (1970). In our direct study on the determination of the visual I-D threshold (Servière et al., 1977a), using three complementary methods, we were able to show that the passage of visual sensation from instantaneous to durable (50% "I" responses, 50% "D" responses) was situated between 60 and 65 msec; for durations shorter than these values, the visual sensation was referred to as being instantaneous. For stimulus durations longer than 140 msec, visual sensation was referred to as durable with certitude; between these two ranges, the subject's responses showed evidence of uncertainty.

Efron (1973b) suggested the existence of an irreducible interval between ON and OFF responses subserving the minimum perceptual duration. His attempt to establish a correlation by recording visual evoked potentials (VEPs) in the cat optic nerve led us to demonstrate electrophysiological correlates of the passage from instantaneous to durable for the same subject under identical experimental conditions.

By examining transcranial VEPs recorded in man, Servière et al. (1977b) found a clear-cut separation of ON and OFF components for stimulus durations longer than 140 msec. Under 125 msec, and as stimulus duration decreased, ON and OFF components showed ever-increasing overlap. By comparing these results with the psychophysical data (Servière et al., 1977a), it was shown that the clear-cut sepration of ON and OFF components coincided with perceptual certainty of durable ($t \geq 140$ msec) and that the progressive overlap of these two components was correlated with subjective uncertainty (30 msec $< t <$ 125 msec) leading to a visual sensation referred to as instantaneous ($t \leq 20$ msec), the I-D threshold (60–65 msec) being situated in the range of uncertainty. By plotting the ON-OFF interpeak interval of the VEPs as a function of stimulus duration, we were further able to show that with stimuli shorter than 80 msec the interpeak interval ceased to decrease proportionally with duration (slope $= -1$). For durations perceived as instantaneous ($t < 32$ msec), the interpeak interval remained constant (slope $\simeq 0$) at a minimum value of approximately 30 msec. Whatever the duration values were under this minimum value, an incompressible interval was obtained.

In humans, the several psychophysical methods which are available give a good approximation of the I-D threshold. In contrast, electrophysiological data can only yield gross activity recorded on associative areas (18-19). We therefore conducted our experiments on the pigeon where access to the primary visual system (optic nerve, tectum) is possible. However, in this case, I-D threshold determinations using complementary methods are more difficult than in man.

The ability to discriminate duration in the animal has been studied for durations on the order of seconds. However, with durations shorter than 1 sec the problem was to get an animal to give significant responses with regard to the determination of I-D threshold.

The two parts of the present study, the psychophysical and the electrophysiological determinations, were conducted in order to get a homogeneous pool of data: (1) psychophysical study—using operant conditioning to determine the conditions of the passage from instantaneous to durable; and (2) electrophysiological study—recording responses evoked in the optic nerve and tectum to study the evolution of ON and OFF components as a function of stimulus duration.

PSYCHOPHYSICAL DATA ON THE RELATION BETWEEN STIMULUS DURATION AND PERCEIVED DURATION

Methods

Subjects. Four experimentally naive Red Carneaux pigeons (*Columba livia*) were maintained at about 75-80% of their free-feeding weights during the experiment.

Apparatus. The rear wall of the chamber contained a rectangular (5 by 8 cm) pecking key (Campden Instruments, No. 444) centered above the opening of the food magazine. Light stimuli were presented by means of a xenon discharge lamp (Osram-XIE 40W/1) monitored by a stroboscopic unit which controlled, independently of the frequency, the total number of impulses in a stimulus train. In order to stimulate well above the pigeon's critical frequency of fusion, the tests were performed using stimuli of 330 elementary flashes per second. In this way, a sequence of impulses was perceived as a continuous flash whose duration was controlled by the number of elementary discharges. The stroboscopic unit made it possible to generate sequences of flashes with durations varying from 50 μsec (duration of an elementary flash) to 1 sec, at a constant luminance level. In order to maximally reduce light-intensity loss, the lamp was placed at the focal point of an optical system providing a parallel beam projected onto the translucent plexiglas key, thus ensuring a uniform illumination. Luminance was modified by interposing graded neutral density filters in the light beam. At the steady rate of 330 flashes/sec and without filtering, the luminance level of the key was 21 cd/m². A steady dim light furnished a constant key-luminance level of 3 cd/m². The interior of the test chamber was illuminated by a 24-V ceiling incandescent lamp. The light diffused through a sheet of white translucent plexiglas and provided an overall chamber illumination of 10 lux (mean luminance level of the walls about 1 cd/m²). In order to isolate the animals from external noise, the experiments were carried out with a steady "white noise" of constant intensity (approximately 30 dB above absolute threshold).

It is known that the perception of duration is dependent on stimulus intensity; thus the intensity factor had to be eliminated. Bearing in mind that the pigeon can easily detect intensity variations (Hodos and Bonbright, 1972), our intention was not to determine the subjective luminance equalization curves, as was the case in man (Servière et al., 1977a). As the stimuli were automatically presented in a random order, it was desirable to randomly place neutral density filters (15, 1, 0.5, 0.1) behind the pecking key. Intervals between each stimulus ranged from 5 to 15 sec. Immediately after the end of a stimulus presentation, an electronic gate opened a 3-sec possibility for pecking, after which pecking was ineffective. Pecks during stimulus application always resulted in a 4-sec period in which the key and chamber lights were turned off. After an average of 20 sessions distributed over 3–4 weeks, the preliminary training was completed and psychophysical sessions were begun.

Psychophysical Test Procedures. Psychophysical sessions were scheduled for 5 days a week. The typical session lasted for 120 positive reinforcements or approximately 1 hr. The procedure adopted was similar to that employed by Hodos et al. (1976). Each session began with a series of 30 "warmup" trials within which two stimuli were presented: a T stimulus equal to 200 msec and a t stimulus of 10 msec duration. This was followed by an assessment period in which the same stimuli were used. If the bird performed at 90% or better on the T, and maximally responded at 15% on the t, the psychophysical testing was continued and the data were compiled. Two psychophysical testing sequences following the "assessment" situation were each carried out in a random order of presentation of durations.

Procedure 1: Eight different durations ranging from 200 to 20 msec were presented with an equal probability of presentation of 0.0625. The ninth duration (t = 10 msec) was presented with an 8 times higher probability of appearance, i.e., 0.5.

Pecking after the presentation of one of the eight durations (from t_1 to t_8) produced a 4-sec period illumination of the food magazine with random access (50%) to the grain hopper. Pecking after the ninth (t)

duration was always followed by negative reinforcement (4-sec black-out period, key and chamber dark, "white noise" cut off). In the latter, no correction procedure was used. After completion of a block of 64 presentations, the initial sequence, including "warmup," was repeated. During the psychophysical testing sequences, four blocks of 64 presentations were performed.

Procedure 2: Two different durations, equal to t (10 msec) and T, changed before each block of around 60 presentations. Each was randomly presented with an equal probability of 0.5. As in the former procedure, pecking after t produced negative reinforcement, whereas pecking after T produced positive reinforcement, with 50% random access to the grain. After a block of presentations (30 times for t and T), "warmup" and assessment sequences were reintroduced before the beginning of another block of presentations in which T had been reduced. In any session, depending on the bird's responses, T was decreased six or eight times. In the different sessions, T was changed according to the following different values: 200, 140, 100, 90, 80, 60, 40, and 20 msec.

Results

Training and Error Rates on Easy Tests. During the training session, the five pigeons gradually learned to peck after the presentation of T (400 msec) and to refrain from pecking after the presentation of t (10 msec). Figure 1 shows the evolution of percentage pecking after T and t during the training sessions for one of the animals. It can be noted that even during the latest training sessions or during "warmup" and assessment periods the animals were able to reach a percentage of responses of only around 10% instead of 0% when the stimulus duration was 10 msec. On the other hand, all birds were able to perform beyond a pecking rate of 98% when the stimulus duration was longer than 100 msec.

Procedure 1. The percentage responses obtained after each of the nine stimulus durations ($t_1, \ldots, t_9$) were plotted as a function of duration to form a psychometric function. These functions are shown in Fig. 2 for four birds. The psychometric function shown in Fig. 2 as a thick-lined curve was obtained by joining the "medians" of the different groups of responses obtained for each duration with the four pigeons. The passage from the lower value of pecking frequency (around 20%) to the upper value (around 100%) is not abrupt; between these two extremes lies a range of progressive transition.

With decision criteria set at 25% and 75%, respectively, the χ^2 test indicates that the probability of the pigeon having obtained a chance

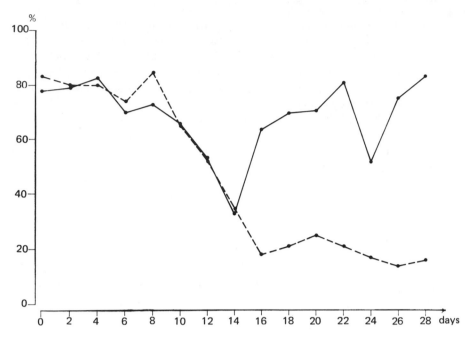

Fig. 1. Evolution of the frequency of the pecking responses during learning of basic conditioning for one of the pigeons. Experimental paradigm: to peck for presentation of a long flash, $T = 400$ msec (●——●), and to refrain from pecking for presentation of a short flash, $t = 10$ msec (●- - -●). Abscissa: percentage of the pecking responses. Ordinate: days (one session every 2 days).

level performance is less than 0.01. The threshold was set at 50% of pecking responses.

The function obtained with the group data shows that frequency pecking stays between 90% and 100% until $T = 100$ msec, thus clearly demonstrating perfect discrimination with respect to t. For shorter values, the pecking rate shifts downward from 75% when T is about 80 msec to 15% when T is about 20 msec.

With a pecking rate of about 20% for a stimulus duration of 10 msec, it can be seen that a null percentage was never obtained with this group of birds after the actual number of 20 sessions. Thus, in order to take into account the inability of pigeons to prevent themselves from pecking, we shall consider that the range of uncertainty discrimination does not lie between 75% and 25%, but between 80% and 40%, the threshold being raised to 60%. With these criteria, the range of perceptual uncertainty lies between approximately between 80 and 30 msec, and the threshold becomes situated around 50 msec.

Procedure 2: In procedure 2, a typical session comprised several different blocks of presentations in which two fixed values of t and T were alternated at random. The percentage responses obtained are plotted as a function of the duration of T in two graphs: the upper one (Fig. 3a) representing the response frequency after T, the lower one representing the response frequency after t (Fig. 3b). The two functions were drawn by joining the means of the four means of data points obtained over 20 sessions. The upper curve exhibits a steady, high level of responses ($\geq 98\%$) until T was decreased to 80 msec. For shorter values of T ($T \leq 50$ msec), the pecking frequency became less than 75% and then rapidly decreased to 40% with T equal to 20 msec. The lower curve exhibits a response level lying under 25% with $T \geq$ 90 msec. For shorter values of T, the frequency of responses rises and oscillates around 25%, reaching 44% with $T = 20$ msec, thus indicating an actual incapability of discrimination between T and t when T is shorter than 60 msec.

In order to take into account the difficulty pigeons have to refrain

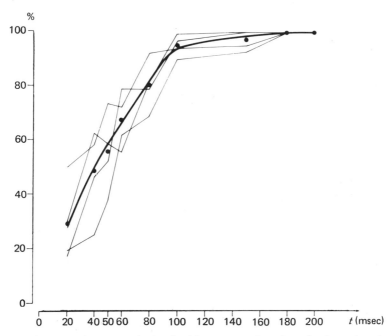

Fig. 2. Psychometric functions obtained with test procedure 1 on the four pigeons. The four thin-lined curves represent the evolution of the percentage of pecking responses as a function of stimulus duration (t_n). The thick-lined curve is obtained by joining the mean frequencies of the four pigeons. In this procedure, pecking for presentation of t_n (from 200 to 2 msec) randomly produced positive reinforcement. Pecking for presentation of $t = 10$ msec always produced punishment.

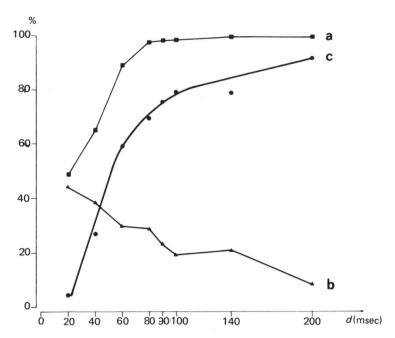

Fig. 3. Evolution of the response frequency obtained with test procedure 2 on the four pigeons. (a) Evolution of the percentage of pecking responses as a function of the duration of T. Pecking for T randomly produced positive reinforcement. (b) Evolution of the percentage of pecking responses for t (10 msec) as a function of the duration of T. Pecking for t always produced punishment. (c) Psychometric function obtained by subtracting the percentage of responses for t (curve b) from the percentage of responses for T (curve a) for each stimulus duration. Points correspond to the mean value of the results obtained on the four animals over 20 sessions.

from pecking, we plotted a third curve obtained by subtracting the frequency of responses on t from the frequency of responses on T for each duration used. The graph of Fig. 3c is a psychometric function similar to the type shown in Fig. 2, but here the range of uncertainty, set between 25% and 75% of pecking frequency, lies between approximately 40 and 90 msec, the I-D threshold settling around 55 msec.

With these decision criteria set at 25% and 75%, the χ^2 test indicates that the probability of the pigeon having attained a chance level of performance is less than 0.01.

Discussion

On the basis of responses given by the animal, one can wonder how the generalization of the basic conditioning is organized (pecking on T produced positive reinforcement, pecking on t produced punishment). In other words, how are the responses distributed as a function of different duration values (t_x) between t and T with $t = 10$ msec and $T = 200$ msec?

The curves of Figs. 2 and 3 indicate that

1. When $t_x \geqslant 100$ msec, the response level is similar to the response level obtained with $T = 200$ msec ("t_x pecking frequency" $\geqslant 90\%$; "T pecking frequency" $= 100\%$).
2. When $t_x < 30$ msec, the response level is not very different from that obtained with $t = 10$ msec ("t_x pecking frequency" $< 40\%$; "T pecking frequency" $\leqslant 20\%$).
3. When $30 < t_x < 80$ msec in procedure 1 and 40 msec $< t_x < 80$ msec in procedure 2, the response level is situated in the range of uncertainty that was previously defined by 40–80% for procedure 1 and 25–75% for procedure 2.

These results indicate the existence of three duration ranges:

1. When $t_x \leqslant 30$ msec, stimulus duration is assimilated to $t = 10$ msec.
2. When $t_x > 100$ msec, stimulus duration is assimilated to $T = 200$ msec.
3. From $t_x = 30$ msec to $t_x = 100$ msec, the response level progresses from a level identical to that obtained with $t = 10$ msec to a level identical to that obtained with $T = 200$ msec.

These values are compatible with those previously obtained in man (Servière et al., 1977a) describing three ranges of duration perception: instantaneous, uncertain, and durable. Further extending the comparison with human perceptual data, it can be seen that for the range of duration in which the pigeon is unable to discriminate stimuli on the basis of their duration the human subject perceived durations as instantaneous. On the other hand, for the range of durations in which the pigeon can easily discriminate stimuli of different durations, the human subject referred to stimuli as durable.

It would be interesting to attempt to clarify the three following points:

1. Concerning the parameter tested, it should be noted that any response based on brightness discrimination or on any other parameter (cf. Methods section) was diminished. Thus we can be assured that pigeons did use duration as the judgment parameter.
2. Concerning the procedure used, the similarity in shape of the

psychometric functions obtained in the pigeon (Figs. 2 and 3c) and in man (Servière et al., 1977a, their Fig. 4) can be interpreted as an indication of the validity of the two procedures employed with regard to the question raised.

3. Concerning the kind of operation performed during the testing procedure of conditioning, did the animal operate under a differential temporal threshold situation or under a "category judgment" situation between two types of temporal perception? On the basis of present data compared with those obtained in man, we can avoid this suspicion. Nevertheless, referring to the determination of a differential temporal threshold in the pigeon for duration values in the order of seconds (Stubbs, 1968; Kinchla, 1970), it is valuable to look for the shortest durations where $\Delta t/T$ can still be determined. Taking into account the existence of an instantaneous range within durations of milliseconds, the hypothesis is that a determination of a $\Delta t/T$ would be impossible.

ELECTROPHYSIOLOGICAL DATA ON THE RELATION BETWEEN STIMULUS DURATION AND PERCEIVED DURATION

Methods

Experiments were carried out on Red Carneaux pigeons (*Columba livia*). The animals were fixed in an apparatus allowing the utilization of the Karten and Hodos (1967) stereotaxic atlas. A continuous perfusion with Flaxedil necessitated forced ventilation, which was assured by an air flow introduced by means of a tracheal nozzle, and brought out by bilateral perforation of posteroaerian sacs. During all of the surgical preparations (tracheotomy, craniotomy, perforation of the aerian sacs, sectioning of the eyelids), the animals were under local xylocaine anesthesia.

Monocular presentation in a Maxwellian view optical system was used. The light source was a glow modulator tube (Sylvania-R 1131C) providing a constant luminance level of the stimulus field (22 deg) of 71,000 cd/m². Stimuli were presented at a frequency of 0.1/sec on a steady, low background with a mean luminance of approximately 5 cd/m². Fourteen different durations were used: 200, 160, 140, 120, 100, 80, 60, 50, 40, 32, 20, 8, 3.2, and 2 msec.

Bipolar recordings of visual evoked potentials (VEPs) were obtained from the optic chiasma (lateral 1.0, anterior 7.0). The concentric steel electrodes had an external diameter of 0.4 mm and an electrical resistance of about 100 kΩ. Responses were amplified (× 500), high- and low-frequency filters set at 500 and 0.3 Hz, respectively, and the signal was recorded on magnetic tape (FM) for later processing. Except for the 320-msec stimulus, the sample time for averaging was 300 msec, using 2000 data points, thus yielding dwell times of 0.15 msec/data point. The averaged potentials were drawn on the X-Y plotter.

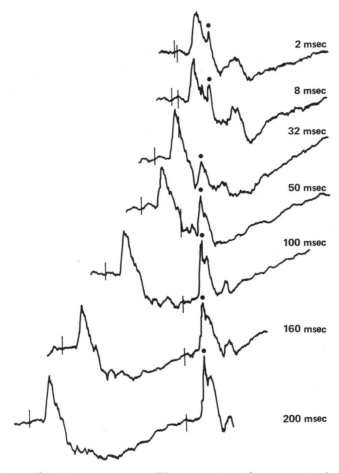

Fig. 4. Averaged optic tract responses (50 presentations) for seven stimulus durations (from 2 to 200 msec) given at a constant luminance level of 7 cd/m². Responses are displayed with the OFF artifacts lined up. The position of the first positive OFF component is indicated by the solid symbol, ●. Total sample time = 300 msec, dwell time = 0.15 msec/data point.

Results

For durations longer than 50 msec, the ON and OFF components of the averaged responses were clearly separated and free of interaction (Fig. 4).

The ON response was composed of a large, stable positive wave (peak latency ~ 29 msec) followed by smaller and more variable oscillations. The OFF response was composed of a large positive wave divided into two peaks of unequal amplitude, the latency of the higher peak being approximately 27 msec. This wave was followed by a second positive peak of much smaller amplitude.

By lining up the OFF artifacts, it was easy to follow the OFF response for flash durations decreasing from 50 to 2 msec. At 50 msec, the OFF response intervened after the latest small oscillations of the ON response. At 32 msec, the OFF response immediately followed the large ON peak. With a further decrease in flash duration, and by bearing in

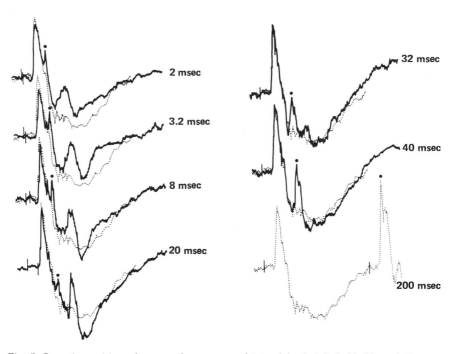

Fig. 5. Superimposition of averaged responses obtained for 2, 3.2, 8, 20, 32, and 40 msec (solid line) with averaged response recorded for 200 msec (dotted line), showing a progressive ascent of the OFF peak along the descending side of the ON component. Responses are averaged over 50 presentations. Total sample time = 300 msec, dwell time = 0.15 msec/data point.

mind the previously observed shift of the OFF response toward the ON response, it is possible to identify the OFF component on the descending phase of the ON peak. This identification is confirmed by the superimposition of responses obtained for 2, 3.2, 8, 20, and 32 msec with the averaged VEP recorded for 200 msec (Fig. 5), which shows the OFF peak progressively ascending along the descending side of the ON peak.

In Fig. 4, where OFF artifacts were lined up, it can be observed that OFF peaks ceased to be aligned for durations under 50 msec, this shift corresponding to a progressive lengthening of the OFF-peak latency.

Peak latencies of the ON and OFF components of the averaged VEPs have been plotted, respectively, in Fig. 6a,b. The peak latency of the ON response (a) remains constant (slope = −0.01) at a mean value of about 30 msec for all stimulus durations. With stimulus presentations ranging from 200 to 60 msec, the peak latency of the off response (b) remains constant (slope = −0.02) around a mean value of 27 msec. At yet shorter flash durations (40–2 msec), the latency is seen to increase (slope = −0.51), reaching 45 msec for a 2-msec flash duration.

By plotting the ON-OFF interpeak intervals (IPI) as a function of stimulus duration, it is shown that these two duration values are equal in the range of 200–50 mscc (slope = 1.00). For the shortest stimulus durations, the IPI reduction ceases to be equal to stimulus duration shortening (slope = 0.64).

Discussion

Recording from the cat optic nerve and employing a constant-intensity light stimulus (3300 cd/m²), Efron (1973b) observed that under a stimulus duration of 48 msec the interval separating ON and OFF components no longer decreased. By looking for an analogous, incompressible, ON-OFF interval at the cortical level in man (VEPs) and employing a constant light stimulus level (160 cd/m² for durable stimuli), we also found that under 50 msec the IPI remained constant.

In the present experiment, using a constant luminance level, it was observed that the slope changed from 1 to 0.64 instead of having a change in slope from 1 to 0.

The discrepancy with Efron's electrophysiological data is at present difficult to explain. The conditions required for producing the phenomenon on incompressibility of the ON-OFF interval are not yet evident.

The same kind of discrepancy is observed for the human transcranial VEPs. We were able to obtain an incompressible interval at this level; however, the phenomenon was not apparent, for example, in the

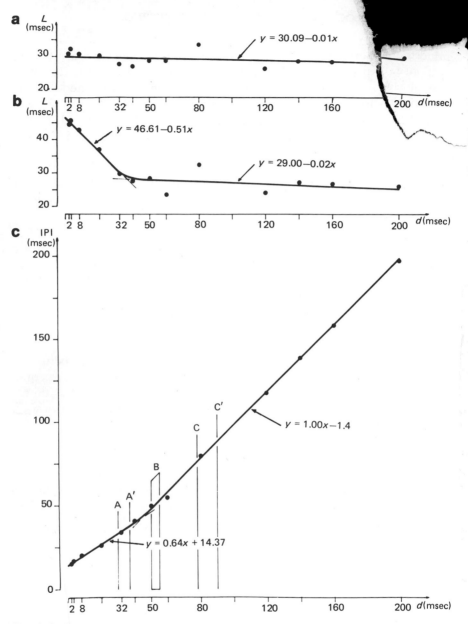

Fig. 6. Peak latencies of the ON and OFF components of the averaged VEPs. The data are derived from the same recordings from which data presented in Fig. 4 are extracted. (a) Latency of the ON peak component as a function of flash stimulus duration. (b) Latency of the OFF peak component as a function of flash stimulus duration. (c) ON-OFF interpeak interval (IPI) as a function of flash duration. Capital letters correspond to results obtained in the conditioning experiments. A and C: durations as determined by procedure 1, representing 40 and 80% pecking responses, respectively. A' and C': durations as determined by procedure 2, representing 25 and 75% pecking responses, respectively. B: zone of durations as determined by the two procedures representing 60 and 50% pecking responses, respectively.

VEP recordings presented by Clynes et al. (1964) in response to stimuli from 250 to 1 msec.

In order to reach a better understanding in this field, further experiments are needed. A number of experiments are in progress using lower luminance levels.

REFERENCES

Clynes, M., Kohn, M., and Lifshitz, K.: Dynamics and spatial behaviour of light evoked potentials, their modification under hypnosis. *Ann. N.Y. Acad. Sci.* **112**:468-508 (1964).

Durup, G., and Fessard, A.: Sur la variation de l'énergie lumineuse et de l'acuité visuelle en fonction de la durée à intensité apparente constante. *Ann. Psychol.* **30**:72-85 (1929).

Efron, R.: The relationship between the duration of a stimulus and the duration of a perception. *Neuropsychologia* **8**:37-55 (1970a).

Efron, R.: The minimum duration of a perception. *Neuropsychologia* **8**:57-63 (1970b).

Efron, R.: Effect of stimulus duration on perceptual onst and offset latencies. *Percept. Psychophys.* **8**:251-254 (1970c).

Efron, R.: The measurement of perceptual durations. *Stud. Gen.* **23**:550-561 (1970d).

Efron, R.: Conservation of temporal information by perceptual systems. *Percept. Psychophys.* **14**:518-530 (1973a).

Efron, R.: An invariant characteristic of perceptual systems in the time domain. In Kornblum, S. (ed.): *Attention and Performance IV*. Academic Press, New York (1973b).

Haber, R., IV, and Standing, L. G.: Direct estimates of the apparent duration of a flash. *Can. J. Psychol.* **24**:216-229 (1970).

Hodos, W., and Bonbright, J. C.: The detection of visual intensity differences by pigeons. *J. Exp. Anal. Behav.* **18**:471-479 (1972).

Hodos, W., Leibowitz, R.W., and Bonbright, J. C.: Near-field visual acuity of pigeons: Effects of head location and stimulus luminance. *J. Exp. Anal. Behav.* **25**:129-141 (1976).

Karten, H., and Hodos, W.: *A Stereotaxic Atlas of the Brain of the Pigeon*. Johns Hopkins Press, Baltimore (1967).

Kinchla, J. Discrimination of two auditory durations of pigeons. *Percept. Psychophys.* **8**:299-307 (1970).

Servière, J., Miceli, D., and Galifret, Y.: A psychophysical study of the visual perception of "instantaneous" and "durable." *Vision Res.* **17**:57-63 (1977a).

Servière, J., Miceli, D., and Galifret, Y.: Electrophysiological correlates of the visual perception of "instantaneous" and "durable." *Vision Res.* **17**:65-69 (1977b).

Stubbs, A.: The discrimination of stimulus duration by pigeons. *J. Exp. Anal. Behav.* **11**:223-238 (1968).

5

Visual Performance of Pigeons

JUAN D. DELIUS and JACKY EMMERTON

INTRODUCTION

Even superficial observation of birds in their natural environment suggests that the performance of their visual system is at least on a par with ours. Many detailed field studies amply confirm this inference. During a 3-year study of free-ranging skylarks (*Alauda arvensis*), circumstantial evidence indicated that their vision was superior to that of the observer in a variety of situations (Delius, 1963). The skylarks could clearly recognize each other individually at a range of 30 m or more purely by visual cues, while the observer could only do so unreliably when aided by a 30× telescope. Skylarks spotted merlins or pigeon hawks (*Falco columbarius*) flying overhead at heights where the observer positively could not resolve them without the aid of 8× binoculars. Perhaps these songbirds' most remarkable performance was the detection of minute, usually camouflaged insect prey in dune sand and vegetation. As hard as the observer tried, helped by a 5× magnifying lens, his hunting success rate was at best only a tenth that of skylarks. Casual observations of free-ranging domestic pigeons (*Columba livia*) indicate that their vision is, if anything, better than that of skylarks. We are thus inclined to believe that the measures of visual capabilities that we obtain in the laboratory are still only a pale reflection of the real performance of the pigeon's visual system.

JUAN D. DELIUS and JACKY EMMERTON • Psychologisches Institut, Ruhr-Universität, Bochum, West Germany. The work reported here has been supported by the Science Research Council and the Deutsche Forschungsgemeinschaft. It was in part carried out while the authors were at the Department of Psychology, University of Durham, England.

The psychophysical techniques must as yet, we feel, be considered far from efficient or optimal in assessing what these animals can do visually. Depending as we do mainly on conditioning procedures, so-called biological constraints on learning could often be the limiting factor (Hinde and Stevenson-Hinde, 1973). Attempts to make psycho-physical measurement pigeon-ergonomic might well prove worth-while. In the case of some other species, such methodological invest-ment has in fact been necessary before measurement was at all possible (Stebbins, 1970).

LEARNING CONSTRAINTS AND PSYCHOPHYSICS

Although we cannot claim to have made a systematic effort in this respect, an experiment of ours gives an indication of what we have in mind (Delius and Emmerton, 1978b). The starting point was an auditory question of whether pigeons could discriminate temporal tone patterns. While this capability could not be demonstrated with appetitive in-strumental techniques (Krasnegor, 1971; Delius, unpublished experi-ments), it proved exceedingly easy to do so with a classical aversive method (Delius and Tarpy, 1974). Conversely, when one of us at-tempted to apply the latter procedure for psychophysical measurements of the color discrimination capabilities of pigeons, the results seemed to indicate that the birds were color-blind! In a specifically designed experiment, we could substantiate the differential effectiveness of the conditioning procedures. We examined discrimination learning of hues and pitch by pigeons with particular versions of two learning para-digms: successive, conditional, food-rewarded, key-pecking condition-ing and classical, shock-reinforced, heart-rate conditioning. In a suit-ably balanced design, the same pigeons were expected to learn to discriminate either broadband white and red diffuse illumination, matched to the same pigeon-subjective brightness, or tones of 1000 and 2000 Hz adjusted to be of nearly equal pigeon-subjective loudness. In the classical conditioning situation, one stimulus of each pair served as the positive conditioned stimulus and was followed by an electric shock as the unconditioned stimulus. The conditioned response re-corded was the relative increase in heart rate during the positive stim-ulus as compared with the negative stimulus. In the instrumental sit-uation, the animals were rewarded with access to grain for pecking either the upper key of a Skinner box in the presence of one stimulus of the pair or the lower key in the presence of the other stimulus. Responses to the incorrect keys resulted in time-out.

The learning curves obtained (Fig. 1) showed that the animals very quickly gave evidence of discriminating the lights in the instrumental situation and the tones in the classical situation. However, there was no evidence of any differentiation of the hues during classical aversive conditioning and of pitch during instrumental appetitive conditioning. Obviously, the former method should be avoided in studies of the pigeon's perception of color. There are indications, though, that this conclusion cannot be extended to include other qualities of visual stimulation: movement or brightness, for example (Kreithen, this volume; Kreithen and Keeton, 1974; Cohen and Trauner, 1969). Experiments by LoLordo and collaborators (see LoLordo and Furrow, 1976) suggest that the variable responsible for this learning asymmetry is not the classical or operant paradigm of conditioning but rather the difference in reinforcement quality, pain or food, is decisive. They showed that in a treadle-pressing task a compound tone–light stimulus comes to exercise control through the light component when food is used as reward and through the tone component when shock is the reinforcement. It seems that pigeons are inherently prepared or counterprepared to associate specific stimulus cues with certain reinforcement qualities (Seligman, 1970). We have argued that the particular constraints can be understood as phylogenetic adaptations to the fact that hues but not tones are associated with food and, conversely, tones but not hues are correlated with pain in the normal environment of pigeons.

Grossly inefficient methods, as aversive cardiac conditioning

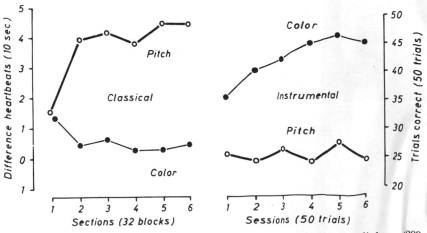

Fig. 1. Mean learning curves of four pigeons discriminating red and white lights or 1000- and 2000-Hz tones both in an appetitive key-pecking and in an aversive heart-rate conditioning situation. Modified from Delius and Emmerton (1978b).

54   JUAN D. DELIUS AND JACKY EMMERTON

turned out to be in the specific context of hue discrimination, are of course rapidly weeded out from the methodological repertoire, but the nagging question is whether the psychophysical procedures we currently use might not be contrary to more subtle constraints of pigeons' specific learning dispositions.

DISCRIMINATION OF LIGHT POLARIZATION PLANE

Associative or learning constraints, which can of course impinge on other contingencies than those between stimuli and reinforcement (Shettleworth, 1972), are certainly not the only ones that interfere with research on pigeon perceptual performance. This is illustrated by our work on this animal's discrimination of the light polarization plane orientation (Delius et al., 1976). In our first experiment, we had hungry pigeons learn to differentiate the changing plane orientation of an overhead light surface in a tall Skinner box. Every second wall of the box was furnished with a response key; pecks to a key aligned in a specified way with respect to the overhead linear polarization were rewarded with access to food; responses to a key not so aligned were punished with a period of darkness. The subjects learned this task easily (Fig. 2), thus confirming and expanding Kreithen and Keeton's (1974) demonstration that pigeons are sensitive to polarization axis changes.

This result, however, contrasted with that of a study by Montgomery and Heinemann (1952). They failed to find evidence of polariza-

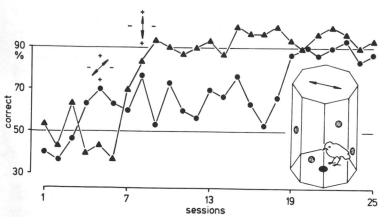

Fig. 2. Learning curves of two pigeons discriminating the polarization plane orientation of an overhead light surface. The insets indicate each subject's task. Unpublished data from a study by Delius et al. (1976).

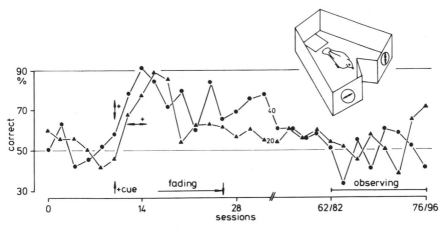

Fig. 3. Learning curves of two pigeons discriminating the polarization plane orientation of a pair of stimuli in a Y-maze. A temporary light cue, then faded off, marked the correct stimulus. Later a prechoice stimulus observing period was enforced. Means of pairs of sessions have been plotted. For simplification, 20 (40) sessions have been left out.

tion axis discrimination by pigeons when presenting the discriminanda on the response key itself. We have argued that this failure might have been due to the location of the stimulus display. Keys are viewed by pigeons in the lower anterior field of vision. In nature, biologically significant stimuli will rarely be recognizable by polarization cues in this field. This is different for the upper field of vision, where the polarization of skylight, dependent on the sun's position (Sekera, 1956), could supplement the pigeon's well-known sun-compass orientation (Schmidt-Koenig, 1958).

A recent experiment of ours appears to confirm that pigeons find it difficult, if not impossible, to learn to discriminate light surfaces of differently oriented stationary polarization planes when these stimuli are placed at eye level. We utilized an automated Y-maze (Fig. 3). The end wall of each goal arm was equipped with a circular surface (diameter 5.5 cm) of linearly polarized light. The plane orientations of the two discriminative stimuli were arranged at right angles to each other, but from trial to trial and while darkened they were quasirandomly either rotated by 90 deg or left stationary (but see use of correction procedure below). A vertical plane orientation was defined as correct for one subject, a horizontal one for another. Approach to a stimulus by the subjects was detected by reed relays sensing small magnets attached to the skulls of the animals with dental cement. Correct choices were rewarded by raising an illuminated food hopper immediately below the stimulus; incorrect ones were followed by a brief period of darkness. The next trial began with the starting end of the maze being illuminated by a lamp. When the animal depressed a weight-sensitive platform, the stimuli came on and remained lit until the subject made a choice. A correction procedure operated to counteract the development of position habits. Following incorrect choices, the polarization plane orientation of the stimuli remained unchanged over the following trials until the animals had made a correct response. These correction trials were of course not scored.

To facilitate acquisition, we initially marked the correct stimulus with an extra light. In later sessions, this cue was progressively dimmed. While the subjects each learned the brightness discrimination, which constituted the initial phase of the fading technique, within less than ten training sessions of 30 trials each, they did not maintain a polarization plane discrimination to a performance level better than about 60% correct over the next 45 trials. In an attempt to improve the performance, a "stimulus-observing" period was enforced during the last 15 trials. The subjects had to remain for at least 5 sec on the starting platform; if they left it prematurely, the stimuli were extinguished and the trial was aborted. There was no steady improvement, but on occasional sessions the animals clearly did not choose at random, yielding scores of 85% correct or, more remarkably, 15% or fewer correct choices (Fig. 3). Although the overall performance might be significantly above chance we are not certain that it is not due to cues other than polarization. Control experiments aimed at removing possible slight parasitic brightness patterns associated with the polarization plane orientation would have to be performed.

It is clear that pigeons are less successful in discriminating the polarization plane orientations in this situation than in our original experiment with overhead stimuli. It could be that the size of the polarized stimuli is a crucial factor. In this latter experiment and in that of Montgomery and Heinemann, the stimuli were relatively small, whereas they were larger in our earlier experiment: the normal stimulus, the sky, is itself an extensive source. We are inclined to believe, however, that the results are explained by the circumstance that the polarization sensitivity of the pigeon is mainly associated with the upper field of vision, much as it has been shown to be in a species of African ant, *Cataglyphis bicolor* (Wehner, 1976).

Support comes from an electroretinographic study of this sensitivity (Delius et al., 1976). Using standard techniques, we have found that the summit of the b-wave of the electroretinogram altered its shape depending on the orientation of the polarization axis of the stimulus flash. This shape difference was fairly small when the stimulus beam fell on the center of the retina but was quite marked when it struck the

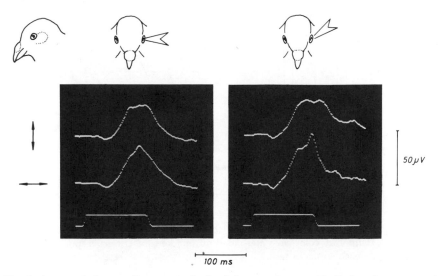

Fig. 4. Averaged electroretinograms obtained from a pigeon with flashes (lower traces) of differing polarization plane orientation and of different angles of incidence. From Delius et al. (1976).

lower portions of the retina (Fig. 4). Which feature of the eye is responsible for this polarization sensitivity of the lower field of vision is not yet certain. We have hypothesized that the double cones, known to be more frequent in the yellow area (posterior and upper field of vision) than in the red area (lower anterior field of vision) of the pigeon retina (King-Smith 1969; Bowmaker, this volume), might be involved. This would agree with Montgomery and Heinemann's failure, but it does not concur so well with our maze results. There the pigeons seemed to observe the stimuli monocularly, that is, presumably with the fovea centralis region, which is part of the yellow field.

An alternative hypothesis is that the pecten might be involved. This structure seems to be particularly well developed in diurnal flying species (Menner, 1938), that is, those that would benefit most from the navigating edge that a polarization plane sensitivity might impart. Current experiments in which we are systematically scanning the various areas of the retina for the electroretinographic polarization effect should help to clarify this issue. However, it seems likely that difficulties with the psychophysics of polarized light have little to do with the constraints of conditioning but rather with the regional specializations of the pigeon's eye.

An experiment using the same tall octagonal Skinner box as in the polarization discrimination study mentioned earlier amplifies this point in a different direction. The pigeons now had to align their responses

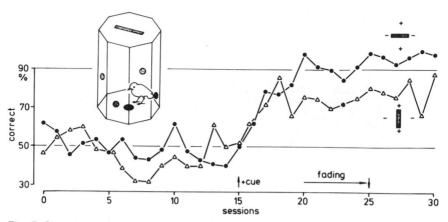

Fig. 5. Learning curves of two pigeons discriminating the orientation of an overhead light bar. A temporary color cue, later faded off, marked the correct response keys. The insets indicate each subject's task.

to the wall keys according to two alternative orientations of an elongated rectangular bar of light projected on the translucent lid of the chamber. Compared with the ease with which pigeons learned the polarization task in the same box, the difficulty they experienced in mastering this nearly equivalent task was surprising. No evidence of acquisition was apparent even after 750 trials, which has to be compared with the less than 400 trials that the subjects in the polarization experiment took to master their task. Only after we aided the birds by introducing an additional cue in the form of red light projected on the correct keys and later fading it off again did they learn to perform this task (Fig. 5). Since similar orientation discriminations certainly present little difficulty for pigeons when the stimuli are displayed on the response key (Zeigler and Schmerler, 1965; but see Delius and Emmerton, 1978a), we are led to assume that the sensory system associated with the upper field of vision is not well adapted for the recognition of brightness pattern orientations. Their ability to orient themselves by the sun in a similar situation (Schmidt-Koenig, 1958), however, suggests that this restriction may be of a very specific nature.

SPECTRUM OF POLARIZATION SENSITIVITY

The polarization of skylight is known to be maximal in the ultraviolet (Sekera, 1956). The polarization plane sensitivity of bees (*Apis mellifica*) is accordingly restricted to their ultraviolet-sensitive mechanisms (Menzel and Snyder, 1974; von Helversen and Edrich, 1974). From both our behavioral and electroretinographic experiments, it is already certain that the polarization sensitivity of pigeons, unlike that of the bee, extends into the visible part of the spectrum. Nonetheless, it might be specially developed in the ultraviolet. We have only begun to look into the effective spectrum of the polarization sensitivity, but there is already good evidence that pigeons can see ultraviolet (Wright, 1972b; see also Huth and Buckhardt, 1972).

One of us has extended the measurement of the spectral sensitivity of the pigeon's retina into the near ultraviolet. Standard electroretinographic techniques supplemented by a transient averager were used to obtain an equal response-amplitude spectrum. Although the optical system did not provide enough energy in the deeper ultraviolet, we could confirm that the pigeon is sensitive to the near ultraviolet. Our results also suggested that a secondary sensitivity peak exists in the deeper UV at or below about 360 nm (Fig. 6) (Emmerton, 1975). Preceding this rise in sensitivity, we found a minimum at 400–420 nm. This agrees reasonably well with the results obtained by Kreithen (this volume) using a spectral threshold determination procedure in conjunction with classical heart rate conditioning. Other spectral sensitivity measurements have also indicated the presence of a secondary maximum at short wavelengths (Blough, 1957; Graf and Norren, 1974; Norren, 1975), but they have positioned the minimum at 440 nm. Furthermore, Graf and Norren report a subsidiary maximum at 400–

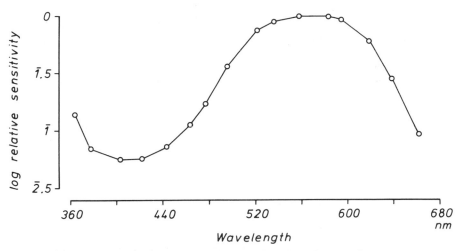

Fig. 6. Electroretinographically measured spectral sensitivity function from two pigeons. Mean of six series of measurements. Criterion amplitude for averaged responses was 32 μV. From Emmerton (1975).

420 nm, and indeed relate these data to the presence of a chromatic mechanism whose response maximum is located in this part of the spectrum. Graf and Norren's electroretinographic measurements showed a shift in the position of the sensitivity minimum from 440 nm to 420 nm, corresponding more closely to our own data, as the electro-retinogram criterion amplitude was increased. In a behavioral experiment designed to remeasure spectral sensitivity in the ultraviolet, we intend to investigate the effect of setting different response criteria and using different adapting conditions on the position of this secondary minimum and on the change in relative sensitivity of short- and longer-wavelength spectral mechanisms which may well occur at "above-threshold" intensity levels.

Our electroretinographic measures were obtained from the central retina; it could be that the lower retina, in connection with the polarization sensitivity, might be especially UV responsive. Incidentally, this ultraviolet sensitivity must depend on a short-wave transparency of the pigeon's ocular media. A recent study (Govardovskii and Zueva, 1977) shows that they indeed transmit wavelengths down to 340 nm. In mammals, it is absorption by the ocular media that precludes an ultraviolet sensitivity (Tan, 1971; Norren and Vos, 1974); such a sensitivity could still be potentially mediated by subsidiary absorption maxima of the photopigments (Dartnall, 1972) or relatively stable breakdown products of the visual pigments (Yoshizawa, 1972) which absorb in this spectral region. A loss with age of short-wave transmittance of the lens of birds, similar to that seen in mammals (Muntz, 1972), does not, however, seem to be averted. This causes a noticeable short-wave sensitivity reduction in older animals (Honigmann, 1921; Thompson, 1971). Thompson, using the same type of ERG technique as in our experiment, compared the spectral sensitivity of juvenile and adult herring and lesser blackbacked gulls (*Larus argentatus* and *Laurus fuscus*), while Honigmann, working with sexually mature and young chickens (*Gallus gallus*), used a behavioral method.

COLOR DISCRIMINATION

The pigeon's capacity for seeing ultraviolet has been independently confirmed in one of the two investigations we made into its spectral wavelength discrimination function (Emmerton and Delius, unpublished results). Here, the animals had to discriminate between two monochromatic patches of light (3 by 3 mm) projected onto two widely separated (9 cm) keys of a Skinner box. The patches differed in wavelength but were adjusted to be of equal pigeon-subjective brightness. One of the patches was kept at a constant wavelength from trial to trial, and responses to it were reinforced by food reward. Responses to the other patch were followed by a waiting period. The positions of re-warded and nonrewarded stimuli on the two keys were quasirandomly alternated between trials. The wavelength of the nonrewarded stimulus was stepwise approximated to that of the other patch depending on the discriminative performance of the pigeon. In the first experiment, such progressive wavelength changes were made between separate sessions until the pigeon's performance gave evidence of its failing to discriminate. In the second experiment, in which discrimination within the near-UV spectral region was investigated, a modified track-ing procedure was used and wavelength changes were made within a session. The wavelength difference between the stimuli at the point at which discrimination was failing (70% of responses correct), or at an equivalent level of performance in the tracking method, was considered the threshold wavelength difference at the corresponding point of the spectrum. Measurements were obtained through the spectrum from 360 nm to 680 nm.

Regarding the ultraviolet, not only did the subjects discriminate quite small wavelength differences but they even seemed to exhibit a minimum in the function at about 360–380 nm (Fig. 7). We are presently extending these delta lambda measurements into the shorter-wave-length region, seeking at the same time to confirm this minimum. In any case, there can be no doubt that pigeons can perceive ultraviolet light.

If we can corroborate the wavelength discrimination minimum in the ultraviolet, the function of the pigeon exhibits four minima (at about 600 nm in the orange, 530 nm in the green, 460 nm in the blue, and 360–380 nm in the ultraviolet regions) as compared with the two minima characterizing the human hue discrimination function (Wright and Pitt, 1934). This would suggest that the pigeon's color vision is at

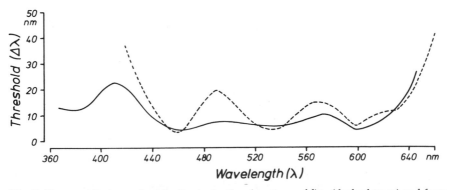

Fig. 7. Mean spectral wavelength discrimination functions of five (dashed trace) and four (continuous trace) pigeons obtained in two different experiments. From Emmerton and Delius (unpublished results).

least pentachromatic! While previous studies indicating that the pigeon's retina contains five morphologically distinguishable cones [four bearing oil droplets of different color (King-Smith, 1969) and one without a droplet, (Cohen, 1963)] would seem to agree with this conclusion, more recent work seems to complicate the picture. Govardovskii and Zueva (1977) conclude, on the basis of an early receptor potential study of the pigeon's isolated retina, that it contains four cone pigments, and state that it possesses seven to eight different-colored oil droplets plus a small number of colorless ones. Bowmaker (this volume), working with microspectrophotometric methods, found three cone pigments and at least five different oil droplets. These findings would indicate a potential complexity of color vision which may not have been fully tapped in these measurements of the pigeon's wavelength discrimination abilities.

There is a further feature of the spectral wavelength discrimination function that needs attention. While comparison of our two separate measurements of this function with those obtained by other authors (Blough, 1972; Riggs et al., 1972; Schneider, 1972; Wright, 1972a; Wright and Cumming, 1971) reveals an approximate agreement regarding the position of the minima in the orange at 600 nm and in the green region of the spectrum at 530–540 nm, there is a peculiar dissension regarding the position of the minimum we located in the blue at 460 nm. While Blough's (1972) results would also seem to indicate that there is a minimum in the blue region, several other authors (Hamilton and Coleman, 1933; Schneider, 1972; Wright, 1972a) have located a minimum in the green-blue, finding in fact a minimum at 500 nm, while conversely Riggs et al.'s (1972) threshold measurements were increasing and our own were at a maximum there. We consider that the variable position of the minimum in the shortwave end of the spectrum is a real phenomenon not due to errors of measurement. A variable that could possibly affect this switch in spectral position is the state of the subject's retina caused by stimulus and/or environmental light intensity that might have been different in the experiments yielding the different minima. In our own experiments, the stimulus intensity level (at 580 nm) was about 1.2 log ft-L in the first experiment, in which the 460-nm blue minimum occurred together with a maximum in the discrimination function at 500 nm in the blue-green, and about 0.7 log ft-L in the second experiment, whose discrimination function was very much flattened in the blue-green. This information would suggest that a decrease in stimulus luminance produces a shift of the minimum toward longer wavelengths. Comparisons of stimulus luminance levels used in the other experiments lead to equivocal conclusions, but any correlation that might have existed would have been confounded by other variations in the conditions of stimulus presentation and testing procedure.

In experiments on spontaneous color preferences of neonate gulls and chickens, there is some indirect evidence that avian color vision in the short-wave region of the spectrum might be particularly sensitive to changes in stimulus intensity and adaptational state (Delius and Thompson, 1970). Incidentally, adult pigeons exhibit a remarkable, strong, spontaneous preference for blue hues (Straka, 1966; Delius, 1968; Sahgal and Iversen, 1975), which could in fact occasionally interfere with psychometric measurements related to hue but which are of interest in their own right. Why blue? That is a functional issue, except that similar blue preferences seem to be of widespread occurrence among vertebrates (frogs *Rana*, e.g., Muntz, 1962), suggesting the persistence of a primitive mechanism.

Another variable that could cause the position switch of the delta lambda minimum in the blue-green section of the spectrum is the geometry of the stimulus display insofar as it might cause the pigeons to view the stimuli in different parts of their visual fields and thus with different retinal areas. While the spectral sensitivity differences between the red and yellow areas are small (Martin and Muntz, this volume; Blough, this volume), there is reason to suspect that the hue discrimination they mediate may differ more markedly. Bowmaker (this volume) shows that the two areas differ in terms of the spectral positioning and bandwidth of the basic mechanisms as determined by the pigment/oil droplet combinations found in the cones of both areas.

In a series of experiments, we have found that stimulus display geometry is indeed a variable that affects the discriminative performance of pigeons when colors but not shapes are involved (Delius, Jahnke-Funk, and Hawker, unpublished results). Some unsystematic observations had indicated that pigeons learn color discriminations in a Skinner box more rapidly when the discriminanda displayed on the response keys are placed one above the other rather than side by side, as is more usual. Accordingly, we equipped a Skinner box with a pair of horizontally and a pair of vertically arranged keys, forming a cross pattern. The keys of each pair were 12.5 cm apart. The subjects had to learn to discriminate the same two broadband colors successively on the vertical and the horizontal pair of keys. A successive conditional method with a correction procedure was used. One or the other color was alternatively presented on either the vertical or the horizontal pair of keys. The unilluminated pair of keys was unresponsive. According to a balanced design, the alternative colors signaled whether the upper or the lower key and the left or the right key was the correct one. Sessions lasted for 32 trials, and each session consisted of two blocks of the "'vertical" task alternating with two of the "'horizontal" task, each block consisting of eight trials. Responses to the correct keys delivered food; pecks to incorrect ones resulted in time-out. Correction trials were disregarded for the performance score but were included in the training-trials count. The cumulative learning curves shown in Fig. 8 indicate that the pigeons learned more rapidly and continued to perform better when the same color discrimination task was laid out on the vertical keys than on the horizontal keys.

The first interpretation we attached to this result was that the pigeons suffer from a left-right confusion much as many humans do (Corballis and Beale, 1976). However, when we replicated the experiment with pattern discrimination tasks instead of a color discrimination one, the effect disappeared. The subjects' performance was nearly identical irrespective of the key geometry. In fact, there is a suggestion that a slight reverse effect might have operated, the horizontal key arrangement yielding a marginally better performance. Since the pattern discrimination should have been as much affected by left-right difficulties as the color differentiation, we have been forced to dismiss the original hypothesis and consider another one.

The binocular field of vision of the pigeon covers a cone-shaped

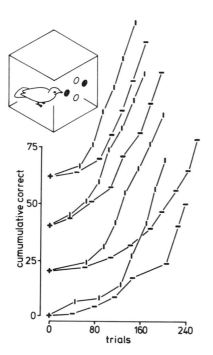

Fig. 8. Cumulative learning curves of four pigeons contemporaneously discriminating the same two colored (orange or red) stimuli arranged on vertical (vertical bars) or horizontal (horizontal bars) pairs of response keys. On the abscissa, the trial count includes correction trials; on the ordinate, it does not. For clarity, the ordinate origins of the pairs of curves have been shifted. From Delius, Jahnke-Funk, and Hawker (unpublished results).

solid angle of lenticular cross-section some 25 deg wide and 90 deg high (estimated from data given by Chard, 1939, and allowing for convergent eye movements) that projects on the red areas of both retinas. In conjunction with the myopia of the binocular field (Catania, 1964; Blough, 1973; Hodos et al., 1976), we assume that the pigeons can simultaneously view the two vertically arranged keys in sharp focus, while they should not be able to encompass the horizontally arranged keys in that way. They have to look at the horizontally arranged keys either successively with the binocular field or simultaneously with one key imaging on the yellow and the other on the red fields of the retinas. Since the performance deficit of the horizontal task has so far proven specific to color cues, we consider that it is the latter viewing style that causes the difficulty; yellow and red fields, as stated earlier, are thought to mediate a different type of color vision. Successive binocular or simultaneous monocular viewing could, of course, also impede discrimination in that they require temporal or interocular integration, respectively. These integration difficulties, however, could be expected to affect both pattern and color differentiation, contrary to our findings. In any case, when the color discrimination experiment was replicated with keys clustered close together (2.5 cm) so that the subjects could presumably also view the horizontal pair of keys binocularly, the performance deficit of the horizontal task was lessened.

It must be kept in mind that the discriminative tasks were of the successive conditional type, identical hues or patterns being displayed on both keys on any given trial. Strictly speaking, viewing only one key of the relevant pair could have been suffecient to solve the problem since no comparison of the stimuli is really necessary unless it be comparison with stored or memorized stimuli seen in previous trials. The suspected chromatovisual differences between the two retinal areas could still have an effect by introducing a subjective hue difference between the two horizontal stimuli, leading the birds to attempt a task solution in terms of a spurious simultaneous discrimination. According to this hypothesis, a more direct and thus more marked stimulus layout effect should become apparent in simultaneous color discrimination experiments which we are presently carrying out. Ultimately, one should expect stimulus layouts allowing, or not allowing, simultaneous binocular or, better, red area viewing to yield differing wavelength discrimination functions. Whether this is the cause of the abovementioned differences in the position of the blue-green delta lambda minimum will have to be specifically investigated. Generally, however, from the point of view of pigeon-ergonomics it seems that horizontally, widely separated presentations of color stimuli may not yield the best hue discrimination performance.

ELABORATION OF PERCEPTUAL CONCEPTS

To close, we want to refer to a more sophisticated level of performance of the pigeon's visual system than we have considered so far. It
is its capacity for elaborating perceptual concepts. Since Koehler's (1955)
early pioneering work and Herrnstein and Loveland's (1964) clear-cut
demonstration, there have been a number of experimental studies that
document this remarkable capacity of birds. We have been concerned
with the concept of symmetry, or, more precisely, bilateral symmetry,
because of the possible role that it may play as a cue for the detection
of camouflaged prey by insectivorous birds (Curio, 1976). Of course,
the pigeon is no such bird, but for the purpose of developing suitable
experimental procedures it has, as a laboratory species, some advan-
tages over more relevant species. As a matter of fact, Morgan et al.
(1976) reported that they could not demonstrate the acquisition of this
concept using a successive instrumental discrimination technique with
free-ranging pigeons visiting a feeding station, although they were
able to teach the same animals a very adaptable concept of the letter A.

Using a conventional, instrumental, simultaneous-discrimination
procedure incorporating correction trials following incorrect choices
and a variable ratio schedule of reinforcement, we taught pigeons to
differentiate 24 symmetrical and asymmetrical stimuli projected on the
keys in various paired combinations for some 5600 trials. In the following 12 sessions, we introduced six new symmetrical and asymmetrical
stimuli assembled in various pair and position permutations under
extinction conditions. All five subjects classified these stimuli, with
which they had no previous experience, in a manner corresponding to
their experience, i.e., those subjects that had been allocated symmetrical stimuli as positive generalized preferentially to the symmetrical
test stimuli, the opposite being true for those trained with the asymmetrical stimuli as positive (Fig. 9). We (Delius and Habers, 1978)
conclude that pigeons are capable of acquiring, or perhaps only learning to apply, the concept of symmetry, thus adding yet another to the
list of concepts they have been shown to master (Herrnstein et al.,
1976). We are presently attempting to establish whether pigeons can
apply the concept to patterns with symmetry axes other than the vertical
that we have used so far. There are reasons to expect that this may not
be so, derived from the fact that the organism's symmetry plane is as
a rule a vertical one (Corballis and Beale, 1976).

This kind of visual performance by pigeons seems to suggest that
when attempting to understand the function of central visual structures
we must unfortunately also consider what, by human standards, are
cognitive processes. And who, to end by taking up an early theme of

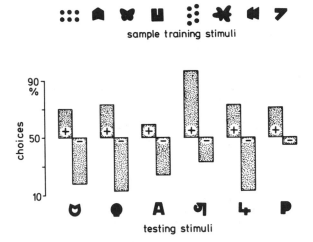

Fig. 9. Generalization of a symmetry/asymmetry concept to a set of novel test patterns under extinction conditions. Five pigeons had been trained with 28 symmetrical and asymmetrical figures (sample shown), two of them with the symmetrical, three with the asymmetrical stimuli positive. Bars marked plus indicate mean choice of given test pattern by subjects for whom the pattern should have been positive; bars marked minus indicate choices by subjects for whom they should have been negative. From Delius and Habers (1978).

this chapter, is to say that the pigeon's cognitive style might not be quite different from ours if it has already been shown that its sensory and learning modes, besides much else, are different. *Evolutio varietates delectat!*

ACKNOWLEDGMENTS. We are grateful to the technical staff and many students in Durham and Bochum for their efficient assistance and collaboration.

REFERENCES

Blough, D. S.: Spectral sensitivity in the pigeon. *J. Opt. Soc. Am.* **47**:827–833 (1957).

Blough, P. M.: Wavelength generalization and discrimination in the pigeon. *Percept. Psychophys.* **12**:342–348 (1972).

Blough, P. M.: Visual acuity in the pigeon. II. Effects of target distance and retinal lesions. *J. Exp. Anal. Behav.* **20**:333–343 (1973).

Catania, A. C.: On the visual acuity of the pigeon. *J. Exp. Anal. Behav.* **7**:361–366 (1964).

Chard, R. D.: Visual acuity in the pigeon. *J. Exp. Psychol.* **24**:588–608 (1939).

Cohen, A. I.: The fine structure of the visual receptors of the pigeon. *Exp. Eye Res.* **2**:88–97 (1963).

Cohen, D. H., and Trauner, D. A.: Studies of avian visual pathways involved in cardiac conditioning. *Exp. Brain Res.* **7**:133–142 (1969).

Corballis, M. C., and Beale, I. L.: *The Psychology of Left and Right.* Lawrence Erlbaum Associates, Hillsdale, N.J. (1976).

Curio, E.: *The Ethology of Predation.* Springer-Verlag, Berlin (1976).

Dartnall, H. J. A.: Photosensitivity. In Dartnall, H. J. A. (ed.): *Handbook of Sensory Physiology, VII/1.* Springer-Verlag, Berlin (1972). Pp. 122–145.

Delius, J. D.: Das Verhalten der Feldlerche. *Z. Tierpsychol.* **20**:297–348 (1963).

Delius, J. D.: Colour preference shift in hungry and thirsty pigeons. *Psychon. Sci.* **13**:273–274 (1968).

Delius, J. D. and Emmerton, J.: Sensory mechanisms related to homing in pigeons. In Schmidt-Koenig, K., and Keeton, W. T. (eds.): *Animal Migration, Navigation and Homing.* Springer-Verlag, Berlin (1978a).

Delius, J. D., and Emmerton, J.: Stimulus-dependent asymmetry in classical and instrumental discrimination learning by pigeons. *Psychol. Rec.* **28**: 425–434 (1978b).

Delius, J. D., and Habers, G.: Symmetry: Can pigeons conceptualize it? *Behav. Biol.* **22**:336–342 (1978).

Delius, J. D., and Tarpy, R. M.: Stimulus control of heart rate by auditory frequency and auditory pattern in pigeons. *J. Exp. Anal. Behav.* **21**:297–306 (1974).

Delius, J. D., and Thompson, G.: Brightness dependence of colour preferences in herring gull chicks. *Z. Tierpsychol.* **27**:842–849 (1970).

Delius, J. D., Perchard, R. J., and Emmerton, J.: Polarized light discrimination by pigeons and an electroretinographic correlate. *J. Comp. Physiol. Psychol.* **90**:560–571 (1976).

Emmerton, J.: The colour vision of the pigeon. Ph.D. thesis, University of Durham (1975).

Govardovskii, V. I., and Zueva, L. V.: Visual pigments of chicken and pigeon. *Vision Res.* **17**:537–543 (1977).

Graf, V., and Norren, D. V.: A blue sensitive mechanism in the pigeon retina: λ_{max} 400 nm. *Vision Res.* **14**:1203–1209 (1974).

Hamilton, W. F., and Coleman, T. B.: Trichromatic vision in the pigeon as illustrated by the spectral hue discrimination curve. *J. Comp. Psychol.* **15**:183–191 (1933).

Herrnstein, R. J., and Loveland, D. H.: Complex visual concept in the pigeon. *Science* **146**:549–551 (1964).

Herrnstein, R. J., Loveland, D. H., and Cable, C.: Natural concepts in pigeons. *J. Exp. Psychol. Anim. Behav. Proc.* **2**:285–311 (1976).

Hinde, R. A., and Stevenson-Hinde, J. (eds.): *Constraints on Learning: Limitations and Predispositions.* Academic Press, London (1973).

Hodos, W., Leibowitz, R. W., and Bonbright, J. C.: Near-field visual acuity of pigeons: Effects of head location and stimulus luminance. *J. Exp. Anal. Behav.* **25**:129–141 (1976).

Honigmann, H.: Untersuchungen über Lichtempfindlichkeit und Adaptierung des Vogelauges. *Pflügers Arch. Ges. Physiol.* **189**:1–72 (1921).

Huth, H.-H., and Burkhardt, D.: Der spektrale Sehbereich eines Violettohr-Kolibris. *Naturwissenschaften* **59**:650 (1972).

King-Smith, P. E.: Absorption spectra and function of the coloured oil drops in the pigeon retina. *Vision Res.* **9**:1391–1399 (1969).

Koehler, O.: "Zählende" Vögel und vergleichende Verhaltensforschung. In Portmann, A., (ed.): *Acta XI Congr. Int. Ornol. 1954.* Birkhäuser, Basel (1955).

Krasnegor, N. A.: The effects of telencephalic lesions on auditory discriminations in pigeons. *Diss. Abstr. Int. B* **31**:502913 (1971).

Kreithen, M. L., and Keeton, W. T.: Detection of polarized light by the homing pigeon, *Columba livia*. *J. Comp. Physiol.* **89**:83-92 (1974).

LoLordo, V. M., and Furrow, D. R.: Control by the auditory or the visual element of a compound stimulus: Effects of feedback. *J. Exp. Anal. Behav.* **25**:251-256 (1976).

Menner, E.: Die Bedeutung des Pecten im Auge des Vogels für die Wahrnehmung von Bewegungen. *Zool. Jahrb, Abt. Allg. Zool. Physiol. Tiere* **58**:481-538 (1938).

Menzel, R., and Snyder, A. W.: Polarised light detection in the bee, *Apis mellifera*. *J. Comp. Physiol.* **88**:247-270 (1974).

Montgomery, K. C., and Heinemann, E. G.: Concerning the ability of homing pigeons to discriminate patterns of polarized light. *Science* **116**:454-456 (1952).

Morgan, M. J., Fitch, M. D., Holman, J. G., and Lea, S. E. G.: Pigeons learn the concept of an "A." *Perception* **5**:57-66 (1976).

Muntz, W. R. A.: Effectiveness of different colours of light in releasing the positive phototactic behaviour of frogs, and a possible function of the retinal projection to the diencephalon. *J. Neurophysiol.* **25**:712-720 (1962).

Muntz, W. R. A.: Inert absorbing and reflecting pigments. In Dartnall, H. J. A. (ed.): *Handbook of Sensory Physiology VII/1*. Springer-Verlag, Berlin (1972). Pp.530-565.

Norren, D. V.: Two short wavelength sensitive cone systems in pigeon, chicken and daw. *Vision Res.* **15**:1164-1166 (1975).

Norren, D. V., and Vos, J. J.: Spectral transmission of the human ocular media. *Vision Res.* **14**:1237-1244 (1974).

Riggs, L. A., Blough, P. M., and Schafer, K. L.: Electrical responses of the pigeon eye to changes in wavelength of the stimulating light. *Vision Res.* **12**:981-991 (1972).

Sahgal, A., and Iversen, S. D.: Colour preferences in the pigeon: A behavioural and psychopharmacological study. *Psychopharmacology* **43**:175-179 (1975).

Schmidt-Koenig, K.: Experimentelle Einflußnahme auf die 24 Stunden Periodik bei Brieftauben und deren Auswirkung unter besonderer Berücksichtigung des Heimfindevermögens. *Z. Tierpsychol.* **15**:301-331 (1958).

Schneider, B.: Multidimensional scaling of colour differences in the pigeon. *Percept. Psychophys.* **12**:373-378 (1972).

Sekera, Z.: Polarization of skylight. In Flügge, S. (ed.): *Handbuch der Physik*. Springer-Verlag, Berlin (1956).

Seligman, M. E. P.: On the generality of the laws of learning. *Psychol. Rev.* **77**:406-418 (1970).

Shettleworth, S. J.: Constraints on learning. *Adv. Study Behav.* **4**:1-68 (1972).

Stebbins, W. C. (ed.): *Animal Psychophysics: The Design and Conduct of Sensory Experiments*. Appleton-Century-Crofts, New York (1970).

Straka, J. A.: Color preferences in pigeons using drinking as a response measure. *Psychol. Rec.* **16**:203-205 (1966).

Tan, K. E. W. P.: Vision in the ultraviolet. Ph.D. thesis, University of Utrecht (1971).

Thompson, G.: The photopic spectral sensitivity of gulls measured by electroretinographic and pupillometric methods. *Vision Res.* **11**:719-731 (1971).

von Helversen, O., and Edrich, W.: Der Polarisationsempfänger im Bienenauge: ein Ultraviolettrezeptor. *J. Comp. Physiol.* **94**:33-47 (1974).

Wehner, R..: Polarized-light navigation by insects. *Sci. Am.* **235**:106-115 (1976).

Wright, A. A. : Psychometric and psychophysical hue discrimination functions for the pigeon. *Vision Res.* **12**:1447-1464 (1972a).

Wright, A. A.: The influence of ultraviolet radiation on the pigeon's colour discrimination. *J. Exp. Anal. Behav.* **17**:325-337 (1972b).

Wright, A. A., and Cumming, W. W.: Colour-naming functions for the pigeon. *J. Exp. Anal. Behav.* **15**:7-17 (1971).

Wright, W. D., and Pitt, F. H. G.: Hue-discrimination in normal colour vision. *Proc. Phys. Soc. London* **46:**459–473 (1934).
Yoshizawa, T.: The behaviour of visual pigments at low temperatures. In Dartnall, H. J. A. (ed.): *Handbook of Sensory Physiology VII/1.* Springer-Verlag, Berlin (1972). Pp. 146–179.
Zeigler, H. P., and Schmerler, S.: Visual discrimination of orientation by pigeons. *Anim. Behav.* **13:**475–477 (1965).

6

Functional Implications of the Pigeon's Peculiar Retinal Structure

PATRICIA M. BLOUGH

INTRODUCTION

The current choice of the pigeon as a subject for behavioral research surely is not based on its presumed visual superiority over other birds. More likely, the popularity of this species is the result of its availability, the convenience of its feeding habits, and the fascination of its navigational skills. These factors must have influenced early researchers in the choice of pigeons for psysiological and behavioral studies. Certainly, convenience more than comparative considerations led B. F. Skinner and his colleagues to develop techniques and equipment that now make pigeons such a tempting behavioral subject in operant laboratories (Skinner, 1958). For those of us who use behavioral techniques to study visually guided behavior, then, it is partly a matter of luck that the pigeon's visual system includes some rather unusual features that make it a useful subject for comparative studies.

RETINAL STRUCTURE

Like most birds, the pigeon is a highly visual species. Its eye and the visual portions of its brain are large and well developed. The eyes,

PATRICIA M. BLOUGH • Department of Psychology, Brown University, Providence, Rhode Island 02912. The author's previously unpublished research, described in the first and last sections of this chapter, was supported by United States Public Health Service Grant MH 02456.

for example, constitute one-half of the weight of the brain according to Chard and Gundlach (1938), and the retina is thick, its several layers rich in cells through both central and peripheral portions. Thus good spatial resolution may not be so dependent on accurate foveal fixation as it is in primates; it is likely that acuity and color vision are good over a large portion of the visual field.

Other characteristics distinguish the pigeon's eye. For example, its shape is not really spherical; rather, the eyeball is somewhat flattened so that the distance from the nodal point of the lens to various portions of the retina is different. The lens is nearly clear (D. Blough, 1957), and there is no yellow macular pigment. Colored oil droplets occur on the outer segments of the pigeon's cones. There seems to be an unusually rich variety of cells in the retina's inner nuclear layer, and it has been suggested (Dowling, 1968) that the bird processes more information at the retinal level than do mammalian species.

Structural Specialization

Despite the relatively even distribution of cells across the pigeon's retina, there still appear to be areas of specialization (Galifret, 1968). A shallow fovea is located almost centrally, slightly ventral to the horizontal median and slightly posterior to the vertical median. Although the fovea itself is marked by depression and although its center contains fewer ganglion cells than the immediately surrounding region, the immediately surrounding areas are relatively high in cell density. Only one foveal depression occurs in the pigeon eye; however, there is a second area of specialization in the posterior dorsal quadrant (Galifret, 1968). This region is also marked by an increase in cell density; its center, about 50 deg superior to the fovea, is almost as rich in cells as the fovea itself. Like the fovea, its center appears to be rod free or nearly so. Galifret has suggested that the central area is used for monocular viewing of targets in the lateral visual field, while the superior dorsal area would view objects located in front of and slightly below the bird. Such objects would be in the binocular field of view, and they would include food that the bird picks up with its beak. It seems likely that pecking keys, used extensively in behavioral experiments, are also viewed with this specialized dorsal region.

The "Red Field"

Perhaps one of the most remarkable features of the pigeon retina is the often-described "red spot" (e.g., van Genderen-Stort, 1887; Galifret, 1968). This spot is easily seen in the freshly excised retina; its bright red color is in sharp contrast to the yellowish appearance of adjacent areas. The colored appearance of both red and yellow fields arises from the presence of colored oil droplets found on the outer segments of the bird's retinal cones. The pigeon's oil droplets, whose wavelength transmission characteristics have been described by King-Smith (1969), are red, orange, yellow, or clear in appearance and have different distributions in different portions of the retina (Bloch and Maturana, 1972). The red field is distinguished by a relatively high density of red and orange droplets. It occupies the superior dorsal quadrant of the retina, its center coinciding approximately with the specialized posterior-dorsal region described above. Oddly, the pigeon appears to be one of the very few bird species to possess a red spot (Galifret, 1968; Muntz, 1972). Oil droplets occur in most birds, but this peculiar distribution is unusual.

We measured the size and position of the red field in five pigeon eyes taken from the White King and White Carneaux breeds used extensively in behavioral research. The eyes were removed from live birds under Nembutal anesthesia and fixed in Sousa'a solution. This procedure preserved the tissue adequately without causing serious discoloration. We prepared flat mounts of three retinas by separating them from the scleral tissue and mounting them on slides. For the remaining two eyes, we made measurements of the attached retinas following removal of the lens and cornea. Two of the preparations came from a single bird; each of the other three came from separate birds.

The red field was clearly demarcated in all five preparations. Viewed through the inner cell layers, this area had an orange appearance that distinguished it easily from its yellowish surround. Viewed more directly from the outer side with the pigment epithelium removed, it was bright red in color and contrasted still more strongly with its surround. The shape of the red field was approximately circular, but it was slightly narrower in the inferior portion than it was at its superior extreme. It occupied almost all of the superior dorsal quadrant of the retina and extended slightly into the ventral quadrant. Its length (along the retina's vertical dimension) averaged 9.0 mm for the five eyes; mean width was 8.4 mm; thus the angle subtended at the posterior nodal point of the lens was approximately 57 deg. The red field extended almost to the fovea. Its inferior edge lay approximately 2.7 mm above the pecten. [The fovea was not visible in this preparation, but it is located about 2 mm above the pecten (Chard and Gundlach, 1938.)]

Although qualitative descriptions of the red field have appeared in the literature from time to time, our findings are noteworthy for two reasons. One is the fact that the red field is present in the highly domesticated breeds used extensively in behavioral research but bred almost entirely for squab. Also of note is the red field's very large size and its proximity to the central fovea. It would appear that this region is involved in many viewing conditions, but especially those for targets below and in front of the bird.

It is clear, then, that the pigeon's retina contains, in addition to a fovea, a second specialized region characterized by its high cell density and the presence of a high proportion of red oil droplets. A recent paper (Clarke and Whitteridge, 1976) suggests that these regions have functional specialization at an early stage of processing. On the basis of recordings from the optic tectum, this report describes two distinct areas of high magnification; that is, at the tectum these two retinal areas have relatively high degrees of spatial representation compared to surrounding regions. It seems reasonable to expect that the pigeon's visually guided behavior would also reflect the peculiar structure of its retina.

VISUAL ACUITY

As would be expected for a diurnal species with a highly developed visual system, the pigeon's visual acuity is good. In a behavioral study of six birds, I found acuity thresholds ranging from 1.4 to 4.0 min of arc (Blough, 1971). A study by Hodos et al. (1976), conducted under quite different conditions, yielded a similar finding when luminance conditions were comparable. Because of the pecularities of the pigeon's retinal structure, however, we might expect acuity to be influenced by viewing conditions.

Refraction

The refractive characteristics of an eye indicate the conditions under which light is focused on the retina. Focusing is affected by the distance of the object from the cornea and lens and by the distance of the cornea and lens from the retina. Because of its flattened shape, various portions of the pigeon's retina have unequal distances from the nodal point of the lens. Figure 1 illustrates this effect, indicating that eccentric portions of the retina are farther from the center of the lens than is the central region. Ray-tracing data (Marshall et al., 1973; Nye, 1973) suggest that the eye's optical system does indeed focus differently at different portions of the retina. Nye's findings indicate that, for good focus, targets viewed peripherally would have to be closer to the eye than ones viewed with the central region of the retina.

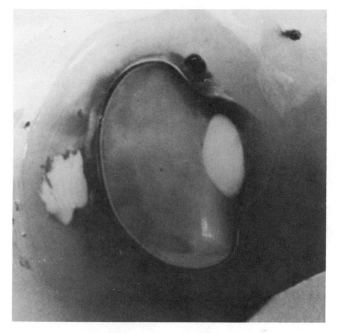

Fig. 1. Cross-section through the center of a frozen pigeon eye sectioned vertically. Reprinted from Millodot and Blough (1971, facing p. 1021).

Analyses such as these must, of course, assume a constant state of accomodation. Although pigeon refraction studies have so far been unable to specify the state of accommodation, we can hope that this condition was constant.

In our laboratory, we attempted to study the refractive characteristics of the pigeon's eye both retinoscopically and electrophysiologically (Millodot and Blough, 1971). Using a retinoscope modified for the pigeon's small eye, Millodot compared readings obtained from an approximately central location with values obtained in regions extending about 30 deg peripherally. Refractive indices obtained in this fashion indicated variation over an approximate two-diopter range. Although specific readings cannot be associated with specific portions of the retina, the values do agree with ray-tracing data to indicate variations corresponding to different portions of the retina.

Our electrophysiological findings also suggested that the pigeon's eye is nonuniform with respect to its refraction characteristics. In this study, we examined the effect of intervening lenses on the photopic ERG response to a 27-deg checkerboard pattern. In human subjects, the ERG's amplitude is very sensitive to the intervention of defocusing lenses (Millodot and Riggs, 1970). In the pigeon, we found that there was also a pronounced focusing effect. However, the function relating lens power to ERG amplitude had two peaks, one when the intervening lens had a negative value of three diopters and one for a positive one-diopter lens. Figure 2 shows this relationship. It is possible that variations in the accommodation of the bird's eye accounted for this double peak. Since the subject was anesthetized, however, it seems more likely that accommodation was constant and that these data also indicate differences in the refractive characteristics of the retinal areas viewing our large stimulus field.

Although the refraction data suggest nonuniformity of the pigeon retina, they do not describe a clear relationship between retinal locus and the eye's refraction characteristics. A number of difficulties stood

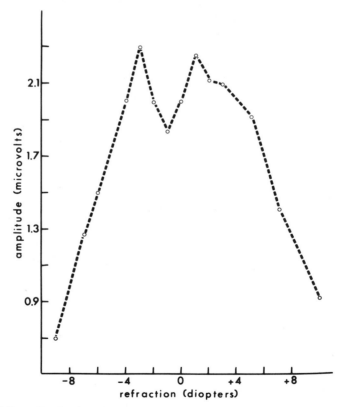

Fig. 2. ERG amplitude plotted against the power of a lens located between the eye and the checkerboard stimulus pattern. Data have been corrected for differences in light transmission by different lenses. Reprinted from Millodot and Blough (1971, facing p. 1020).

in the way of seeking such a relationship: it is difficult to achieve full pupil dilation in the pigeon; it is difficult to locate the fovea because of the absence of blood vessels used as "landmarks" in primates; and ordinary optometric tools, ophthalmoscopes and retinoscopes, require special adjustments to compensate for the eye's small size. For further clarification of the eye's acuity characteristics, then, we decided to approach the problem using behavior techniques.

Behavior Assessments of Visual Acuity

Visual acuity is of course a function of many variables, including target luminance, size, and contrast, the type of stimulus and the techniques used to determine threshold. Another factor is the distance between the subject and the target; if this distance is less than the subject's near point or greater than the far point of accommodation, the target will be out of focus. The position of the near and far points depends on the eye's refraction characteristics. In the myopic eye, the far point is closer than normal; in hypermetropia, the near point is abnormally far from the subject.

The possibility that the pigeon's eye contains different refractive systems was first suggested by Catania (1964). Noting that birds appeared unable to make spatial discriminations among stimuli located close up in the lateral visual field, Catania suggested that the pigeon's lateral vision is hypermetropic. Since the birds discriminate well when the stimuli are on the pecking keys, the frontal field could be myopic.

We attempted to test this notion by investigating the relationship between visual acuity and target distance (Blough, 1973). The relationship would indicate myopia if acuity declined with increasing target distance. Hypermetropia and/or emmetropia would be indicated in cases where acuity was constant over a range of large target distances but declined for near targets as they moved within the near point. (It would, however, be difficult to distinguish between hypermetropia and emmetropia with this technique since they would be revealed only by absolute distances for the near point, and we do not know what the "correct" distance is.)

We conducted this study in a special apparatus designed to control the subject-target distance while maintaining good stimulus control. The bird's task was to enter one of two alleys. At the end of one alley was a blank target; at the end of the other was a striped target of variable spatial frequency. Location of the two targets varied randomly. A food reward was available for entrances to the alley leading to the striped key. By varying the length of the alley, we could manipulate target distance. We assessed the visual acuity of three pigeons at target distances ranging from 13 to 73 cm. We made these measurements for both free-viewing conditions and conditions where vision was restricted to the frontal field of view. In the latter case, the birds wore special goggles designed to prevent lateral viewing but allowing frontal vision over a wide range (Catania, 1963; Mello, 1967).

We found the relationship between visual acuity and target distance for frontal viewing conditions to be different from what it was when free viewing was allowed. Figure 3 summarizes the findings. For two birds, acuity clearly improved with distance when the visual field was unrestricted. For frontal viewing conditions, however, acuity improved slightly (bird 2) or not at all (bird 144) with increasing distance. The third subject, bird 194, showed constant acuity over the three greater target distances for free-viewing conditions, and there was an improvement as distance became short. This bird did not work well with goggles, and we were able to obtain only one threshold under restricted viewing conditions. This value, shown by the open circle, indicated poorer acuity at the 73-cm target distance for frontal viewing than for free-viewing conditions. This finding agrees with comparable data for the other two subjects.

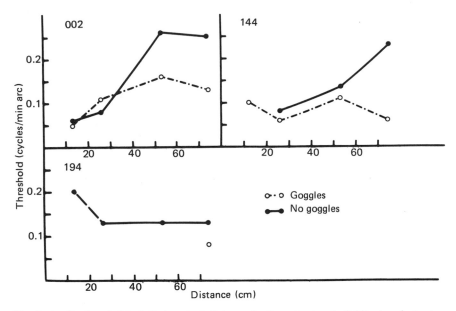

Fig. 3. Acuity threshold plotted against distance for free viewing (solid line) and viewing restricted to the frontal field (dashed line). Most points were obtained by interpolation from functions describing percent correct responses plotted against spatial frequency. For bird 194, however, the point at 13 cm was obtained by extrapolation from an incomplete psychometric function. Reprinted from Blough (1973, p. 338).

The interaction between target distance and viewing conditions suggests that the data reflect the activity of different refractive systems. When viewing was unrestricted, acuity clearly improved with distance. These findings are consistent with those of Chard (1939), who measured this relationship over a narrower range and concluded that the pigeon was hypermetropic. The decline in acuity for near targets does indeed suggest that these stimuli were inside the birds' near point and thus out of focus. Since field of view was uncontrolled in this phase of the study, we cannot definitely associate this relationship with a retinal locus. However, extensive observations of the birds revealed a clear tendency for lateral orientation at the greater target distances.

When vision was restricted to the frontal field, acuity was clearly poorer at the greater target distances, but thresholds for the two viewing conditions became similar as target distance decreased. These findings suggest that the goggles occluded a hypermetropic system that allowed acuity to improve with target distance. A frontal myopic system would be seen as an improvement in acuity at very short distances whether or not the birds were goggles. Although we were unable to collect many data for close targets, the performance of bird 194, shown in Fig. 4 and described more fully in our report (Blough, 1973), revealed a definite improvement as the target moved in from 26 to 6 cm. The good agreement between our distance acuity thresholds and recently reported thresholds for near acuity (Hodos et al., 1976) also suggests that we would have seen an improvement for very near targets.

To clarify further the acuity-distance relationship, it will be necessary to make additional threshold assessments at near distances. The present findings suggest, however, that the pigeon's eye does indeed have two refractive systems and that these systems may not overlap. The hypermetropic system involving lateral vision permits good acuity at large distances. A myopic system, probably frontal, may take over at close distances, but there appears to be an intermediate range where neither system achieves best focus.

Worth a note here is the role of the foveal depression in visual acuity. The fovea is located in the central portion of the pigeon retina and probably is involved only when lateral viewing is permitted. In another acuity experiment, we compared acuity for distance viewing before and after destruction of the fovea by a laser beam. The results showed little or no effect of foveal lesions on the function relating performance to spatial frequency of a striped pattern. Only in one out of five cases did performance deteriorate following the lesions, and in this case the lesion did not destroy the fovea itself. Other studies with pigeons have also failed to find an effect of foveal lesions on pattern discrimination (Goodson, 1969; Yarczower, 1964). It appears that the

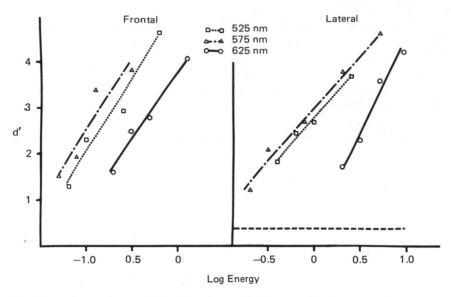

Fig. 4. Sample psychometric functions for bird 194 in an experiment on the pigeon's sensitivity to lights of varying wavelengths. The left-hand panel shows data obtained under frontal viewing conditions; the data in the right-hand panel are for lateral viewing. The data points, showing sensitivity (d') plotted against log stimulus energy, have been fitted by a straight line using the least-squares method. The horizontal line at the bottom of the right-hand panel shows the d' level obtained when the stimulus lamp was turned off. Each point is based on 100 stimulus presentations.

availability of foveal vision is not responsible for good distant acuity when lateral vision is permitted.

COLOR VISION

Distribution of Oil Droplets

With its high cone density and its nearly rod-free area, the superior portion of the pigeon's dorsal retina is surely specialized for good acuity. But why is it red? Many explanations draw on an analogy to a red filter. Walls (1942), for example, suggested that oil droplet filters heighten hue and luminance contrasts. Galifret (1968) pointed out the usefulness of a red filter in contrasting food objects against the greens in nature; in an analagous vein, he and Walls suggested that the yellow oil droplets enhance contrasts against the blue sky. Because they appear to cut out short wavelengths, oil droplets may also improve acuity by reducing stray light and chromatic aberration. As Wolbarsht (1976) reminded us, the yellow macular pigment and the slight yellow color of the lens and ocular media serve this function in humans. Pigeons do not have such pigmentation, and perhaps the oil droplets act as a replacement. This function would, of course, apply to all colored oil droplets, but the red ones would cut out a wider range of the spectrum.

It is incorrect to draw close analogies between the pigeon's "red fields" and "yellow fields" and solid color filters such as those used in photographic work. All portions of the pigeon's retina contain a mixture of oil droplet and pigment types (Govardovskii and Zueva, 1977; Bowmaker, this volume). The two fields appear to differ in the proportions of oil droplet types (Bloch and Maturana, 1972) and in the details of their transmission spectra (King-Smith, 1969; Bowmaker, this volume). The red field may be further distinguished by the presence of "microdroplets" (Pedler and Boyle, 1969). These very small bodies are similar in structure to the larger oil droplets and occur only in cones that contain the larger red globule.

The Red Field and Color Vision

The red field, then, is not a solid filter, but rather a multicolored one whose appearance is somewhat misleading. Because there are differences in the relative numbers of the various oil droplet types, however, we might expect the red field to have different color-discriminating characteristics than the surrounding yellow region. Recent spectral sensitivity data provide some support for this conclusion. An unpublished report by King-Smith (Muntz, 1972) describes the spectral sensitivity of tectal recordings from the retina's red and yellow fields. The data show a clear depression in the red field's sensitivity to light in the 500–600 nm region; that is, sensitivity was relatively greater in the recordings from the yellow field in this wavelength region. A behavioral study (Romeskie and Yager, 1976; Yager and Romeskie, 1975) is also suggestive. A comparison of their findings with those of an earlier spectral sensitivity study (D. Blough, 1957) shows, in the Romeskie and Yager function, a marked suppression in the 500–600 nm region. These authors have suggested that their data, based on stimuli located at the response key, reflect the sensitivity of the retina's red field. Since D. Blough's procedure involved an above-key stimulus, they suggest that his work reflects the response of the yellow field.

These findings are intriguing because they are among the few that relate oil droplet distribution to behavior. They also have important practical implications: if spectral sensitivity differs according to viewing condition, then studies that attempt to control luminance must take viewing condition into account. We felt an explicit study of spectral sensitivity in the two fields of view would be useful. In our work, we held constant adaptation conditions and all other variables that we would expect to affect spectral sensitivity. We attempted to confine the stimulus to one or the other fields of view by using brief (200–400 msec) flashes of light and a small (3-mm) stimulus area. The flash was produced by a key peck; thus the bird's head was in an approximately constant position at the time the stimulus occurred. In one portion of the study, the stimulus was frontal; that is, it was located on the response key. In the other phase, it was lateral and slightly superior; here the target was located on a panel at right angles to and slightly above the response key.

To assess sensitivity, we used a threshold procedure. The birds learned to peck at the upper of two keys until a flash occurred. Following a flash, a switch to a lower key was reinforced occasionally with food. We measured performance over a series of gradually decreasing energy values. Figure 4 shows psychometric functions relating our performance measure, d', and stimulus energy. As expected, d' (Swets, 1964) decreased with decreasing stimulus energy. Assessments of this relationship were made at three wavelengths. These values, 525, 575, and 625 nm, were selected because they should best reveal the expected effect. Each point on the psychometric function represents the mean over five sessions meeting a predetermined stability criterion. A single session lasted about 1 hr and included 20 flash presentations at each energy value. A set of functions was acquired at each wavelength, in the order 625, 525, and 575 nm. This series was then repeated, and the two psychometric functions at each wavelength were averaged. Thus final psychometric data were based on ten sessions and 200 presentations of each energy value.

Figure 5 compares sensitivity to lights of different wavelengths in two fields of view. The data are for two White Carneaux pigeons, 2–3 years of age. Relative sensitivity values come from interpolation on functions like those in Fig. 4. Each point on the present graph indicates stimulus energy at which a criterion performance level occurred. We are showing the findings for three criterion values since the psychometric functions varied in slope, a fact that affects to some extent the curves shown here. In no case, however, was sensitivity relatively higher to the shorter wavelengths when the stimulus was lateral. For bird 164, in fact, viewing conditions had little or no effect on relative sensitivity. For bird 702, relative sensitivity was slightly higher to short wavelengths in the frontal field of view. This finding fails to support the hypothesis that relative sensitivity to short wavelengths is greater in the lateral field of view than it is in the frontal field.

These results suggested that viewing conditions are not so impor-

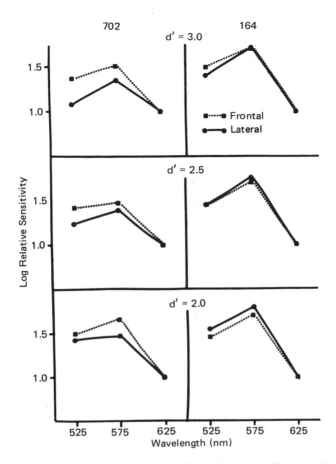

Fig. 5. Sensitivity for lights of three wavelengths for frontal and lateral viewing conditions. The two columns show data for two birds; the three rows show the functions separately for separate threshold criteria. In all cases, sensitivity is shown relative to its value at 625 nm, where it is set at the arbitrary value of 1.0. Each point is based on interpolation from psychometric functions like those shown in Fig. 6.

tant as one might expect. However, their precise implications for the comparison between the red and yellow fields are less clear. Although the procedure tried to differentiate between retinal areas, there was no way to be sure that the frontal and lateral viewing conditions corresponded, respectively, to the red and yellow fields. Further, since dim (6-V) tungsten light illuminated the subject chamber, it was difficult to compare the details of these data with other studies, most of which used more neutral adaptation conditions. In a recent experiment, we assessed relative sensitivity under explicitly frontal viewing conditions. To increase the probability of stimulating the pigeon's red field, the position of the stimulus key was quite low, just 10 cm above the food tray and 10 cm below the usual location of a pecking key. The study was designed to facilitate comparison with other research by presenting stimuli in darkness, maintaining photopic adaptation with dim, neutral lights turned on between trials.

This experiment used three White Carneaux pigeons 2–4 years of age. They were trained on a trialwise procedure to respond differentially to the presence or absence of a monochromatic light. Between trials, the subject chamber was illuminated with dim (approximately 10.5 d/m²) tungsten light filtered by Wratten 78AA ("daylight") filters. A trial was signaled by the offset of this light. During a trial, a peck on the low, observing key produced a 500-msec flash of light with a probability of 0.5. The light was a 3-mm spot located just behind this key. The peck also dimly illuminated two choice keys located above the observing key. Pecks on the left choice key were correct and occasionally reinforced following a stimulus flash; pecks on the right choice key were correct and occasionally reinforced when observing responses did not produce the stimulus. Varying the energy of the light yielded psychometric functions relating stimulus energy to probability of a correct choice. Such functions were obtained for three wavelengths, 525, 575, and 625 nm. These wavelengths again were chosen because relative sensitivity to them should reflect the differential transmission characteristics of the different types of oil droplets.

Thresholds were determined by interpolation on psychometric functions similar to those in Fig. 4. For this study, however, the ordinate represented the normalized probability of a response to the left key. Each point on the function was the mean over four sessions meeting a predetermined stability criterion. A single session consisted of 240 trials, half of which were presentations of darkness and the other half were presentations of one of five predetermined energy values. A randomized block design determined stimulus order. Thus final psychometric functions were based on 96 presentations of each of five energy values.

Figure 6 summarizes these findings. Interpolation on lines fitted to the psychometric functions yielded the data points here. These points are for a threshold criterion of 0.5; that is, they reflect the energy required for the subject to detect the light flash half of the time. If the criterion had been set at a higher probability of seeing the 525-nm point would have been depressed slightly for two of the birds. If criterion probability had been less, this point would have been slightly elevated for those subjects. Although the individual data (top panel) indicate some variability, there is good agreement between the group findings and those of other studies (bottom panel). Indeed, the simi-

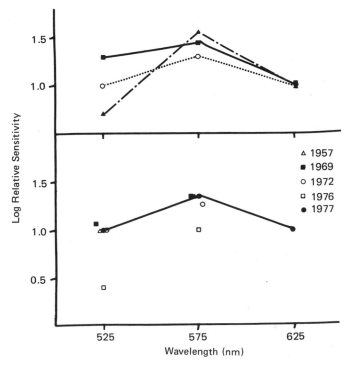

Fig. 6. Sensitivity at three wavelengths for lights located in the lower portion of the frontal field of view. The upper panel shows individually the data for the three birds in the present study. The lower panel plots the means of those points (filled circles) and compares them to the data of D. Blough (1957), Graf (1969), P. Blough et al. (1972), and Romeskie and Yager (1976). As a visual aid, some of the points are moved slightly along the abscissa. In all cases, sensitivity is shown relative to its value at 625 nm, where it is set at the arbitrary value of 1.0.

larities among these data are quite remarkable considering the large procedural differences involved. Graf's (1969) behavioral procedure used flicker photometry and an on-key target; Blough et al. (1972) used photopic electroretinographic techniques and a lateral stimulus; D. Blough (1957) used a behavioral photopic threshold measure and an above-key target; and the present study used stimuli explicitly confined to the lower portion of the frontal field. Our findings do not agree with those of Romeskie and Yager (1976), however, and recent data of Martin and Muntz (this volume) also indicate a slight depression in sensitivity in the lower relative to the upper portion of the pigeon's visual field.

The notion that different visual fields are associated with different spectral sensitivities comes from the assumption that stimuli in the frontal and lateral fields fall on the retina's red and yellow areas, respectively. In all studies cited, this assumption is tenuous, since in no case have viewing conditions been arranged to ensure this correlation. The experiments we have just described attempted to investigate stimulus location by controlling its physical relation to the response key. However, as the anatomical data indicate, the red field is large; in fact, it extends almost to the fovea, which is usually associated with lateral viewing. It is unclear what, if any, conditions in nature confine a stimulus to the pigeon's yellow field. It does seem likely, however, that food objects fall on the retina's red field.

If the separation of the pigeon's retina into red and yellow areas does have functional significance, the function may not be to enhance luminance contrasts but rather to enhance hue contrasts. A comparison of differential wavelength sensitivity data provides some support for this notion. Wavelength discrimination studies of P. Blough (1972) and of Wright (1972) used frontal viewing conditions and indicate maximum sensitivity in the region about 600 nm. An electroretinographic study by Riggs et al. (1972) used lateral viewing and found maximum sensitivity to contrasts in the region of 525 nm. Figure 7 compares the data of these experiments. Note that the ERG function of Riggs et al. has its minimum around 525 nm, while those of Blough and of Wright have theirs around 600 nm. In humans, ERG and psychophysical techniques agree with respect to regions of best wavelength discrimination (Riggs, 1976). Involvement of different retinal areas could account for the discrepancy in the pigeon data.

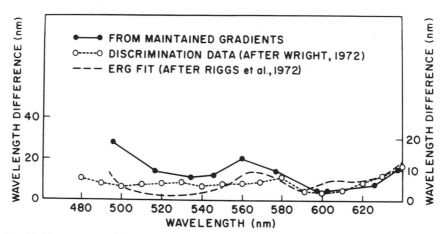

Fig. 7. Comparison of three "wavelength discrimination" functions obtained with different methods. Maintained gradient data (P. Blough, 1972) are scaled on the left ordinate; Wright (1972) data are scaled on the right. ERG data have arbitrary scales and are adjusted to facilitate comparison. Reprinted from Blough (1972, p. 346).

The anatomical evidence for specialization in the pigeon retina is clear. Less clear are the functional correlates of the anatomically distinct areas. We have offered some support for the notion that the pigeon views distant objects laterally and monocularly, and that its frontal, binocular field of view is adapted for nearby objects. We suspect, however, that acuity is relatively good across the entire retina—that, unlike primates, the pigeon detects many of its natural targets without having to achieve the precise fixation we require. The functional role of the red field remains a mystery. We do not believe that its high concentration of red and orange oil droplets affects spectral sensitivity, but the possibility remains that hue discrimination is different in this region. Again, however, the effects appear to be subtle. Perhaps the peculiar structure of the pigeon retina is adapted for more complex tasks as well. Surely there is much to be learned from the way in which the visual system integrates the spatial and color information coming in from many portions of the wide visual field.

ACKNOWLEDGMENTS. Priscilla A. Furth made the red field measurements; Bonnie L. Zeigler ran portions of the study that compared frontal and lateral spectral sensitivities. The author is indebted to Donald S. Blough for his suggestions in all phases of the research described here.

REFERENCES

Bloch, S., and Maturana, H.: Colour discrimination—Lack of correlation with oil droplet distribution in the pigeon retina. *Nature (London) New Biol.* **234**:284 (1972).

Blough, D. S.: Spectral sensitivity in the pigeon. *J. Opt. Soc. Am.* **47**:827–833 (1957).

Blough, P. M.: The visual acuity of the pigeon for distant targets. *J. Exp. Anal. Behav.* **15**:57–67 (1971).

Blough, P. M.: Wavelength generalization and discrimination in the pigeon. *Percept. Psychophys.* **12**:342–348 (1972).

Blough, P. M.: Visual acuity in the pigeon. II. Effects of target distance and retinal lesions. *J. Exp. Anal. Behav.* **20**:333–343 (1973).

Blough, P. M., Riggs, L. A., and Schafer, K. L.: Photopic spectral sensitivity determined electroretinographically for the pigeon eye. *Vision Res.* **12**:477–486 (1972).

Catania, A. C.: Techniques for the control of monocular and binocular viewing in the pigeon. *J. Exp. Anal. Behav.* **6**:627–629 (1963).

Catania, A. C.: On the visual acuity of the pigeon. *J. Exp. Anal. Behav.* **7**:361–366 (1964).

Chard, R. D.: Visual acuity in the pigeon. *J. Exp. Psychol.* **24**:588–608 (1939).

Chard, R. D., and Gundlach, R. H.: The structure of the eye of the homing pigeon. *J. Comp. Psychol.* **25**:249–272 (1938).

Clarke, P. G. H., and Whitteridge, D.: The projection of the retina, including the "red area," on to the optic tectum of the pigeon. *Q. J. Exp. Physiol.* **61**:351–358 (1976).

Dowling, J. E.: Synaptic organization of the frog retina: An electron microscopic analysis comparing the retinas of frogs and primates. *Proc. R. Soc. London Ser. B* **170**:205–228 (1968).

Galifret, Y.: Les diverse aires fonctionelles de la rétine du pigeon. *Z. Zellforsch. Mikrosk. Anat.* **86**:535–545 (1968).

Goodson, J. E.: Optokinetic responses in the pigeon. Unpublished doctoral dissertation, George Washington University, 1969.

Govardovskii, V. I., and Zueva, L. V.: Visual pigments of chicken and pigeon. *Vision Res.* **17**:537–543 (1977).

Graf, V. A.: A spectral luminosity function in the pigeon determined by flicker photometry. *Psychon. Sci.* **17**:282–283 (1969).

Hodos, W., Leibowtiz, R. W., and Bonbright, J. C.: Near-field visual acuity of pigeons: Effects of head location and stimulus luminance. *J. Exp. Anal. Behav.* **25**:129–141 (1976).

King-Smith, P. E.: Absorption spectra and the function of the coloured oil drops in the pigeon retina. *Vision Res.* **9**:1391–1399 (1969).

Marshall J., Mellerio, J., and Palmer, D. A.: A schematic eye for the pigeon. *Vision Res.* **13**:2449–2453 (1973).

Mello, N. K.: A method for restricting stimuli to the frontal or lateral visual field of each eye separately in pigeon. *Psychon. Sci.* **8**:15–16 (1967).

Millodot, M., and Blough, P.: The refractive condition of the pigeon eye. *Vision Res.* **11**:1019–1022 (1972).

Millodot, M., and Riggs, L. A.: Refraction determined electrophysiologically. *Arch. Ophthalmol.* **84**:272–278 (1970).

Muntz, W. R. A.: Inert absorbing and reflecting pigments. In Dartnall, H. J. A. (ed.): *Photochemistry of Vision.* Springer-Verlag, Berlin (1972).

Nye, P. W.: On the functional differences between frontal and lateral visual fields of the pigeon. *Vision Res.* **13**:559–574 (1973).

Pedler, C., and Boyle, M.: Multiple oil droplets in the photoreceptors of the pigeon. *Vision Res.* **9**:525–528 (1969).

Riggs, L. A.: Human vision: Some objective explorations. *Am. Psychol.* **31**:125–134 (1976).

Riggs, L. A., Blough, P. M., and Schafer, K. L.: Electrical responses of the pigeon eye to changes in wavelength of the stimulating light. *Vision Res.* **12**:981–991 (1972).

Romeskie, M., and Yager, D.: Psychophysical studies of pigeon color vision. I. Photopic spectral sensitivity. *Vision Res.* **16**:501–505 (1976).

Skinner, B. F.: Reinforcement today. *Am. Psychol.* **13**:94–99 (1958).

Swets, J. A.: *Signal Detection and Recognition by Human Observers.* Wiley, New York (1964).

van Genderen-Stort, A. G. H.: Über Form und Ortsänderungen der Netzhautelelemente unter Einfluss von Licht und Dunkel. *Graefes. Arch. Klin. Exp. Ophthalmol.* **33**:229–292 (1887).

Walls, G. L.: *The Vertebrate Eye and its Adaptive Radiation.* Hafner, New York (1942) (reprinted 1963).

Wolbarsht, M. L.: The function of intraocular color filters. *Fed. Proc.* **35**:44–49 (1976).

Wright, A. A.: Psychometric and psychophysical hue discrimination functions for the pigeon. *Vision Res.* **12**:1447–1464 (1972).

Yager, D., and Romeskie, M.: On the proper control of luminance cues in pigeon color vision experiments. *J. Exp. Anal. Behav.* **23**:293–295 (1975).

Yarczower, M.: The development of a behavioral system to evaluate visual performance in animals. Report for Institute of Behavior Research, August, 1964.

7

Color-Vision Psychophysics: A Comparison of Pigeon and Human

ANTHONY A. WRIGHT

INTRODUCTION

Light as a physical stimulus can be characterized in terms of its wavelength(s) and intensity, but when it impinges on the visual system it creates a sensory experience with the psychological properties of hue, brightness, and saturation. Various psychophysical tests on humans have allowed us to infer some of the transduction mechanisms of the physical to the psychological. What have we learned about the pigeon's visual system from the large number of visual psychophysical tests performed on it? The human eye perceives the continuum of light wavelengths as a colored spectrum composed of several discrete categories or hues. Does the pigeon perceive wavelengths of light in distinct groups or hues as humans do? More generally, are the interrelationships of the psychophysical functions the same for pigeons as they are for humans? Other than man and monkey, the pigeon has received more visual psychophysical study than any other organism. The purposes of this chapter are to draw together much of the color-vision pyschophysical data on the pigeon, show the interrelationships of the psychophysical functions, compare and contrast these interrelationships with those of man, and attempt some conclusions about what these interrelationships imply about the pigeon's color-vision mechanisms.

ANTHONY A. WRIGHT • The University of Texas Health Science Center at Houston, Graduate School of Biomedical Sciences, Houston, Texas 77025. Preparation of this chapter was partially supported by Grants MH25593, BNS 78-07253, and EY01256 to the author.

HUE PERCEPTION AND HUE DISCRIMINATION

Color Naming

Results of color-naming experiments demonstrate the perception of color. Figure 1 shows the results from a human color-naming experiment by Beare (1963). In her experiment, subjects were shown various wavelengths of light and were allowed to use the color names violet, blue, green, yellow, orange, or red to describe them. The intersection points of these gradients are at the hue transition points. We could compare points of hue transition of humans to those of pigeons by conducting a color-naming experiment with pigeons, and this comparison of hue transition points would tell us something about the similarities or differences in the human and pigeon color vision systems.

One cannot ask a pigeon to introspect on its sensations from spectral stimulation, or indeed to verbally name colors. In pigeon color-naming experiments (Wright and Cumming, 1971), operant conditioning techniques were used to ask a pigeon which of two hues was more similar to a test wavelength. A variety of supporting tests showed the

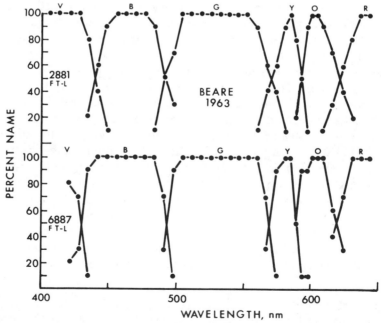

Fig. 1. Two sets of human color-naming functions at two different luminance levels. After Beare (1963).

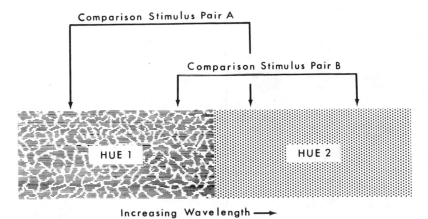

Fig. 2. Method used to identify a hue boundary by changing the pair of training stimuli in a hypothetical color-naming experiment.

point of equality of judgment to be the hue transition point. Perhaps the best way to introduce the pigeon color-naming procedure is to make an analogy to human color perception. Consider a boundary between two hues as schematically shown in Fig. 2. A subject (human or pigeon) is shown test wavelengths of light, one by one, and asked whether its color is more like the member from hue 1 of the comparison stimulus pair A or like the member from hue 2. To the left of the hue boundary the subject would say it looks more like hue 1, because the test wavelength and the comparison from hue 1 are the same color. To the right of the hue boundary it would appear more like hue 2; thus the transition from calling the test wavelengths more like hue 1 than hue 2 to calling them more like hue 2 than hue 1 identifies the hue transition point or boundary. The same argument holds for comparison stimulus pair B. The spectral point identified as a point of hue transition will be the same for the second pair as it was for the first pair; this demonstrates that the results are not dependent on the particular members of each hue chosen. This invariance in the point of hue transition also serves to ensure against the members of comparison pair both being from the same hue. The hue boundaries identified from the following color-naming experiment have since been supported by the results from other psychophysical color-vision studies on the pigeon.

The color-naming procedure was a three-alternative matching-to-sample procedure. In this simultaneous matching procedure, the center stimulus was present during the display of the side stimuli. The pigeons were first trained to match hues in the procedure shown in Fig.

TRAINING TRIAL

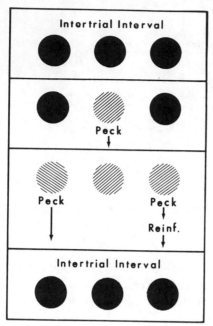

Fig. 3. Sequence of stimuli and contingencies during a training trial in a matching-to-sample experiment.

3. Monochromatic light transilluminated the center key, and a single response or a peck on this center key produced monochromatic light behind two side keys. A peck to the side-key wavelength which matched the center-key wavelength produced access to mixed grain. When the six pigeons performed well on this task, 17% of the trials were changed to test trials. A test trial is schematically shown in Fig. 4. A wavelength intermediate between two of the training wavelengths appeared behind the center key. A peck on the center key produced the two training wavelengths, one on each of the side keys. There was no physical match between any two of the three stimuli, and no reinforcement was ever available on test trials. The object was to test whether the subjects would report a test wavelength as more like training wavelength 1 rather than training wavelength 2.

Mean results for the six pigeons are shown in Fig. 5. The functions intersect at a wavelength slightly more than 540 nm and at a wavelength slightly less than 600 nm. That is, as the test wavelength is increased, the chances that the pigeon will choose 572 nm as opposed to 512 nm increase, and at a wavelength slightly greater than 540 nm the pigeon reports that the test wavelength appears more like 572 nm

TEST TRIAL

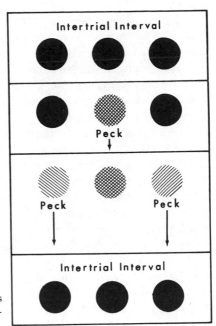

Fig. 4. Sequence of stimuli and contingencies during a trial to test the pigeon's color naming.

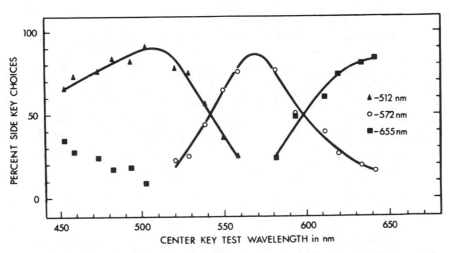

Fig. 5. Average of six pigeons' color-naming results from the first test. Each curve is the percentage of choices to that training wavelength appearing on one of the side keys as a function of center key test wavelength.

than like 512 nm. Similar arguments hold for the 600 nm intersection point.

In the second test, the training wavelengths were changed to 473, 555, and 633 nm. These results are shown in Fig. 6; interpretation is the same as for the first test. Note that these functions, too, intersect at a wavelength slightly greater than 540 nm and at a wavelength slightly less than 600 nm. The correspondence is clearly shown in Fig. 7 by the superimposed gradients. This close correspondence is evidence that the pigeons were choosing the training wavelengths based on their apparent hue. Otherwise, the 20 nm or so decrease in training wavelengths from experiment 1 to experiment 2 would have shifted the intersection point to a shorter wavelength for experiment 2 relative to experiment 1. It seems that any member of the set of wavelengths composing the hue can represent it. Said in human color terms, the subject will match a green test stimulus to a green training stimulus no matter whether the green training stimulus is bluish green or yellowish green. Its greenness places it with the set of "green" wavelengths, and test wavelengths which appear green are judged more similar to it than an alternative yellow training wavelength. Thus the gradients intersect at the boundary between green and yellow, and will intersect at this boundary no matter which specific green and yellow are used as training wavelengths. A third test (results not shown) showed that the wavelengths of the hue transitions were ambiguous as to which hue they represented.

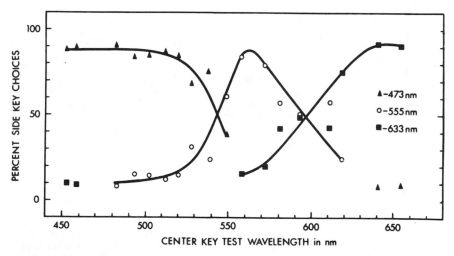

Fig. 6. Average of six pigeons' color-naming results from the second test. Interpretation of the figure is the same as in Fig. 5.

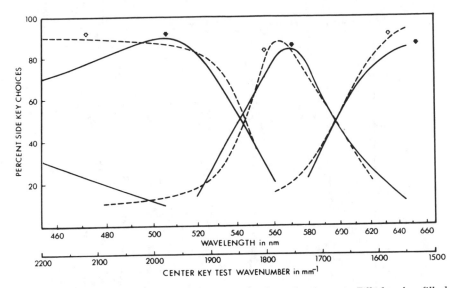

Fig. 7. Superimposition of the color-naming results from the two tests. Filled and unfilled arrows indicate training wavelengths from first and second tests, respectively.

Hue Discrimination

Hue-discrimination experiments on humans and pigeons corroborate the finding from the color-naming experiments that the intersection points identify hue boundaries. The close relationship between color naming and hue discrimination is a very reasonable one, and is clearly stated by W. D. Wright (1947): "the part of the spectrum where a minimum exists must obviously occur where there is a rapid change of hue; thus in the yellow where the color turns redder on one side and greener on the other, in the blue/green where it turns bluer on one side and greener on the other and in the violet where it becomes redder or bluer minimum steps would be expected" (p. 167).

Figure 8 shows a comparison between Beare's (1963) human color-naming functions and a hue-discrimination function for the human obtained by Laurens and Hamilton (1923). These particular hue-discrimination results were chosen because they show detailed features. Similar functions have been previously shown (Steindler, 1906; Jones, 1917). This figure shows that four of the five color-naming intersection points correspond to the minima of the hue-discrimination function.[1]

---

[1] The status of orange as a hue is a bit questionable. The human color-naming procedures cannot distinguish "true" from "pseudo" hues in the same way that the invariance of the intersection points of the pigeon color-naming functions serves to substantiate the spectral location of pigeon hue boundaries.

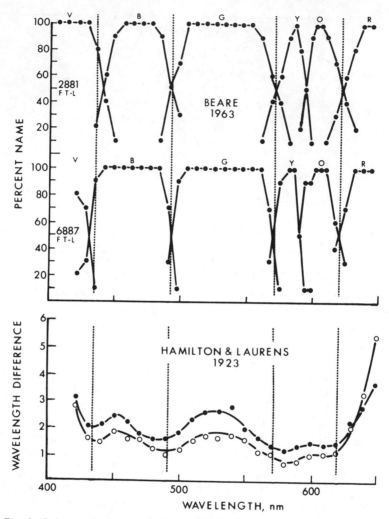

Fig. 8. Comparison of human color naming and human hue discrimination.

The pigeon's hue-discrimination results, like those for the human, show best hue discrimination at the hue boundaries and validate the previously described color-naming procedure. The pigeon hue-discrimination study was conducted over a 3½-year period (see Wright, 1972b, 1974, for a more complete description). In this study, three pigeons judged whether two halves of a split field were equal in hue or different in hue. This procedure is shown in Fig. 9. They pecked the center key behind which was the split field, and then pecked the appropriate side key (right or left) to indicate whether the split field was different or equal in hue, respectively. A 600-trial session was divided among five wavelength differences and a wavelength equal (100 trials each). During the 15 sessions at each reference wavelength, the pigeon's bias toward making right-side key pecks vs. left-side key pecks was manipulated in order to extract bias-free indices of discriminability (see Wright, 1972b). These bias-free discriminability measures allowed the true shape of the psychometric function to be revealed (Wright, 1974).

The psychometric functions from one of the pigeons in this experiment are shown in Fig. 10. A steep sloping function indicates good discriminability, whereas a shallow sloping function indicates poor discriminability. Note that the functions are linear (median correlation coefficient of 0.99) and have essentially a zero intercept.

A collection of hue-discrimination functions (sometimes referred to as "wavelength-discrimination functions," elsewhere referred to as "relative sensitivity functions," Wright, 1974) were derived from the psychometric functions of Fig. 10 by intersecting them at different

EQUAL WAVELENGTH TRIAL   UNEQUAL WAVELENGTH TRIAL

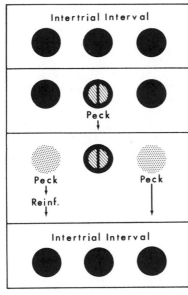 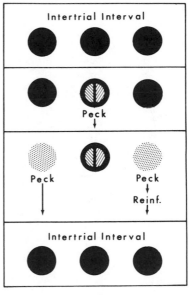

Fig. 9. Sequence of events and contingencies during a trial where the two halves of the split field were equal in wavelength and during a trial where the two halves of the split field were unequal in wavelength in the Wright (1972b, 1974) hue-discrimination experiment.

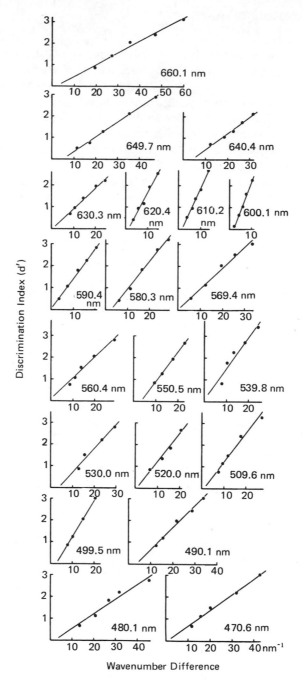

Fig. 10. Psychometric hue-discrimination functions for pigeon 287, one of three subjects in the hue-discrimination experiment. The d' values were computed at the line of equal bias and are plotted as a function of wavenumber (wavelength reciprocal) difference between the two halves of the split field.

values of the discrimination index and plotting the resulting wavelength difference at the spectral point of the reference wavelength.

Figure 11 shows the hue-discrimination results compared to the color-naming results. Note that the intersection points of the color-naming functions correspond to two of the three points of best hue discrimination. There is no intersection point of the color-naming functions at the 500 nm minimum of the hue-discrimination functions, but this is not surprising because there was no combination of training stimuli in the color-naming experiments which should have revealed such an intersection point.

Several other studies (Shepard, 1965; D. Blough, 1961; Schneider, 1972; P. Blough, 1972) support these results on the pigeon's color perception and hue discrimination. These constitute a substantial amount of evidence from a variety of procedures, and they agree with one another as well as (if not better than) the human hue-discrimination results (see Judd, 1932).[2] Figure 12 shows the results from three of these experiments bounded by the previously mentioned color-naming and hue-discrimination results.

The Schneider experiment (1972) was similar in many respects to the previously discussed hue-discrimination experiment (Wright, 1972b, 1974). Pigeons observed a split field and made judgments as to whether or not the two halves of the field were equal in hue or different in hue. One difference between the Schneider and Wright experiments is that in the Schneider experiment the pigeons were confronted with many more different pairs of stimuli. In one of Schneider's experiments, the pigeons saw each of 105 stimulus pairs each session. Schneider performed an unusual and interesting analysis on his data. He rank-ordered the stimulus pairs according to their discrimination difficulty and then used only their rank order to position them in a two-dimensional color perception space for the pigeon. Since every stimulus was judged against every other stimulus, the rank-order information was sufficient to constrain the position of a wavelength in a two-dimensional space. The two-dimensional space was similar to a color circle. Easy-to-discriminate pairs were widely spaced on the circle, and difficult-to-discriminate pairs were closely spaced. The distance between Schneider's stimuli was measured along the perimeter of his color circle, and was normalized in arbitrary units per wavelength. The results are plotted in Fig. 12 at the mean wavelength between the stimulus pair. They are plotted so that a dip in the function will be a

[2] The pigeon hue-discrimination results from the Hamilton and Coleman (1933) study are at odds with all more modern results. There were severe procedural problems with this study (see Wright, 1972b, for explanation) and so these experimental results will not be considered in this chapter.

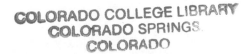

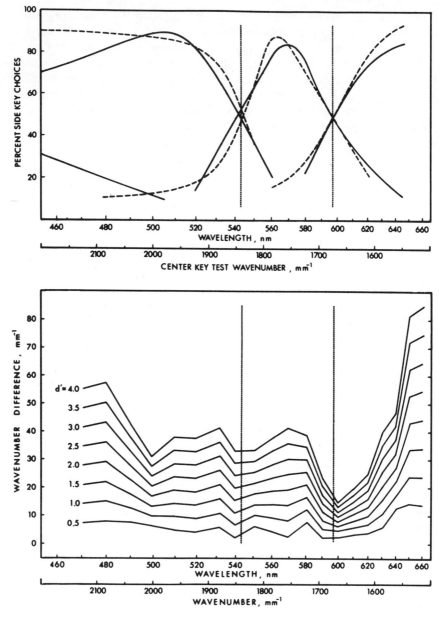

Fig. 11. Comparison of pigeon color-naming functions and hue-discrimination functions. The hue-discrimination functions were derived from those of Fig. 10 and the psychometric functions for the other two subjects of this experiment by horizontally sectioning the psychometric hue-discrimination functions at eight values of the discrimination index and plotting the resulting wavenumber differences at the appropriate reference wavenumber.

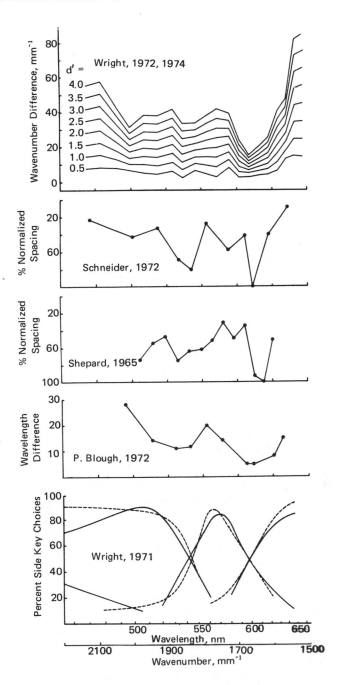

Fig. 12. Comparison of the results of two pigeon hue-discrimination experiments (upper two panels) and three pigeon generalization experiments (lower three panels).

point of best hue discriminability, and so that the dips and humps of
the function can be related to the hue-discrimination study (Wright,
1972b). The two hue-discrimination functions relate rather well. There
is a point of best hue discriminability at 600 nm, a point of good hue
discriminability at 540–550 nm which is somewhat less good than that
at 600 nm, and a hint of good hue discriminability in the 500 nm
region. Results from these two hue-discrimination studies relate well
to the results in the lower three panels, which, by the nature of their
procedure, may be described as generalization rather than discrimination.

Tests of generalized behavior reveal hue boundaries because subjects conditioned to respond to a particular wavelength will generalize
these responses to other wavelengths which are members of the same
hue. Said in human color terms, if the subject is conditioned to respond
to a yellow stimulus, it will generalize its responses to other yellow
stimuli whether they be yellow-green or yellow-red, and these responses will generalize very little across hue boundaries to the green
stimuli or to the red stimuli.

The function in the third panel from the top in Fig. 12 is based on
an analysis of the slopes of the generalization gradients collected from
different groups of pigeons trained at different spectral points. Shepard
(1965) analyzed the classical data of Guttman and Kalish (1956) in order
to determine the appropriate transformation of the wavelength scale to
render all the generalization gradients to the same shape. The large
overlap of the gradients constrained this analysis to produce a unique
solution to this problem. Where the slope of the generalization gradient
was shallow, the wavelengths had to be pushed a little closer together
in order to steepen the gradient. Where the slope of the generalization
gradient was steep, the wavelengths had to be spread apart a little in
order to make the gradient more shallow so that all the gradients would
be of the same shape and symmetrical. One can think of the process
as a search for a scalar transformation of wavelength so that each unit
change along the transformed scale would produce an equal change in
hue and consequently an equal change in the degree to which the
subjects generalize their responses. The distance along the transformed
scale is plotted in Fig. 12. A large distance indicates a point of least
generalization. These distance values are normalized and plotted at the
mean of the two measured wavelengths. An inverted scale is used so
that the interpretation of the humps and dips will be the same as the
previously discussed functions. The correspondence to the discrimination functions is quite good. Points of least generalization correspond to points of best hue discriminability. The point of best hue
discriminability, 600 nm, is very close to the point of least generali-

zation. The 540–550 nm point of good hue discriminability corresponds to a somewhat broad area of least generalization, the trough of which is located at about 535 nm as opposed to 545 nm. The 500 nm point of good hue discriminability corresponds also to a point of minimal generalization.

The fourth function from the top of Fig. 12 is from an experiment by P. Blough (1972). She trained pigeons in a maintained generalization procedure. Pigeons were occasionally reinforced for pecks to a particular wavelength, and interspersed among these training trials were presentations of other wavelengths. She determined the wavelength difference necessary to obtain 50% of the S+ response rate. If the pigeons were trained in a spectral region where hues were changing rapidly, a large wavelength change would be necessary to reduce the generalized response rate to 50% of its S+ value. Thus a small wavelength difference plotted in Fig. 12 indicates a region where hue is changing rapidly and a comparatively large wavelength difference indicates one where hue is changing slowly. P. Blough's results also suggest that pigeons have a hue boundary at 600 nm and another in the vicinity of 540 nm. There is no suggestion in this study of a hue boundary at 500 nm.

The previously discussed color-naming study, shown in the lowest panel of Fig. 12, is essentially a study of hue generalization and is included for comparison.

The correspondence among the discrimination and generalization data for the pigeon is quite remarkable. All of the hue-discrimination and generalization results show best hue discrimination at 600 nm and 540 nm. There is some controversy as to whether 500 nm is a point of best hue discrimination. The two hue-discrimination procedures (Wright, 1972b; Schneider, 1972) showed 500 nm to be a point of best hue discrimination; these studies used a split-field stimulus. Two other procedures (P. Blough, 1972; Delius and Emmerton, this volume) showed 500 nm to be a point of poor hue discrimination; they used a single stimulus and two widely separated stimuli, respectively. This difference in stimulating conditions may have something to do with the discrepancy in the shape of the hue-discrimination functions. One repeated topic of discussion at the Delaware Conference concerned the pigeon's two visual fields, referred to as the "yellow field" and the "red field" because of the preponderance of yellow and red oil droplets, respectively. Most of the evidence concerning differences between these two fields (see section on spectral sensitivity) indicates that if the pigeon "looks" with its red field as opposed to its yellow field, very different psychophysical results are produced. Perhaps a split field encourages the pigeons to use a different retinal field than when they view a single, uniform stimulus. The two retinal fields are sufficiently different in their photopigments, oil droplets, and photopigment–oil droplet combinations (Bowmaker, this volume) to account for these differences in hue discrimination. The problem of different psychophysical results produced by viewing with different retinal fields is discussed more thoroughly in the next section on spectral sensitivity, where attempts have been made (P. Blough, this volume) to directly manipulate which field the pigeon is using to view the stimulus.

SPECTRAL SENSITIVITY

Spectral sensitivity is related to hue discrimination in that both psychophysical functions are a reflection of the underlying color-vision processes. Hue discrimination is dependent on spectral sensitivity in that the stimuli in the hue-discrimination experiment must be made equally bright so that subjects will not use brightness differences to cue their discriminations, but must depend on hue differences only. The problem is that any contribution of brightness differences to performance will be incorrectly attributed to hue discriminability.

Experimenters working with humans and animals regularly equate the luminance of the colored stimuli before conducting a hue-discrimination experiment. They also should occasionally vary the luminance of their stimuli as a test (cf. Wright, 1972b) to document that subjects are under control of hue differences, not brightness ones. Frequently, researchers (Wright and Cumming, 1971; Wright, 1972b; Schneider, 1972; P. Blough, 1972) use a spectral sensitivity function from a different group of pigeons in a different apparatus (e.g., D. Blough, 1957) to equate the brightness of the stimuli. This is often a practical necessity because many hue-discrimination experiments entail several years of research, and an equally carefully conducted spectral sensitivity experiment itself would likely require several years of research. One notable example is an experiment by Romeskie and Yager (1976a,b), where spectral sensitivity functions were obtained on individual pigeons, and these individual spectral sensitivity values were used to equate the luminance of the stimuli before conducting a saturation discrimination experiment.

The human's spectral sensitivity function is the well-known unimodal, bell-shaped function with its mode at 555 nm; it will not be discussed further here. In contrast to the human function, the pigeon's spectral sensitivity function is bimodal, and the shape of the function may vary depending on which retinal field the pigeon uses to view the stimulus.

There are at least two different pigeon spectral sensitivity functions. The difference between the functions is not due to chance variation. A substantial amount of behavioral evidence (D. Blough, 1957; Graf, 1969; Romeskie and Yager, 1976a; Kreithen, this volume; P. Blough, this volume; Delius and Emmerton, this volume) directly or indirectly supports this difference. Typical of these two different functions for the pigeon are the spectral sensitivity results shown in Fig. 13. Results from experiments by D. Blough (1957) and Graf (1969) are typical of one type. Results from the experiment by Romeskie and Yager (1976a) are typical of the other type. These three spectral sensitivity experiments used instrumental behavioral procedures: D. Blough (1957) used a tracking method where the intensity of the stimulus was under the pigeon's control; Graf (1969) used a go/no-go behavioral response in conjunction with a flicker photometric procedure; Romeskie and Yager (1976a) used a discrete-trial, two-key, forced-choice procedure.

There are several ways in which the Romeskie and Yager function differs from that of Graf and D. Blough: (1) The Romeskie and Yager function shows maximum sensitivity of wavelength slightly longer than that shown by Graf and D. Blough. (2) The shape of Romeskie

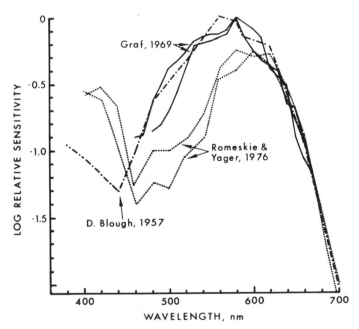

Fig. 13. The pigeon's light-adapted spectral sensitivity functions from three different experiments. The function from D. Blough is an average of three subjects; the other functions are for individual pigeons.

and Yager's spectral sensitivity function for wavelengths shorter than the peak wavelength is very different from that shown by Graf and D. Blough. There is somewhat less sensitivity than shown by Graf and D. Blough between the maximum sensitivity and the short-wavelength inflection point. The short-wavelength inflection point occurs at a wavelength slightly longer than shown by Graf and D. Blough. Sensitivity at wavelengths shorter than the short-wavelength inflection point is greater than that shown by Graf and D. Blough.

There seem to be at least two causes for these different spectral sensitivity functions: (1) differences in the state of the subjects' adaptation and (2) different retinal areas used to make the discriminations. Romeskie and Yager speculated that their pigeons were using their "red" retinal field whereas D. Blough's pigeons were using their "yellow" retinal field. This speculation of Romeskie and Yager appears to be largely correct at this time, although there are several puzzling questions which remain to be answered. Why did Romeskie and Yager's pigeons use their red field whereas D. Blough's and Graf's pigeons used their yellow field? A related question is, what are the conditions conducive to using one field as opposed to the other? The pigeon is completely free in these behavioral settings to turn its head, stretch its neck, squat down, etc., and so it seems unlikely that anything as simple as the height of the pecking key from the chamber floor would produce such a difference in retinal focus (cf. Romeskie and Yager, 1976a). Pigeons in a behavioral setting where they can move freely will probably view the stimulus in such a way to always maximize their likelihood of detecting the stimulus and hence maximize their chances for reinforcement. It will be of some importance to learn which facets (if any) of the task are critical in determining which field the pigeon will use to view the stimulus. To this point, it may be of some note that D. Blough's and Graf's pigeons could always stand directly in front of the stimulus and peck the response key, whereas Romeskie and Yager's pigeons had to compare two stimulus displays and pick the one containing the stimulus.

The adapting light in the Romeskie and Yager study was different from the adapting lights used by D. Blough and Graf. Romeskie and Yager used an adapting light which was filtered (Kodak 79) to produce approximately uniform intensity across the visible spectrum (color temperature of about 5400°K) so that this "white" adapting light would uniformly adapt all the chromatic processes. By contrast, Graf (personal communication) and most likely D. Blough used an unfiltered tungsten light resulting in a ramp function across the visible spectrum (likely about 3200°K). This ramp function would adapt the long-wavelength processes more than the short ones, and would tend to change the form of the spectral sensitivity function in the same way that the Graf and D. Blough functions differ from Romeskie and Yager's.

Two chapters in this volume (Bowmaker; P. Blough) shed some light on this spectral sensitivity issue. P. Blough has shown some changes in spectral sensitivity with changes in color temperature of the adapting light; these measurements were made in the same apparatus on the same subjects. Bowmaker has modeled spectral sensitivity using oil droplet and photopigment MSP measurements for the red field and the yellow field. Bowmaker's model of the different retinal fields and P. Blough's difference in adaptation conditions separately account for only a part of the difference between the two types of spectral sensitivity functions. It seems reasonable that both retinal location and adaptation conditions are responsible for the two types of spectral sensitivity functions shown in Fig. 13.

The difficulty for experimenters who wish to equate the brightness of their colored stimuli will be to select the appropriate spectral sensitivity function for equating the stimulus luminance. My suggestion is that, if colored stimuli are to be presented on a single key, then experimenters should use D. Blough's spectral sensitivity coefficients and adapt with tungsten light. If colored stimuli are presented on multiple keys, then experimenters should use Romeskie and Yager's spectral sensitivity coefficients and adapt with a filtered (Kodak 79) tungsten light.

ULTRAVIOLET SENSITIVITY OR FLUORESCENCE?

The spectral sensitivity functions in Fig. 13 show that the pigeon's sensitivity increases with wavelengths shorter than 420 nm. This is a very reliable finding. Recently, Kreithen (this volume) tested spectral sensitivity down to about 310 nm and showed the pigeon to have a bimodal spectral sensitivity function: the usual long-wavelength mode around 550–560 nm and a secondary mode around 350 nm. His pigeons were almost a log unit more sensitive at this secondary mode than they were at the more usual long-wavelength mode. This finding is unusual because before 1972 (Wright, 1972a) it was not known that pigeons (or any other birds, apparently) were ultraviolet sensitive.

In three separate experiments, Wright (1972a) showed that pigeons are very sensitive in the near-ultraviolet region, wavelengths of about 350 nm. The pigeon's ultraviolet sensitivity is interesting and at the same time puzzling. For example, what is the survival value of ultraviolet sensitivity?

I have frequently been questioned as to whether the pigeon really

sees ultraviolet light or whether structures in the pigeon's retina flu-
oresce and the pigeon perceives this fluorescence which is of wavelengths known to be in the normal sensitive range. An important but
unfortunately complicated experiment which I reported in 1972 answers
this question, I believe. A split-field stimulus was used. Wavelengths
from the more standard visible region illuminated the separate halves
of the split field and the pigeons reported whether the two halves of
the field were equal or different in wavelength. When a UV stimulus
was added to one-half of the split field, the subjects' discrimination
performance substantially changed. If ultraviolet light from the one half
of the split field had fluoresced preretinal structures in the pigeon's
eye, e.g., the lens, then this fluorescence would not be confined to the
retinal image of one half of the split field, and should not have changed
the pigeon's discrimination performance. But there were changes in
the pigeon's discrimination performance. Thus, this test excludes the
possibility that the discrimination performance changes were due to
preretinal fluorescence, but it does not exclude the possibility that they
were due to retinal fluorescence. However, this latter possibility can
be excluded on the basis that the pigeon is a full order of magnitude
more sensitive in the UV (Kreithen, this volume) than at its other
sensitivity mode. If the UV light were transformed (through fluorescence) to a "visible wavelength", then the sensitivity in the UV ought
to be somewhat less than the sensitivity at the transformed wavelength
because the same photoreceptors are being used in both cases and
because the fluorescence conversion, like all energy conversions, is not
a perfect one. Thus, we are left, I believe, with the only remaining
possibility: that the pigeon has bona fide ultraviolet receptors.

SATURATION DISCRIMINATION

Brightness and hue are only two of the three psychological dimensions of color perception. The third is saturation. Like the problem of
brightness differences among the stimuli, a hue-discrimination task
should not involve saturation differences among the stimuli in order
to ensure that the subjects are basing their discriminations on hue
differences, not saturation ones. Experimenters conducting hue-discrimination studies routinely ignore any contamination by saturation
differences among the spectral stimuli. Indeed, it has been speculated
(Hurvich and Jameson, 1955; Hecht and Shlaer, 1936) that hue discriminability by dichromats is largely the result of saturation discrimination except at the transition point between the two dichromatic hues.
A mathematical model by Hurvich and Jameson (1955) predicts per-

formance in the hue-discrimination task as a sum of a hypothetical hue-discrimination process and a hypothetical saturation-discrimination process. Figure 14 shows a comparison of the human's saturation-discrimination function to its hue-discrimination function. The human hue-discrimination function is a compilation of data from eight different hue-discrimination experiments.[3] The saturation-discrimination function is from an experiment by Priest and Brickwedde (1938) and the essential features of this saturation-discrimination function shown in Fig. 14 have been confirmed in other experiments (Wright and Pitt, 1937; Nelson, 1937). Technically, these experiments are colorimetric purity experiments, not saturation experiments, because monochromatic stimuli are not equally saturated. Colorimetric purity is measured by determining the energy in a spectral light which is just visible against a background of white light, and this energy is divided by the sum of the energies of the white light and the spectral light. Figure 14 shows that the spectral region of least colorimetric purity, that region which is least saturated, corresponds to a spectral region of good hue discrimination. Furthermore, this spectral region is the region where there is the greatest rate change in saturation discrimination. Hurvich and Jameson (1955) say that performance in the hue-discrimination task is enhanced according to how rapidly saturation discrimination is changing.

Results of two experiments which bear on the pigeon's saturation discrimination are compared to the pigeon's hue-discrimination function in Fig. 15. In one experiment by Romeskie and Yager (1976b), pigeons were required to choose the achromatic stimulus from a two-stimulus display containing a monochromatic and an achromatic stimulus of equal luminance. The experimenters found the stimulus energy necessary to produce 75% correct discriminations and subtracted from it the energy necessary for detection (spectral sensitivity) at the same spectral point. A photochromatic interval function resulted, which is shown in Fig. 15. The human photochromatic interval function is closely related to the human colorimetric purity function (Graham and Hsia, 1969).

The pigeon's colorimetric purity function shown in Fig. 15 is from an experiment by P. Blough (1975). Her colorimetric purity experiment was a go/no-go maintained generalization experiment. Pigeons were trained to peck a key when it contained only achromatic light and to refrain from pecking when it contained any amount of monochromatic

---

[3] Most any hue-discrimination function would be adequate for the purposes of this comparison. This collection of functions shows the agreement among investigators that the spectral point of least saturation is one of best hue discriminability.

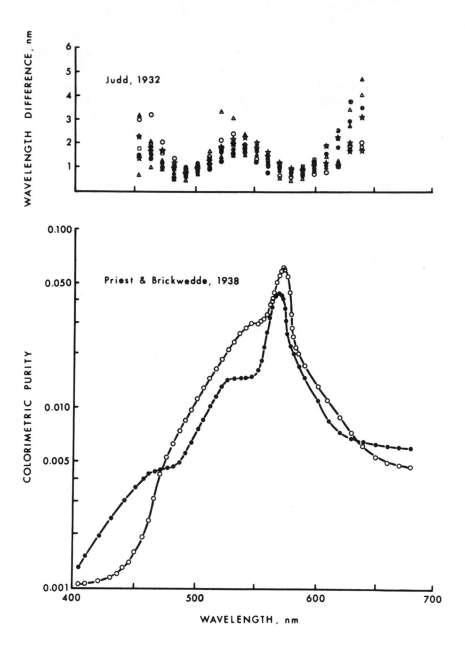

Fig. 14. Comparison of human saturation discrimination and human hue discrimination. The different hue-discrimination points correspond to eight different observers and are taken from an article by Judd (1932).

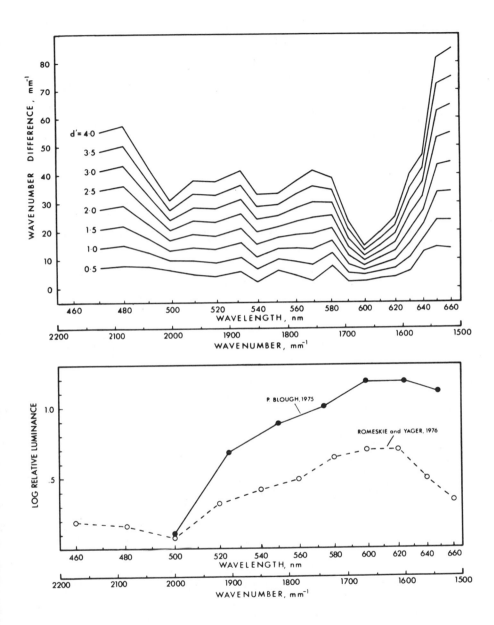

Fig. 15. Comparison of pigeon saturation discrimination to pigeon hue discrimination. One saturation-discrimination function is from a colorimetric purity experiment (P. Blough, 1975). The other is from a photochromatic interval experiment (Romeskie and Yager, 1976b).

light, however small, mixed with the achromatic light. The values shown in Fig. 15 are monochromatic light energies necessary in the mixture to produce a response probability equal to one-half the response probability to the positive achromatic stimulus.

Figure 15 shows that, similar to the human relationship between saturation and hue discrimination, a point of good hue discriminability (600 nm) corresponds reasonably well to the point of maximal spectral desaturation. The pigeon and the human are quite different, however, in that the human shows a very rapid change in colorimetric purity and achromatic interval at its point of maximal desaturation, whereas the pigeon does not show such a rapid change at its point of maximal desaturation. The difference in rate change may be an important comparative relationship with regard to models of hue discrimination that consider the rate change of saturation an important attribute in hue discrimination experiments.

INTERACTION BETWEEN BRIGHTNESS AND HUE

Hue, saturation, or brightness can serve as the basis for a discrimination. It is somewhat unfortunate for the advancement of color-vision science that these three psychological dimensions do not operate independently. As the luminance of a monochromatic light is varied, there is a change in the hue of the light as well as in its brightness. Thus a change in the brightness of one of two monochromatic patches of light will in most cases change the hue difference between the two patches of light. In some cases it will make the hue difference less, and in other cases it will make the hue difference greater. Such interactions make the analysis of the color-vision system quite complicated. It is likely that there are interactions of each pair of psychological dimensions: hue and brightness, hue and saturation, brightness and saturation. The only interaction which has been extensively studied has been the hue–brightness interaction, known as the Bezold–Brücke hue shift.

The human hue-shift function is shown in Fig. 16 along with the human hue-discrimination function. The essential features of this function are quite reproducible (van der Wildt and Bouman, 1968; Larimer et al., 1974, 1975; Boynton and Gordon, 1965; Jacobs and Wascher, 1967, Smith et al., 1967; Luria, 1967; van der Horst and Muis, 1969). At the spectral extremes, the contours converge with increasing intensity. As brightness varies, the hue is thought to shift toward spectral regions of invariant hue. These are convergent points. At very high intensities, all wavelengths longer than about 505 nm appear yellow, equivalent to

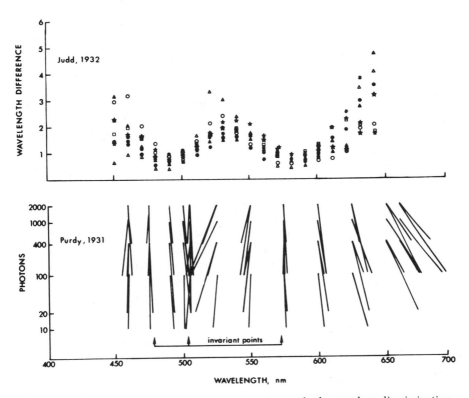

Fig. 16. Comparison of the human hue-shift function to the human hue-discrimination function.

a wavelength of about 575 nm at more moderate intensities, and all wavelengths shorter than about 505 nm appear blue, equivalent to a wavelength of about 480 nm. As brightness decreases, the shorter wavelengths converge to a green of about 505 nm (supposedly there is a red convergence point somewhere at very long wavelengths). The hue of these convergence points allegedly does not change with brightness changes, and these points have a critical role in certain theories of color vision. For instance, Hurvich and Jameson's (1955) theory says that the spectral points of invariant hue are the "pure" hues. Since the spectral points of invariant hue were thought to be "pure" hues, there should be one invariant point for each of the human hues of blue, green, yellow, and red. Figure 16 shows the relationship between the human hue-discrimination and the hue-shift function. The hue-discrimination function, as we have seen, identifies spectral points of hue transition and thereby identifies the boundaries of each hue. Note that near the blue-green transition point of about 495 nm there are two spectral points of invariant hue very close to this hue transition point. The third spectral point of invariant hue occurs at the other minimum of hue-discrimination function. This is the invariant hue for the yellow hue; there are not separate minima for the green-yellow and yellow-red transition points because the yellow hue is so narrow.

Some human hue-shift experiments (Purdy, 1931; van der Wildt and Bouman, 1968; van der Horst and Muis, 1969; Cohen, 1975) required human subjects to match hues of two color patches of light while disregarding any brightness differences between them. Such verbal instructions may or may not be interpretable to human subjects, but certainly would be difficult to convey to animal subjects through the contingencies of reinforcement.

The Bezold–Brücke hue-shift function for the pigeon was obtained in an experiment (Wright, 1976) conducted concurrently with the previously mentioned hue-discrimination experiment (Wright, 1972b, 1974). Pigeons had extensive experience judging whether the two equal-luminance halves of the split field were of the same hue or of different hues before they were tested for brightness–hue interaction. Infrequent tests were made of the brightness–hue interaction by increasing and then decreasing the luminance of one of the five comparison stimuli during the last two sessions at each spectral point. All indications were that the pigeons continued to respond on the basis of hue difference during these infrequent tests of luminance change.

Figure 17 shows how the hue shifts were calculated from changes in the subjects' hue-discrimination performance. The subjects' results were in close agreement and the procedure proved to be quite sensitive.

The mean hue-shift function is shown in Fig. 18 along with the mean hue-discrimination function for the same pigeons. Several differences are apparent when the pigeon hue-shift function is compared to the human hue-shift function. Human and pigeon hue-shift functions move in opposite directions at the extreme spectral points used in testing. At the red end of the spectrum, which approaches the long-wavelength visibility extreme for pigeons and humans, the pigeon hue-shift function diverges with increasing intensity whereas the human's converges with increasing intensity. At the blue end of the spectrum, the pigeon hue-shift function again diverges with increasing intensity, whereas the human's converges. The shortest-wavelength blue light used in testing the pigeon certainly does not push the limits of the pigeon's blue sensitivity; the pigeon is sensitive to at least 320 nm (Kreithen, this volume).

The invariant points for the pigeon are very different from those for the human. The invariant points for humans are located at 480, 505,

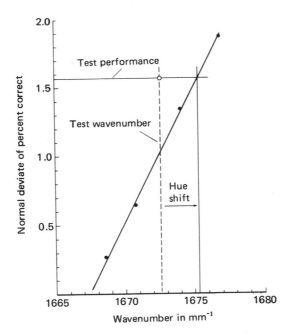

Fig. 17. Example of hue-shift calculation from a session by one pigeon. The four filled data points are for performance in the four spectral stimuli, photometrically equated for the pigeon's sensitivity. The unfilled point is for performance in a stimulus brightened by 0.30 log unit. Hue of the brightened test stimulus was defined equivalent to the wavenumber of the intersection of a horizontal line through the test performance with the least-squares linear function. The hue shift was calculated as the difference between this calculated wavenumber and the actual wavenumber of the test stimulus.

and 575 nm, and a red of indeterminate wavelength. The pigeon has one invariant point located at a long wavelength of about 630 nm and another at a wavelength of 530 nm. The spectral location of these two convergence or invariant points is quite clear. There is at least one other convergence point between these two. Because of the slant of the functions between the 530 and 630 nm convergence points, there will be an odd number of convergence points between 530 and 630 nm. A case for only one convergence point between 530 and 630 nm could be made because the previously discussed hue-discrimination, generalization, and color-naming data indicate that there is only one hue from 540 to 600 nm; consequently, there should be only one point of "pure" hue (Hurvich and Jameson, 1955) identified by the convergence point. It is most likely located in the vicinity of 550 nm. The nearly vertical hue-shift function at about 595 nm was previously identified as an invariant point (Wright, 1976), but the hue-shift functions for shorter

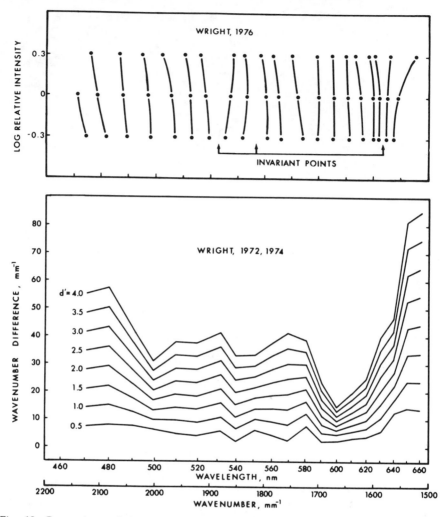

Fig. 18. Comparison of the pigeon's mean hue-shift function (Wright, 1976) to the pigeon's mean hue-discrimination functions (Wright, 1972b, 1974).

wavelengths do not converge on this point. The vertical hue-shift function at 595 nm may be due to the particularly keen hue discrimination at this spectral point. The brightness changes at this spectral point may have caused a substantial hue change, but the wavelength change corresponding to this hue change was so small as not to tilt the hue-shift function very much. At 600 nm, where hue discrimination is so very good, a small wavelength change creates a comparatively large hue change, or, conversely, a moderate hue change is a very small change in wavelength or wavenumber.

The human hue-shift function (Fig. 16) shows that the hue-shift functions converge on the blue and the yellow invariant points with increasing intensity. These invariant points are thought to be the "pure" hues of one of the two (excitatory–inhibitory) processes (Hurvich and Jameson, 1955). The assumed red invariant point and the green invariant point are similarly thought to be the "pure" hues of the other opponent process pair. Returning now to Fig. 18, the pigeon's hue-shift function shows convergence points at 530 and 630 nm as intensity is decreased. Thus this pair of convergence points is likely to identify an opponent process pair just as the yellow and blue points do for humans. The opponent member for the 550 nm convergence point is likely to be at wavelengths shorter than those investigated in the Wright (1976) hue-shift experiment. In all of my investigations and in those of others which I have seen, there has never been any hint of an improvement in hue discriminability above 660 nm; there is only a further deterioration.

Two of the pigeon's invariant points, 530 nm and 550 nm, are very close to a point of hue transition, 540 nm. If these invariant points represent "pure" hues, then these pure hues are skewed with respect to the wavelength range representing the hue, and are closely located on either side of the hue boundary. The same situation is found with humans (Fig. 16), where the "pure" green is located at 505 nm, representing a wavelength range from 495 to 565 nm. The opposing "pure" blue hue (480 nm) is just on the other side of the blue-green transition point (495 nm). The 630 nm pigeon invariant point is located well away from any hue transition point.

Thus the pigeon and human differ in many details of their color vision but are similar in many of their general relationships. The next section will bring some of these details together within a theoretical framework so that they can be more thoroughly scrutinized.

THEORETICAL CONSIDERATIONS

Many of the similarities and differences between pigeon and human color vision which have been previously discussed in this chapter are summarized in the remainder of this paragraph. The color-naming boundaries between hues and the minima of hue-discrimination functions are located at different spectral points for pigeons and humans; in both cases, color-naming boundaries occur at the points of best hue discrimination. The pigeon's spectral sensitivity is not too different from the human's at moderate and long wavelengths; at short wavelengths, however, the pigeon shows a resurgence of sensitivity and thus reveals a bimodal spectral sensitivity function. The point of maximum desaturation for pigeons and humans occurs at different spectral points, but in both cases this point of maximum desaturation corresponds to the point of best hue discriminability. The pigeon's saturation discrimination function is not so steep as the human's function. This difference in steepness is particularly apparent at the spectral point of maximum desaturation, where the human function rises to a sharp peak and the pigeon's function is broad. This difference in rate change of saturation discrimination may become more important when it is considered within the context of a color vision theory. The hue-shift functions for human and pigeon are quite different in the spectral location of their invariant points and differ in their direction of convergence with increasing and decreasing intensities. They are similar in that they produce convergence points and that the relationship of the convergence points to the hues seems to be one to one in both cases.

What do these similarities and differences imply about the underlying color mechanisms for pigeons and humans? And are the basic mechanisms and interactions among these mechanisms the same for the pigeon and human, in spite of any differences in specifics such as the shape and spectral location of photopigment absorptions? To definitively answer these questions, we need to know the true form of the underlying mechanisms for humans and pigeons, and unfortunately neither is known at this time. We can approximate an answer to these questions by hypothesizing a set of mechanisms which adequately accounts for human color vision and then see if these same mechanisms will adequately account for pigeon color vision. This exercise is useful in itself because it is a vehicle to draw together the diverse psychophysical functions within a framework in which they are interrelated. One such set of mechanisms was proposed by Hurvich and Jameson (1955). I have chosen this theory because it adequately and quantitatively accounts for most human psychophysical color-vision functions, and it deals with the different psychophysical functions which have been obtained on the pigeon. This chapter will deal only with the chromatic aspects of Hurvich and Jameson's theory and will be concerned primarily with the elements leading up to the hue discrimination function.

Hurvich and Jameson's (1955) derivation began with what they termed the chromatic response functions. "The chromatic responses ($Y - B$ and $R - G$) do not represent the total initial responses of the whole visual apparatus to the stimulus light. Rather, in the opponent-colors theory, they are assumed to result from differences in excitation of opponent visual processes that are excited, in turn, by the action of light on the retinal photosensitive materials" (p. 602). An example of the chromatic response curves or chromatic valence curves, as they are often called, is shown in the top panel of Fig. 19. These curves are actually the average color mixture values for the CIE standard observer (Judd, 1951), but they can be obtained from a chromatic cancellation experiment (Jameson and Hurvich, 1955). "To measure the amount, say, of yellow chromatic response evoked by a spectral test stimulus perceived as yellow, whether pure yellow, red-yellow, or green-yellow, the experimenter adds to the test stimulus a variable amount of blue stimulus (e.g., 467 mμ) until the observer reports that the yellow hue of the test stimulus is exactly canceled. In other words, the observer's endpoint is a hue (or a neutral sensation) that is neither yellow nor blue" (p. 548). These chromatic response curves form the basis, along with several reasonable assumptions, for the derivation of the human hue-shift function and hue-discrimination function. The following four paragraphs briefly describe these derivations.

The chromatic response curves shown in the upper panel of Fig. 19 are given by the following expressions:

$$y_\lambda - b_\lambda = k_1(Y_\lambda - B_\lambda) \tag{1}$$

$$r_\lambda - g_\lambda = k_2(R_\lambda - G_\lambda) \tag{2}$$

where k_1 and k_2 are free variables. The B, G, Y, and R are related to the tristimulus values according to the following four equations:

$$B_\lambda = 13.0682\bar{y}_\lambda + 0.2672\bar{z}_\lambda \tag{3}$$

$$G_\lambda = 0.6736\bar{x}_\lambda + 14.0018\bar{y}_\lambda + 0.0040\bar{z}_\lambda \tag{4}$$

$$Y_\lambda = 0.0039\bar{x}_\lambda + 13.4680\bar{y}_\lambda - 0.1327\bar{z}_\lambda \tag{5}$$

$$R_\lambda = 0.3329\bar{x}_\lambda + 13.0012\bar{y}_\lambda - 0.0011\bar{z}_\lambda \tag{6}$$

The opponent processes depicted by the chromatic response function produces a hue sensation, reasoned Hurvich and Jameson, according to the ratio of each separate chromatic response to the sum of all chromatic responses at a given wavelength. They call this function a "hue-coefficient function." The hue-coefficient function is thus derived from the following expression:

$$h_\lambda = \frac{(|y - b|)_\lambda}{(|y - b| + |r - g|)_\lambda}$$

or

$$\tag{7}$$

$$h_\lambda = \frac{(|r - g|)_\lambda}{(|r - g| + |y - b|)_\lambda}$$

and is shown in the middle panel of Fig. 19.

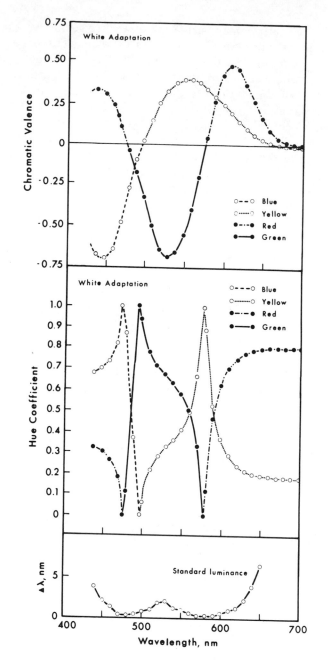

Fig. 19. A human hue-discrimination function (bottom panel) derived from hypothetical hue-coefficient functions (middle panel) which are derived from chromatic response functions (top panel). See text for details. After Hurvich and Jameson (1955).

Two psychophysical functions which can be derived from the hue-coefficient function and which will be considered here are the hue-shift function and the hue-discrimination function. The hue-shift function is derived by assuming that different luminance levels will change the coefficients k_1 and k_2 of equations (1) and (2). By substituting different k_1's and k_2's in those equations and producing chromatic response functions for each pair of k_1 and k_2, Hurvich and Jameson computed those wavelengths which gave identical hue coefficients for each k_1 and k_2 pair corresponding to the different luminance levels. The resulting hue-shift data from their model corresponded well to Purdy's experimental results. Note that a change in the constants k_1 and k_2 will not change the zero crossing points of the chromatic response functions; zero crossing points occur when either equation (1) or equation (2) is zero. Hence, at these zero crossing points, the hue-coefficient function will be one (or zero) independent of the change in k_1 or k_2. The hue coefficients at these points likewise will not change with luminance changes because changes affect only k_1 and k_2, and hence these points will show no hue shift.

Hue discrimination was hypothesized to be a function of the rate change of the hue-coefficient function, its slope. They further hypothesized that saturation discrimination would contribute to hue discrimination and that the rate change of the hue-coefficient function and the rate change of the saturation discrimination function would contribute equally to hue discriminability. The resulting expression for hue discrimination is

$$2\Delta\lambda = \Delta h_\lambda \left[\frac{\Delta\lambda}{\Delta(\,|y-b|\,)/(\,|y-b|+|r-g|\,)} \right] \tag{8}$$
$$+ \Delta\sigma \left[\frac{\Delta\lambda}{\Delta(\,|y-b|+|r-g|\,)/(\,|y-b|+|r-g|+|w-bk|\,)} \right]$$

(after Graham, 1965) and the resulting hue-discrimination function is shown in the lower portion of Fig. 19. It corresponds quite well to the experimental data.

The chromatic response functions cannot be derived directly for the pigeon as they were for the human. The tristimulus values used for the human chromatic response functions came from color-mixture experiments which have not been performed on the pigeon. Of course, nothing comparable to Hurvich and Jameson's cancellation experiment could ever be performed on the pigeon, or on any infrahuman organism for that matter. Instead of beginning with the chromatic response functions, I will begin with the pigeon's hue-discrimination function and its Bezold–Brücke hue-shift function and work in the opposite direction to derive a workable pair of chromatic response functions. I will attempt to show that these chromatic response functions are not entirely arbitrary, but rather are considerably constrained by the pyschophysical data.

Consider for a moment the constraints that the hue-discrimination and Bezold–Brücke hue-shift functions place on the form of the chromatic response functions. The pair of chromatic response functions must show zero crossings at 530, 550, and 630 nm because these are the invariant points identified from the pigeon's hue-shift function. Furthermore, because the hue lines converge on the 530 nm and 630 nm invariant points with decreasing intensity, these two invariant points must be the zero crossing points of the same chromatic response function. That is, either $r - g$ or $y - b$ must contain both the 630 nm and the 530 nm zero crossing points. The other chromatic response function will show a zero crossing point at 550 nm.

The hue-discrimination function imposed considerable constraint on the form of the chromatic response functions. First, note that human hue discrimination is best in the vicinity of the zero crossing points of the chromatic response function. This is no accident; the ratio of one chromatic response to the sum of both chromatic responses is changing most rapidly when one chromatic response function passes through zero. Hence the hue-coefficient function will naturally be steepest in the vicinity of zero crossings of the chromatic response functions and will result in a prediction of best hue discrimination at these spectral points. The pigeon's 540 nm point of good hue discriminability is located between the 530 nm and 550 nm invariant points, and so this point of good hue discriminability will be close to two zero crossing points of the chromatic response functions. Many different chromatic response functions with these zero crossing points will account for the good hue discriminability at 540 nm. The other points of good hue discriminability, and those of comparatively poor hue discriminability, are not so easily accounted for by chromatic response functions with zero crossing points at 530, 550, and 630 nm. Wavelengths just shorter than 530 nm, just longer than 550 nm, and in the vicinity of 630 nm are all areas of comparatively poor hue discriminability, but these are regions adjacent to the zero crossing points of the chromatic response functions. There is also the problem of accounting for the comparatively good hue discriminability at 500 nm and at 600 nm, which are areas where there are no zero crossing points of the chromatic response functions. The areas of poor hue discriminability, located adjacent to zero crossings of the chromatic response functions, dictate that the chromatic response function must be very shallow in these regions in order to produce a comparatively slight change in the hue coefficients at these points. In order to produce rapid changes in hue coefficients at spectral regions where there are no zero crossings of the chromatic response function, the chromatic response functions must be quite steep and changing in opposite directions; one must change toward a smaller chromatic valence. The top panel in Fig. 20 shows a set of chromatic response functions which comes quite close to fulfilling the above requirements. The resulting hue-coefficient function is shown in the middle panel, and the derived hue-discrimination function is shown by the solid line in the bottom panel. The unfilled points in the

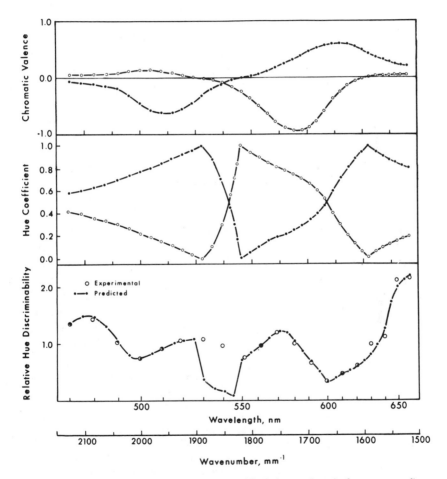

Fig. 20. Pigeon hue-discrimination results (unfilled data points in bottom panel) compared to a predicted hue-discrimination function (filled points on line in bottom panel). The hypothetical pigeon hue-coefficient function (middle panel) and hypothetical chromatic response function (top panel) were derived by a trial-and-error procedure using the pigeon's hue-discrimination function and its hue-shift function. See text for details.

bottom panel are experimentally obtained measures of the pigeon's hue discriminability from the previously discussed hue-discrimination experiment (Wright, 1972b, 1974).[4] The derived hue-discrimination function fits the data quite well except for the region of 540 nm, where somewhat better hue discriminability is predicted than is actually obtained. The intricacies of the curve-fitting procedure allow the derived hue-discrimination function to be fitted to the obtained data for the region 530–550 nm or for the region 550–630 nm, but not to both regions at the same time.

Hurvich and Jameson, in their theory, gave equal weight to changes in the saturation coefficients and changes in the hue coefficients. The contribution of saturation discrimination to the performance of the pigeon in the hue-discrimination task may be minimal. The present account of the pigeon's hue discrimination is based solely on changes in the hue coefficients. Furthermore, taking saturation into account would only complicate matters where the pigeon is concerned. Any contribution of saturation discrimination in the manner of Hurvich and Jameson would make the fit between the predicted and the obtained hue discrimination slightly worse.

The theory of Hurvich and Jameson provides us with the framework to bring together the psychophysical information and to compare these two color-vision systems. This model may not be valid in the final analysis, but it is a convenient organizational scheme and provides a good vantage point from which to compare these systems. The model of Hurvich and Jameson can be extended to account for other pigeon psychophysical data such as spectral sensitivity and saturation discrimination (cf. Romeskie and Yager, 1976b). Another useful extension would be to relate the chromatic response functions to the pigeon's receptor processes (preretinal absorptions, oil droplets, photopigments). All of these relationships would be useful in establishing the validity of the chromatic response functions and would allow other

[4] The particular hue-discrimination function chosen was a plot of the slope reciprocals of the psychometric functions. This measure of hue discriminability is possible because the psychometric functions from the 20 spectral points tested were linear and of zero intercept. The slope, then, summarized the psychometric function. The slope reciprocals proportional to the threshold and is the appropriate measure of relative sensitivity (Wright, 1974). There are two reasons for using the slope reciprocal function instead of one of the hue-discrimination functions shown in Fig. 20: first, there is no rational basis for choosing one of the functions shown in Fig. 20 as opposed to any other one; second, the predicted hue-discriminability measure from the hue-coefficient function is very similar to the slope reciprocals of the psychometric functions. The hue-discriminability measure from the hue-coefficient function is the rate change of this function, which is its slope. The slope reciprocal is used here, too, because this slope is directly related to the threshold; steeper slopes produce smaller thresholds.

predictions to be made, but no individual extension would be conclusive in itself. Initially, Hurvich and Jameson (1955) related their chromatic response functions to hypothetical receptor substances which differed only very slightly in extent and peak wavelength. Later, it was shown (Brown and Wald, 1964; Marks et al., 1964) that these assumed receptor substances were incorrect. Jameson and Hurvich (1968), however, showed how their chromatic response functions could also be derived from these new visual pigment data. Such flexibility means that there are too many free variables in this fitting procedure for this relationship to be a definitive test of the theory. It, of course, would have been noteworthy if there had been no combination of relative weightings of the photopigment data which would have accounted for Hurvich and Jameson's chromatic response functions. One difficulty in assessing the uniqueness and value of a theory such as Hurvich and Jameson's is to determine to what degree all of the various predictions combine to constrain the theory and make the predictions more unique than they would be individually.

Psychophysical investigations provide only a portion of the information necessary to formulate a truly robust theory of color vision; the same can be said for the biological investigations. One needs a bit of both, the psychological and the physiological, to generate a reasonably unique solution with regard to the underlying mechanisms and to generate some reasonable predictions. Physiological, biophysical, and biochemical evidence provides some of the inputs to these solutions such as the shape and spectral location of the photopigment distributions, and the spectral sensitivity data and hue-discrimination data constrain the way in which these photopigments and resulting excitations must interact.

REFERENCES

Beare, A. C.: Color-name as a function of wavelength. *Am. J. Psychol.* **76**:248–256 (1963).

Blough, D. S.: Spectral sensitivity in the pigeon. *J. Opt. Soc. Am.* **47**:827–833 (1957).

Bough, D. S.: The shape of some wavelength generalization gradients. *J. Exp. Anal. Behav.* **4**:31–40 (1961).

Blough, P. M.: Wavelength generalization and discrimination in the pigeon. *Percept. Psychophys.* **4**:342–348 (1972).

Blough, P. M.: The pigeon's perception of saturation. *J. Exp. Anal. Behav.* **24**:135–148 (1975).

Boynton, R. M., and Gordon, J.: Bezold-Brücke hue shifts measured by color naming technique. *J. Opt. Soc. Am.* **55**:78–86 (1965).

Brown, P. K., and Wald, G.: Visual pigments in single rods and cones of the human retina. *Science* **44**:45–51 (1964).

Cohen, J. D.: Temporal independence of the Bezold-Brücke hue shift. *Vision Res.* **15**:341–351 (1975).

Graf, V. A.: A spectral luminosity function in the pigeon determined by flicker photometry. *Psychonom. Sci.* **17**:282–283 (1969).

Graham, C. H.: Color: Data and theories. In Graham, C. H. (ed.): *Vision and Visual Perception.* Wiley, New York (1965). P. 437.

Graham, C. H., and Hsia, Y.: Saturation and the focal achromatic interval. *J. Opt. Soc. Am.* **59**:993–997 (1969).

Guttman, N., and Kalish, H. I.: Discriminability and stimulus generalization. *J. Exp. Psychol.* **51**:79–88 (1956).

Hamilton, W. F., and Coleman, T. B.: Trichromatic vision in the pigeon as illustrated by the spectral hue discrimination curve. *J. Comp. Physiol. Psychol.* **15**:183–191 (1933).

Hecht, S., and Shlaer, S.: The color vision of dichromats. *J. Gen. Physiol.* **20**:57–93 (1936).

Hurvich, L. M., and Jameson, D.: Some quantitative aspects of an opponent colors theory. II. Brightness, saturation, and hue in normal and dichromatic vision. *J. Opt. Soc. Am.* **45**:602–616 (1955).

Jacobs, G. H., and Wascher, T. C.: Bezold-Brücke hue shift; further measurements. *J. Opt. Soc. Am.* **57**:1155–1156 (1967).

Jameson, D., and Hurvich, L. M.: Some quantitative aspects of an opponent-colors theory. I. Chromatic responses and spectral saturation. *J. Opt. Soc. Am.* **45**:546–552 (1955).

Jameson, D., and Hurvich, L. M.: Opponent-response functions related to measured cone photopigments. *J. Opt. Soc. Am.* **58**:429–430 (1968).

Jones, L. A.: The fundamental scale for pure hue and retinal sensibility to hue differences. *J. Opt. Soc. Am.* **1**:63–67 (1917).

Judd, D. B.: Chromatic sensibility to stimulus differences. *J. Opt. Soc. Am.* **22**:72–108 (1932).

Judd, D. B.: Basic correlates of the visual stimulus. In Stevens, S. S. (ed.): *Handbook of Experimental Psychology.* Wiley, New York (1951). Pp. 811–867.

Larimer, J., Krantz, D. H., and Cicerone, C. M.: Opponent-process additivity. I. Red/green equilibria. *Vision Res.* **14**:1127–1140 (1974).

Larimer, J., Krantz, D. H., and Cicerone, C. M.: Opponent process additivity. II. Yellow/blue equilibria and nonlinear models. *Vision Res.* **15**:723–731 (1975).

Laurens, H., and Hamilton, W. F.: The sensibility of the eye to differences in wavelength. *Am. J. Physiol.* **65**:547–568 (1923).

Luria, S. M.: Color-name as a function of stimulus-intensity and duration. *Am. J. Psychol.* **80**:14–27 (1967).

Marks, W. B., Dobelle, W. A., and MacNichol, E. F.: Visual pigments of single primate cones. *Science* **143**:1181–1183 (1964).

Nelson, J. H.: The color-vision characteristics of a trichromat. *Proc. Phys. Soc. London* **49**:332–337 (1937).

Priest, I. G., and Brickwedde, F. G.: The minimum perceptible colorimetric purity as a function of dominant wavelength. *J. Opt. Soc. Am.* **28**:133–139 (1938).

Purdy, D. M.: Spectral hue as a function of intensity. *Am. J. Psychol.* **43**:541–559 (1931).

Romeskie, M., and Yager, D.: Psychophysical studies of pigeon color vision. I. Photopic spectral sensitivity. *Vision Res.* **16**:501–505 (1976a).

Romeskie, M., and Yager, D.: Psychophysical studies of pigeon color vision. II. The spectral photochromatic interval function in the pigeon. *Vision Res.* **16**:507–512 (1976b).

Schneider, B.: Multidimensional scaling of color difference in the pigeon. *Percept. Psychophys.* **12**:373–378 (1972).

Shepard, R. N.: Approximation to uniform gradients of generalization by monotone transformation of scale. In Mostofsky, D. I. (ed.): *Stimulus Generalization*. Stanford University Press, Stanford, Calif. (1965). Pp. 94–111.

Smith, V. C., Pokorny, J., Cohen, J., and Perera, T.: Luminance thresholds for the Bezold-Brücke hue shift. *Percept. Psychophys.* **3**:306–310 (1967).

Steindler, O.: Die Farbenempfindlichkeit des normalen und farbenblinden Auges. *Sitzber. Wien. Akad. Wiss. Math-Naturwiss. Kl.* **15(IIa)**:39–62 (1906).

van der Horst, G. J. C., and Muis, W.: Hue shift and brightness enhancement of flickering light. *Vision Res.* **9**:953–963 (1969).

van der Wildt, G. J., and Bouman, A. M.: The dependence of Bezold-Brücke hue shift on spatial intensity distribution. *Vision Res.* **8**:303–313 (1968).

Wright, A. A.: The influence of ultraviolet radiation on the pigeon's color discrimination. *J. Exp. Anal. Behav.* **17**:325–337 (1972a).

Wright, A. A.: Psychometric and psychophysical hue discrimination functions for the pigeon. *Vision Res.* **12**:1447–1464 (1972b).

Wright, A. A.: Psychometric and psychophysical theory within a framework of response bias. *Psychol. Rev.* **81**:322–347 (1974).

Wright, A. A.: Bezold-Brücke hue shift functions for the pigeon. *Vision Res.* **16**:765–774 (1976).

Wright, A. A., and Cumming, W. W.: Color-naming funcitons for the pigeon. *J. Exp. Anal. Behav.* **15**:7–17 (1971).

Wright, W. D.: *Researches on Normal and Defective Color Vision*. Mosby, St. Louis (1947).

Wright, W. D., and Pitt, F. H. G.: The saturation-discrimination of two trichromats. *Proc. Phys. Soc. London* **49**:329–331 (1937).

8

Four Spectral Mechanisms in the Pigeon (*Columba livia*)

VIRGIL A. GRAF

INTRODUCTION

The pigeon is known to have color vision at photopic luminance levels (Hamilton and Coleman, 1933; Bough, 1972; Wright, 1972, 1976). Consequently, there must be at least two spectral mechanisms in the pigeon's visual system that have different action spectra. However, the number and characteristics of mechanisms underlying color vision in the pigeon have not been resolved, although physiological, electrophysiological, and behavioral studies have suggested a variety of candidates.

Wald (1958), using retinal extracts, reported a cone photopigment with λ_{max} at 560 nm, and Bridges (1962), with a similar technique, observed a cone photopigment with λ_{max} at 544 nm. Liebman (1972), using a microspectrophotometer, reported a cone pigment with λ_{max} at 562 nm. None of these data takes into account the absorption spectra of the three classes of oil droplets which are interposed between the incoming light and the receptor photopigment (Strother, 1963; King-Smith, 1969). Combining each oil droplet with each of the known pigments noted above provides at least six possibilities. In addition, Cohen (1963) showed that some cones have no oil droplets associated with them.

VIRGIL A. GRAF • Department of Psychology, Dartmouth College, Hanover, New Hampshire 03755. The research reported here was supported by PHS Grant EY-00355.

Electrophysiologically, a variety of spectral mechanisms have been reported. Granit's (1942) early optic nerve recording showed only a photopic dominator with λ_{max} at 580 nm. However, Donner (1953) found narrowband units in the pigeon optic nerve with λ_{max} at 480 nm, 600 nm, and 620 nm. Ikeda's (1965) data from an electroretinographic (ERG) study of spectral sensitivity was broadband, with λ_{max} at about 545 nm. However, a second mechanism with λ_{max} at about 605 nm was noted. More recent electrophysiological studies show photopic sensitivity maximal at about 580 nm (Blough et al., 1972). In addition to the 580 nm peak, Graf and Norren (1974) observed a very-short-wavelength-sensitive mechanism with λ_{max} at about 400 nm. Norren (1975) reports spectral mechanisms with λ_{max} at 415 nm, 480 nm, and 580 nm. Granda and Yazulla (1971) reported single units in the pigeon's nucleus rotundus with peaks at 540 nm and 600–620 nm. Finally, Yazulla and Granda (1973) have demonstrated that there are opponent units in the nucleus rotundus with maximal excitatory response at 420 nm and 530 nm, and maximal inhibitory response at 570 nm and 440 nm, respectively. Taken together, there is evidence for spectral mechanisms with λ_{max} at 420 nm, 480 nm, 540 nm, 560 nm, 580 nm, 600 nm, and 620 nm.

It is natural to ask which, if any, of the above mechanisms is reflected in the behavior of the animal. Psychophysical studies of spectral sensitivity (Blough, 1957; Graf, 1969; Romeskie and Yager, 1976) show broadband curves with peak sensitivity at about 580 nm. Bough's data show a secondary peak at short wavelengths which is consistent with the short-wavelength mechanism seen in Graf and Norren's and in Norren's ERG data. Romeskie and Yager suggest a model of spectral sensitivity and saturation discrimination based on mechanisms with λ_{max} at 415 nm, 570 nm, 590 nm, and 620 nm. The long-wavelength mechanisms were derived by screening a 562 nm pigment by "yellow," "orange," and "red" oil droplets.

There seems to be general agreement between electrophysiological and behavioral studies that there is a mechanism with λ_{max} at very short wavelengths (400–415 nm). However, no corresponding visual pigment has been observed in this part of the spectrum. There is also good agreement between electrophysiological and behavioral studies in the declining portion of spectral sensitivity curves in the long-wavelength end of the spectrum. Furthermore, there is a corresponding visual pigment in this part of the spectrum. Although Romeskie and Yager note a modest shoulder in their data at about 480 nm, there does not seem to be a clear behavioral correlate to the 480 nm mechanism that is observed electrophysiologically. This is true also of the mechanism in the 545 nm region which has been noted with retinal extracts and electrophysiologically.

The experiments to be reported here were designed to provide additional data for assessment of the underlying spectral mechanisms which exist in the pigeon visual system. Behavioral spectral sensitivity was measured by determining the pigeon's increment threshold for small chromatic stimuli (2 deg) superimposed on large backgrounds (20 deg) which were either "white," "red," "yellow," or "blue."

METHOD

Subjects

The subjects were five male White Carneaux pigeons (*Columba livia*) obtained from the Palmetto Pigeon Plant, Sumpter, South Carolina. They were $1\frac{1}{2}$ years old at the beginning of the experiments and had had previous experience in a form discrimination task.

Apparatus

A schematic of the apparatus is shown in Fig. 1. The pigeon shown viewing the stimulus-response key (RK) was actually in a Leigh Valley test chamber (model 132-02). It was 34 cm high, 34 cm wide, and 30 cm deep. The front panel consisted of a single RK (2.5 cm diameter) located 25 cm above the floor. Two side keys were occluded. There was a grain hopper located 12 cm below RK.

The optics shown in Fig. 1 projected the stimuli onto the RK. The

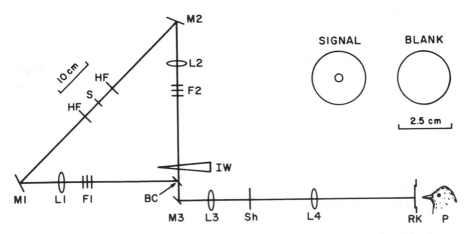

Fig. 1. Schematic of the apparatus drawn to scale (10 cm). The inset on the right shows the two classes of stimuli the pigeon saw, also drawn to scale (2.5 cm).

source was a 500-W CZX projection lamp run at 4.2 A. The current was adjusted manually with a Variac and monitored visually. The channel at the left of the source provided the background beam, and the channel on the right provided the test stimulus beam. A beam-splitting cube (BC) combined the background and test stimulus channels, and the final lens (L4) projected a superimposed image of the planes of L1 and L2 onto the plane of RK. A filter box between L1 and BC held color and neutral density filters in the background channel. Blue backgrounds were obtained with a Kodak 47B filter and Corning 497 to suppress unwanted long-wavelength sidebands. Yellow was obtained with a Corning 3482 (1.5 mm thick) and red with a Kodak 29. The neutral white background was obtained by placing an annulus in the plane of L1. When projected onto RK, its outer diameter was 2.0 cm and it was about 0.25 cm thick. The ring was white (approximately 4800°K).

The chromatic test stimuli were obtained by passing light through a Schott (Veril S200) interference wedge (IW). It had a half bandwidth of 15 nm under the conditions used here. A stop in the plane of L2 determined the projected dimensions of the test stimuli (2 deg). The luminance of both the background and the test stimulus was controlled with calibrated Kodak 96 neutral density filters.

The luminance of the background was measured with a Tektronix J16 digital photometer and J6503 luminance probe. The relative radiance of the test spot was measured with the Tektronix instrument and a J6502 radiometric probe.

Procedure

Each pigeon was trained to eat food from the food hopper and peck the background-illuminated RK with conventional shaping methods. When the pigeons were pecking RK readily, the training procedure was started.

Each subject received 120 trials/day. On half the trials the background light was presented alone, and on half the trials a small spot of light was superimposed on the background. A trial started when an electromechanical shutter opened.

On trials on which the background alone was presented, a single peck to RK produced 4-sec access to the grain hopper. This was considered a correct response. If the subject did not respond within 4 sec of trial onset, the shutter closed and a 6-sec time-out (TO) period was started. This was considered an error. When the TO period ended, a 4-sec intertrial interval (ITI) was started. At the end of the ITI the shutter opened and the subject had another opportunity to earn a grain reward. The trial sequence programmer was not advanced until the subject made a correct response.

On trials during which the small test stimulus was superimposed on the background, a pecking response was considered an error. The error contingencies described above were in effect. If the subject did not respond for 4 sec, this was considered correct. However, in this case, grain reinforcement was not delivered. Instead, the ITI was started after which the next trial in the sequence was begun.

After the subjects had learned to respond appropriately, they were started on a partial reinforcement schedule. At the final stage, subjects were rewarded on 50% of the background-alone trials. Of course, subjects were never rewarded for correct response on background-plus-signal trials. The only payoff for correct performance on background-plus trials was advancement of the trial sequence programmer. On background-alone trials in which no reinforcement was programmed, the reward cycle was bypassed altogether. The ITI started immediately and the trial sequence advanced. Thus the contingencies on correct nonreinforced background-alone trials were the same as on correct background-plus-signal trials. The testing sequence was not begun until the subjects performed to a criterion of 90% correct or better on both kinds of trials for 2 consecutive days.

During the testing phase of the experiment, there were 60 background-alone trials and 60 background-plus-signal trials in the daily 120-trial sequence. Forty-four of the background-alone trials were reinforced and the rest were not. Twelve of the background-plus-signal trials were given with the test-spot radiance set at the same level that was used in training, and the contingencies were the same as described above. For purposes of description, these are referred to as "training trials." The remaining 48 background-plus-signal trials had test spots with lower radiances and were defined as test trials. Twelve were attenuated 0.20 log unit relative to the radiance of that used in training, 12 were attenuated 0.40 log unit, 12 were attenuated 0.60 log unit, and 12 were attenuated 0.80 log unit. The contingencies associated with test trials were different from those defined as training trials. If a response occurred on a test trial, it was treated in the same way as nonreinforced background-alone trials. The ITI was started immediately and the trial sequence programmer was advanced to the next trial.

Trial sequence was random, with the restriction that no more than three background-alone or background-plus-signal trials occur consecutively and no background-plus-signal trials of the same radiance occur consecutively. The subjects were maintained at 80% of their free-feeding weight during the course of the experiment.

RESULTS

The results are shown in Figs. 2, 3, 4, 5, and 6. On each figure, the data points represent the mean sensitivity of five pigeons. The vertical bars are the standard errors associated with each data point.

Figure 2 shows the data for the neutral white background condition. A case can be made that there are four peaks of sensitivity. One is in the very-short-wavelength end of the spectrum at about 400–420 nm, a second peak appears at about 480 nm, a third peak in the region of 550 nm, and the fourth peak at about 615 nm. The foregoing is admittedly speculative and, in fact, anticipates the discussion in which a model that deals with all the data is considered. Although there may be some question as to the peaks of sensitivity in these data, the deep trough at 450 nm is to be noted.

Figure 3 shows the data for the red background. In this case, there

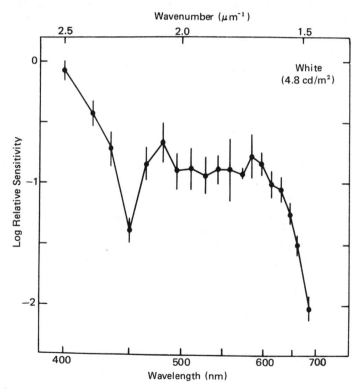

Fig. 2. Mean relative spectral sensitivity of five pigeons on a neutral white (annulus) background (4.8 cd/m²). The vertical bars represent 1 standard error of the mean for each data point. Sensitivity is based on a quantum spectrum.

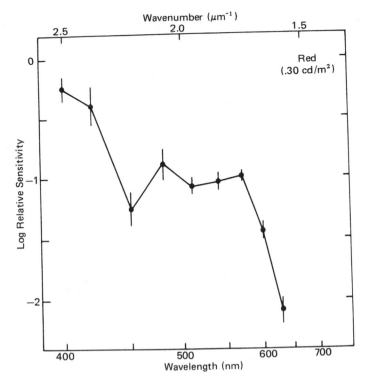

Fig. 3. Mean relative spectral sensitivity of five pigeons on a red (Kodak 29) background (0.30 cd/m²).

seem to be only three peaks: one at a very short wavelength, another at about 480 nm, and a third at about 570 nm. The trough at 450 nm is evident once again.

Figure 4 shows the data for the yellow background. Again, there seem to be four peaks of sensitivity. The short-wavelength peaks are clearly evident: one in the 400–420 nm region and the other at 480 nm. There is a deep trough at 450 nm also. In the long-wavelength portion of the spectrum, there is a modest shoulder in the 540–570 nm region, and there is a clear peak at 615 nm. Note that there appears to be a trough at about 600 nm.

Figures 5 and 6 show the data for two levels of the blue background. Figure 5 represents the data for a 0.11 cd/m² blue background. In these data, only three peaks are apparent: one at a very short wavelength, one in the 540–570 nm region, and the third at about 615 nm. There may be a modest shoulder at about 480 nm as well. Figure 6 shows the results with a 0.26 cd/m² blue background. In these data,

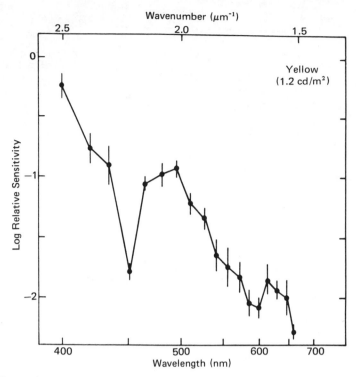

Fig. 4. Mean relative spectral sensitivity of five pigeons on a yellow (Corning 3482) background (1.2 cd/m²).

only two peaks are seen: one in the 540–570 nm region and the other at about 630 nm.

DISCUSSION

All of the data taken together support the hypothesis that there are at least four mechanisms which contribute to spectral sensitivity measured in these experiments. Although there is some variability in the placement of the peaks from experiment to experiment, an overall picture is fairly clear.

There is a mechanism which has maximum sensitivity at a very short wavelength. This can be reasonably fitted by a Dartnall nomogram with λ_{max} at 400 nm. A photopigment at such a short wavelength has not been observed in vertebrates, and it may be argued that there is no short-wavelength-sensitive pigment at all. That is, the very-short-wavelength sensitivity might be due to the interaction of two or more spectral mechanisms that are maximally sensitive to longer-wavelength light. It has been shown (Naka and Rushton, 1966; Sirovich and Abramov, 1977) that the action spectrum of a visual pigment can be mimicked by the interaction of two other spectral mechanisms. This does not seem a likely explanation of the very-short-wavelength-sensitive system in the pigeon. Graf and Norren (1974) and Norren (1975) have shown that the sensitivity of the very-short-wavelength-sensitive mechanism measured electroretinographically is reduced by about 0.30 log unit with a chromatic background which reduces sensitivity of the long-wavelength-sensitive mechanisms by about 2.50 log units. This selective loss of sensitivity argues against the likelihood that the very-short-wavelength sensitivity is the consequence of an interaction of longer-wavelength mechanisms. The selective loss of sensitivity also reduces the likelihood that these results are due to an artifact such as fluorescence or scattered light. Furthermore, the observation that the

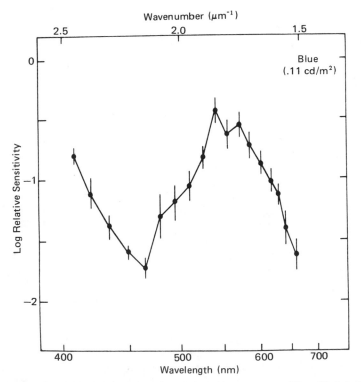

Fig. 5. Mean relative spectral sensitivity of five pigeons on a blue (Kodak 47B and Corning 497) background (0.11 cd/m²).

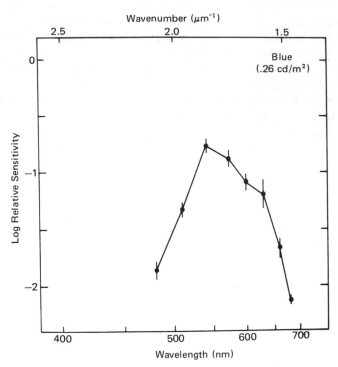

Fig. 6. Mean relative spectral sensitivity of five pigeons on a blue (Kodak 47B and Corning 497) background (0.26 cd/m²).

short-wavelength-sensitive mechanism is suppressed with short-wavelength background light lends added support to a visual pigment hypothesis.

A second short-wavelength-sensitive mechanism has maximal sensitivity at about 480 nm. This corresponds to Donner's (1953) narrowband optic nerve unit, and Norren (1975) observed a similar peak in his ERG study of pigeons, chickens, and daws. On the assumption that the peak observed here is not an interaction effect or an artifact, what might be the underlying mechanism? A reasonably good fit to all the data is achieved by choosing a 460 nm nomogram and multiplying it by the large yellow oil droplet measured by King-Smith. It should be noted that a 480 nm nomogram screened by either an orange or red oil droplet fits nearly as well. In any case, as with the very-short-wavelength-sensitive mechanism, a pigeon visual pigment with λ_{max} at 460 nm or 480 nm has not yet been reported.

The data for neutral, red, and yellow backgrounds all show a trough at 450 nm. This appears to reflect a subtractive interaction between the very-short-wavelength mechanism and the mechanism which has a peak at 480 nm.

In the long-wavelength end of the spectrum, the data support the hypothesis that there is a mechanism with λ_{max} in the 550–570 nm region and another one with λ_{max} at about 610–620 nm. The former is evident in the spectral curves for all conditions. All of the data points in this portion of the spectrum can be fitted quite well by choosing a nomogram with λ_{max} at 530 nm and multiplying it by King-Smith's (1969) orange oil droplet. The 620-nm mechanism is fitted by a nomogram with λ_{max} at 560 nm multiplied by the absorption spectrum of King-Smith's red oil droplet.

The yellow background data show a clear trough at 600 nm. This is consistent with a subtractive interaction between the 620 nm mechanism and the other long-wavelength system. The neutral white and blue backgrounds show a slight notch at about 600 nm as well. If there is a subtractive interaction between the two long-wavelength mechanisms, it appears that it is dependent on the adaptation level of the contributing mechanisms. When the adaptation level of the long-wavelength mechanism is high, as in the yellow-background condition, then the interaction is apparent. When the adaptation level is relatively low, as with neutral white and blue backgrounds, then the interaction is not clearly seen. Sperling and Harwerth (1971) have noted interactions between spectral mechanisms which contribute to primate increment threshold that are adaptation-level dependent.

Figure 7 shows a composite of all the data along with theoretical curves based on the prospective mechanisms indicated above, namely, a 400 nm pigment with no oil droplet, a 460 nm pigment screened by the large yellow oil droplet, a 530 nm pigment screened by the orange oil droplet, and a 560 nm pigment screened by the red oil droplet. The normalized relative sensitivities of these mechanisms are shown in Fig. 8, labeled a, b, c, and d, respectively. The smooth curves in Fig. 7 represent the envelope of the most sensitive mechanism as determined by the following expression:

$$S_\lambda = \begin{vmatrix} k_1 a_\lambda - k_2 b_\lambda \\ k_3 b_\lambda - k_4 a_\lambda \\ k_5 c_\lambda - k_6 d_\lambda \\ k_7 d_\lambda - k_8 c_\lambda \end{vmatrix} \tag{1}$$

The parameters k_1–k_8 were chosen to provide the best overall visual fit under each condition.

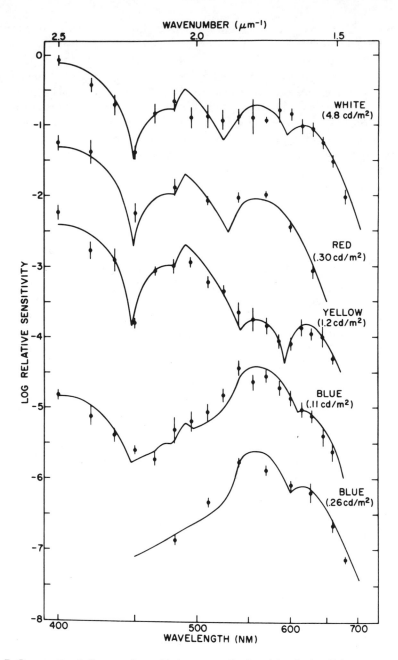

Fig. 7. Composite of all spectral sensitivity curves displaced for clarity. Relative to white, red is displaced −1 log unit, yellow is displaced −2 log units, 0.11 cd/m² blue is displaced −4 log units, and 0.26 cd/m² blue is displaced −5 log units. The smooth curves are theoretical curves (see text for details).

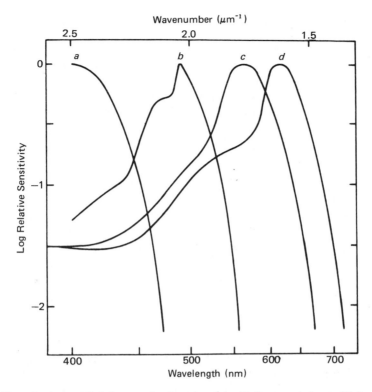

Fig. 8. Hypothetical underlying mechanisms used to fit the spectral sensitivity data. Mechanism a represents the normalized quantal sensitivity of Dartnall nomogram with λ_{max} at 400 nm. Mechanism b is a 460 nm nomogram screened by King-Smith's large yellow oil droplet. The nomogram was multiplied by the absorption spectrum of the oil droplet, and the product was normalized and expressed as log relative sensitivity. Mechanism c is a 530 nm nomogram screened by King-Smith's orange oil droplet. Mechanism d is a 560 nm nomogram screened by King-Smith's red oil droplet.

The top curve in Fig. 7 shows the data from the neutral background and the envelope of the mechanisms a, b, c, and d with coefficient k_1 = 1, k_2 = 0.405, k_3 = 0.405, k_4 = 0.303, k_5 = 0.253, k_6 = 0.063, k_7 = 0.126, and k_8 = 0.0. The data are displaced arbitrarily for clarity. The second curve is fitted to the red background data, the third curve is for the yellow background data, the fourth curve is for the less intense blue background data, and the fifth curve is for the more intense blue background data. Table 1 shows the coefficients for k_1–k_8 which were used to fit the data in each case.

If the coefficients for the neutral background data are used as the referent, the effect of various chromatic backgrounds on each coefficient is qualitatively correct; that is, blue backgrounds suppress the shorter-

Table 1. Coefficients Used to Fit the Empirical Data for Each Background

Background	Coefficient							
White	1.0	0.405	0.405	0.303	0.253	0.063	0.126	0.0
Red	0.633	0.253	0.253	0.190	0.113	0.0	0.0	0.0
Yellow	0.506	0.253	0.253	0.190	0.025	0.015	0.023	0.015
0.11 Blue	0.190	0.038	0.076	0.190	0.494	0.063	0.110	0.0
0.26 Blue	0.0	0.0	0.0	0.0	0.253	0.063	0.095	0.0

wavelength mechanisms ($k_{1,2,3,4}$) more than the long-wavelength ones ($k_{5,6,7,8}$), and intense blue backgrounds suppress the short-wavelength mechanisms more than weak blue backgrounds do. The red and yellow backgrounds have the opposite effect; the long-wavelength mechanisms are suppressed more than the short-wavelength ones. However, it should be noted that the red and yellow backgrounds also have the effect of partly suppressing the sensitivity of the short-wavelength mechanisms. The data reported here are not sufficient to determine the source of this sensitivity loss.

While the model represented by equation (1) provides a fairly good description of the data, there are some additional points to be noted. One is that for neutral, red, and yellow backgrounds the data are fitted best if the ratio of coefficients k_2 and k_3 is 1. However, this does not hold when fitting the weak blue data. These data are best fitted if the k_2/k_3 ratio is 0.5. Similarly, the neutral, red, and yellow background data are fitted best if the ratio of coefficients k_1 and k_4 is about 0.3, except with the weak blue background, in which case k_1/k_4 is 1. It appears that the extent to which the a mechanism subtractively interacts with the b mechanism and vice versa depends on the adaptation level of one or both of them. However, the effect of adaptation level is opposite for the a and b mechanisms. The extent to which the b mechanism subtracts from the a mechanism decreases if the short-wavelength coefficients are small, but the extent to which a subtracts from b interaction increases if short-wavelength coefficients are small.

Interaction between the long-wavelength mechanisms appears to be adaptation level dependent, too. The coefficient k_8 is always 0 except with the yellow background, when it is 0.015. It seems that the c mechanism does not interact with the d mechanism until the coefficient k_5 is at least less than 0.113 and/or the coefficient k_7 is less than 0.095. The interaction of the d mechanism on the c mechanism does not indicate any clear adaptation-level-dependent component. The ratio of the coefficient k_6 to coefficient k_7 varies between 0.5 and 0.75 in an unsystematic manner.

The mechanisms proposed here are consistent with most but not all previous work. The most notable departure is the requirement of a

530 nm pigment screened by the orange oil droplet to fit the data in the middle of the spectrum (540–600 nm). One would have expected the most likely candidate in this portion of the spectrum to be the 544 nm or 560 nm pigment screened by one or more of the yellow, orange, or red oil droplets. A wide range of pigment–oil droplet combinations was tried, including weighted averages of two or more oil droplets with the same pigment. None provided a satisfactory approximation of the data. The 530 nm mechanism was the only one that consistently fit the data.

The other mechanisms are in better accord with previous findings. The short-wavelength mechanism (400–420 nm) is similar to that observed in Graf and Norren's (1974) and Norren's (1975) ERG work. In addition, this mechanism fits Bough's (1957) short-wavelength peak as well as Romeskie and Yager's (1976) short-wavelength data. The 460-nm pigment screened by the yellow oil droplet (peak 480 nm) is similar to that observed by Norren, and agrees with Donner's (1953) observations. The long-wavelength mechanism at 620 nm, achieved by choosing a 560 nm pigment and screening it by a red oil droplet, agrees with all of the spectral data that the author is aware of.

The mechanisms proposed to fit the data reported here are not the same as those proposed by Romeskie and Yager to fit their behavioral spectral sensitivity data. Although they chose a pigment with λ_{max} at 415 nm and here a 400 nm pigment was chosen, the difference is minor. The main difference is that they selected one pigment with λ_{max} at 562 nm and assumed it to be screened by each oil droplet in turn. In the model proposed here, three different pigments are screened by three different oil droplets. The mechanisms proposed here do fit Romeskie and Yager's spectral sensitivity data fairly well, but their mechanisms do not fit the data reported here. Direct evidence bearing on these alternatives is lacking. However, it has been shown that in the chicken retina different classes of oil droplet are associated with particular morphological classes of cone (Morris, 1970). If it is assumed that morphology is correlated with photopigment spectra, and that the pigeon retina is like the chicken retina, then a scheme such as the one proposed here is plausible. Each of three cone classes (460 nm, 530 nm, or 560 nm) is screened by a different oil droplet (yellow, orange, or red), and one cone class (400 nm) has no oil droplet associated with it.

REFERENCES

Blough, D. S.: Spectral sensitivity in the pigeon. *J. Opt. Soc. Am.* **47**:827–833 (1957).
Blough, P. M.: Wavelength generalization and discrimination in the pigeon. *Percept. Psychophys.* **12**:342–348 (1972).

Blough, P. M., Riggs, L. A., and Schafer, K. L.: Photopic spectral sensitivity determined electro-retinographically for the pigeon eye. *Vision Res.* **12**:477–485 (1972).

Bridges, C. D. B.: Visual pigments of the pigeon *(Columba livia). Vision Res.* **2**:125–137 (1962).

Cohen, A. I.: The fine structure of the visual receptors of the pigeon. *Exp. Eye Res.* **2**:88–97 (1963).

Donner, K. O.: The spectral sensitivity of the pigeon's retinal elements. *J. Physiol. (London)* **122**:524–537 (1953).

Graf, V. A.: A spectral luminosity function in the pigeon determined by flicker photometry. *Psychonom. Sci.* **17**:282–283 (1969).

Graf, V., and Norren, D. V.: A blue sensitive mechanism in the pigeon retina: λ_{max} 400 nm. *Vision Res.* **14**:1203–1209 (1974).

Granda, A. M., and Yazulla, S.: The spectral sensitivity of single units in the nucleus rotundus of pigeon *(Columba livia). J. Gen. Physiol.* **57**:363–384 (1971).

Granit, R.: The photopic spectrum of the pigeon. *Acta Physiol. Scand.* **4**:118–124 (1942).

Hamilton, H. F., and Coleman, T. B.: Trichromatic vision in the pigeon as illustrated by the spectral discrimination curve. *J. Comp. Psychol.* **15**:183–191 (1933).

Ikeda, H.: The spectral sensitivity of the pigeon *(Columba livia). Vision Res.* **5**:19–36 (1965).

King-Smith, P. E.: Absorption spectra and function of the coloured oil drops in the pigeon retina. *Vision Res.* **9**:1391–1401 (1969).

Liebman, P. A.: Microspectrophotometry of photoreceptors. In Dartnall, H. J. A. (ed.): *Handbook of Sensory Physiology VII/1.* Springer-Verlag, Berlin (1972). Pp. 481–528.

Morris, V. B.: Symmetry in a receptor mosaic demonstrated in the chick from the frequencies, spacing, and arrangement of the types of retinal receptor. *J. Comp. Neurol.* **140**:359–398 (1970).

Naka, K. I., and Rushton, W. A. H.: An attempt to analyse colour perception by electrophysiology. *J. Physiol. (London)* **185**:556–586 (1966).

Norren, D. V.: Two short wavelength sensitive cone systems in pigeon, chicken and daw. *Vision Res.* **15**:1164–1166 (1975).

Romeskie, M., and Yager, D.: Psychophysical studies of pigeon color vision. I. Photopic spectral sensitivity. *Vision Res.* **16**:501–505 (1976).

Sirovich, L., and Abramov, I.: Photopigments and pseudopigments. *Vision Res.* **17**:5–16 (1977).

Sperling, H. G., and Harwerth, R. S.: Red-green cone interactions in the increment threshold spectral sensitivity in primates. *Science* **172**:180–184 (1971).

Strother, G. K.: Absorption spectra of retinal oil globules in turkey, turtle and pigeon. *Exp. Cell Res.* **29**:349–355 (1963).

Wald, G.: Retinal chemistry and the physiology of vision. In *Visual Problems of Color.* 8th Symp. Nat. Phys. Lab. H.M.S.O., London (1958). Pp. 7–61.

Wright, A. A.: Psychometric and psychophysical hue discrimination functions in the pigeon. *Vision Res.* **12**:1447–1464 (1972).

Wright, A. A.: Bezold-Brücke hue shift functions for the pigeon. *Vision Res.* **16**:765–774 (1976).

Yazulla, S., and Granda, A. M.: Opponent-color units in the thalamus of the pigeon *(Columba livia). Vision Res.* **13**:1555–1563 (1973).

9

Spatial Interactions in the Visual Receptive Fields of the Nucleus Dorsolateralis Anterior of the Pigeon Thalamus

D. JASSIK-GERSCHENFELD, J. TEULON,
and O. HARDY

INTRODUCTION

It has been well known for a long time that birds possess a major visual pathway that reaches the telencephalon through the optic tectum (OT) and the nucleus rotundus (Cowan et al., 1961; Karten and Hodos, 1970; Karten and Revzin, 1966). The large size of this system led to the assumption that, in birds, all the visual information passing from the retina to the telencephalon is coded and transmitted by the OT, whose receptive field properties have been studied by many workers (Hughes and Pearlman, 1974; Jassik-Gerschenfeld and Guichard, 1972; Jassik-Gerschenfeld et al., 1970). Recently, however, another well-organized visual path which connects the retina to the nucleus dorsolateralis anterior (DLA) of the contralateral thalamus and goes from there to the hyperstriatum of the telencephalon has been traced in birds (Cowan et al., 1961; Hunt and Webster, 1972; Karten et al., 1973; Karten and Nauta, 1968; Meier et al., 1974; Repérant et al., 1974). This second visual path has been thought to be similar to the retinogeniculocortical

D. JASSIK-GERSCHENFELD, J. TEULON, and O. HARDY • Laboratoire de Psychophysiologie Sensorielle, Université Pierre et Marie Curie, 75230 Paris Cédex 05, France. This study was supported by CNRS Grant ERA No. 333 and by INSERM Grant No. 76.1.042.6.

path of mammals; thus the DLA may be considered homologous to the lateral geniculate body. The visual properties of the receptive fields in the hyperstriatum have been analyzed in the pigeon (O'Flaherty and Invernizzi, 1971; Revzin, 1969) and in the owl (Pettigrew and Konishi, 1976), and some of their functional characteristics resemble those of the mammalian visual cortex.

In a recent paper, we analyzed the visual properties of DLA receptive fields in pigeons (Jassik-Gerschenfeld et al., 1976), compared them with our previous results in OT (Jassik-Gerschenfeld and Guichard, 1972, Jassik-Gerschenfeld et al., 1970), and showed that the two separate paths from the eye to the telencephalon do not strictly convey the same visual information. In the DLA, 56% of the cells sampled were ON center or OFF center cells (in many of them the activity generated at the field center was inhibited by surround stimulation), 16% of the DLA cells were ON-OFF cells, and 28% responded exclusively to motion. In the OT, we found that 7% of the cells were ON center or OFF center cells, 52% were ON-OFF cells, and 20% responded only to movement. The remaining 21% of the tectal units were directionally selective cells which, like the avian directional retinal ganglion cells (Maturana, 1962; Maturana and Frenk, 1963; Miles, 1972; Pearlman and Hughes, 1976), respond preferentially to one of the directions of motion and do not respond or are inhibited by movement in the opposite direction. Interestingly, we failed to find any directional selective units in the DLA. We feel that this implies that if these types of neurons are present in the DLA they are there in very small numbers, in contrast to the situation in the OT. Furthermore, it is clear from our results that the great majority of ON center and OFF center retinal ganglion cells project to the thalamus. A similar dichotomy of the visual information has been described in the ground squirrel (Michael, 1972, 1973).

It is well known that the properties of the receptive fields of cells in the mammalian visual system vary considerably with the level of the visual system examined. One feature of the visual message which changes at the geniculate level is the center–surround interaction (Hubel and Wiesel, 1961; Jacobs and Yolton, 1970; Maffei and Fiorentini, 1972; Singer and Creutzfeldt, 1970; Wiesel and Hubel, 1966). Therefore, the experiments to be reported in this chapter were designed to investigate the ON center and OFF center cells of the pigeon DLA from two points of view: (1) the modification of the center discharge by inclusion of the surround area and (2) the spatial distribution of both the center and the surround regions in the field. We found evidence suggesting that visual information is greatly modified at the pigeon's thalamic relay, the DLA.

METHODS

All experiments were performed in adult Red Carneaux pigeons. Under local anesthesia (xylocaine), the trachea and a wing vein were cannulated for artificial respiration by unidirectional airflow and continuous intravenous infusion of Flaxedil (14 mg/ml; 0.95 ml/hr) for immobilization. Particular care was taken to block conduction of nociceptive impulses by using local anesthetics at all pressure points and incisions. The body temperature was maintained at 41–42°C using an electric heating pad. The pigeon was placed in a head holder providing standard head fixation for stereotaxic manipulation. The right side of the telencephalic portion of the skull and the dura were removed and the telencephalon was exposed. The eyelid and the nictitating membrane of the left eye were removed. A contact lens protected the cornea and focused the eye for a distance of 0.5 m. The animals viewed a translucent spherical screen (∅ 1 m). The location of the area centralis was found by indirect ophthalmoscopy and projected onto the screen.

Stimulation

Two tungsten-filament projectors were used to explore the receptive fields. Light pulses were obtained by an electronic shutter placed in the light beam. Visual stimuli were projected onto the back of a spherical projection screen. The second beam was added to provide a spot together with a concentric annulus. Their intensities could be varied independently. The spots were superimposed on a background luminance of 6 cd/m². Stimuli luminances were 60–80 cd/m².

Recordings

Extracellular action potentials were recorded with glass micropipettes with resistances of about 20 MΩ. The microelectrodes were filled with a solution of methyl blue in 1 M potassium acetate. At some stage in each penetration, two or more marks were made by passing anodic current through the microelectrode (3 μA for 3 min) (Thomas and Wilson, 1966). One of the marks was always placed at the end of the penetration. The micropipettes were placed in the dorsolateral thalamus according to the coordinates given by Karten and Hodos (1967): anterior 7.5–6.25, lateral 2.0–3.5. In the course of an experiment, the electrode was slowly advanced and the retina was continuously stimulated by moving patterns or flashes of light. The number of units studied in a single penetration was thus not limited to spontaneously active elements. The action potentials were led through a cathode follower and preamplifier to a cathode-ray oscilloscope and loudspeaker. The records were stored on tape and later photographed if necessary. Poststimulus-time histograms (PSTH) of the responses to 20 stimuli were obtained from a small computer (Didac 4000, Intertechnique); such histograms give the time density of impulses (ordinate) as a function of the time after stimulus onset (abscissa). The bin width for PSTH was 20 msec. To avoid the cumulative effects of stimulation, a delay of 4–10 sec was used between successive stimuli.

Histological Localization of Recording Sites

At the end of each experiment, the brain was removed from the skull, serially sectioned in the frontal plane, and stained with fuchsin. The sections containing the marks were used to reconstruct the electrode tracks and identify the recording sites. Estimates of brain shrinkage during fixation were made by measuring the distance between two marks in a section and comparing it with the distance calculated from the depths at which the two marks were made. The positions of different cells along the electrode track were then determined by taking the micrometer depth readings corresponding to each unit in the track and calculating the distance to these points from one or more marks made in the penetration.

RESULTS

The present study concerns the receptive fields of 80 units which were shown by histological reconstruction to be in the DLA. The quantitative analysis, however, was limited to the 34 ON center and 9 OFF center cells, which were held for a sufficiently long time to complete the study (at least 2 hr and as long as 5 hr). During this time, there were no changes in receptive field characteristics. Twenty-three cells were sustainedlike and 20 cells transientlike as characterized, respectively, by their continuous or phasic responses to a spot of light. The receptive field of each cell was determined by a light spot located at various positions along two meridians of the field. The type of response to light onset or offset was judged by listening to a loudspeaker and checked by recording poststimulus-time histograms (PSTHs) for some of the most critical positions of the stimulus. Afterward, the center-surround interaction was studied by (1) simultaneous stimulation of the center and surround at threshold and suprathreshold intensities,

(2) isolated stimulation of the surround, and (3) mapping of the receptive fields with a small static spot of light.

SIMULTANEOUS STIMULATION OF THE CENTER AND THE SURROUND

Threshold Intensity

Area sensitivity curves were obtained by plotting the logarithmic sensitivity of a unit (logarithm of the reciprocal of the threshold intensity for a criterion response) as a function of the size of the stimulus. With increases in spot size, the sensitivity usually increased, indicating summation. When the stimulus became so large that it included the surround as well as the center, the sensitivity of the center-type response decreased as more of the periphery was included. Figure 1 gives a representative sample of three ON cells, which represent three different classes of interaction between the center and the surround.

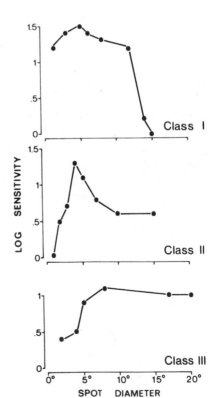

Fig. 1. Changes in sensitivity of center responses with area of illumination. Three different classes of center-surround interaction, measured for three ON cells, are presented (see text).

For the class I cell, there was a summation of the center response up to 5 deg, i.e., its center area was about 5 deg in diameter. For the class II cell, the center response summed over 4 deg, while for the class III unit the size was about 8 deg in diameter. Since the spot sizes were varied in rather coarse steps, these results may not accurately reflect the sizes of the receptive field areas, although it is clear that the center areas must be quite different in size. The antagonistic influence of the periphery of the receptive field on the center can also be seen in Fig. 1. There was a rise in the threshold of the center responses as more of the surround was included in the area of illumination. The amount of this peripheral suppression of the center response varied from one cell to another. In the class I cell, the difference in sensitivity for a spot of 5 deg in diameter, illuminating only the center, and a 15 deg spot, covering the whole receptive field, was about 1.5 log units. Cells with a surround effect this strong were not frequently found. Class II cells showed less peripheral suppression, and class III cells with the largest center showed only a small difference in sensitivity between the center and whole-field illumination.

Suprathreshold Intensity Stimulation

Another indication of center–surround interaction can be obtained from suprathreshold stimulation (1.0–1.5 logarithmic units above threshold) by comparing the amplitude of the response produced by a spot stimulus which covers only the center region to a stimulus that covers the whole receptive field. As before, the cells can be divided into three different classes according to the degree of peripheral suppression. Illustrations of such comparisons appear in Fig. 2, where PSTHs are shown for three ON center cells representing the three classes of interactions. In each case, the responses of the unit to a centered spot (CT) and to a stimulus covering the entire receptive field (WF) are compared. For the class I cell depicted there, the stimulation of the entire field produced a decrease in firing rate to the spontaneous level. In the class II unit, stimulation of the entire field substantially diminished the response. The class III cell showed a small reduction in amplitude between the stimulation of the center and of the entire field. Within our sample, we found five class I cells, 20 class II cells, and 18 class III cells.

So far, in describing our results, we have considered only the action of the surround on the center-type discharge, i.e., the amount of reduction of the ON response for ON center units and of the OFF discharge for OFF center units. However, some of the cells are apparently heavily balanced in favor of the surround and yield a surround-

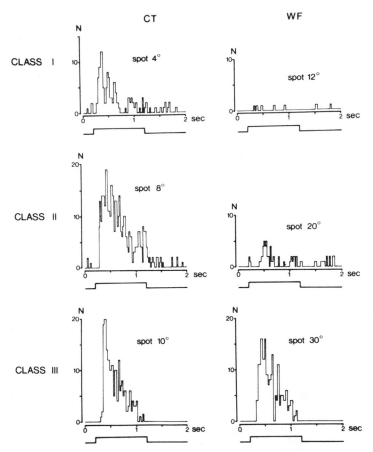

Fig. 2. Three classes of center–surround interaction to suprathreshold stimulation for three different cells. In this and following figures, responses were to stimuli flashed on for 1 sec (each PSTH is the collected output of 20 sweeps). Bin width is 20 msec. Abscissa shows time in seconds; ordinate shows the number of spikes. At the bottom of each PSTH, the upward deflection of the trace signals the onset of light. CT, Center stimulation; WF, whole-field stimulation. Class I cells give no responses to whole field stimulation, class II cells give weak responses, and class III cells give responses to whole-field stimulation almost as large as that obtained by center stimulation.

type response to whole-field stimulation. That is to say, in an ON center unit an OFF discharge might develop as the periphery of the field is invaded, and vice versa for OFF center cells. Figure 3 gives examples of cells of classes I, II, and III which develop surround-type responses to whole-field stimulation. As in Fig. 2, the responses in Fig. 3 of each unit to a centered spot (CT) and to a stimulus covering the whole field (WF) are compared. Class I and class III cells are ON center cells; class

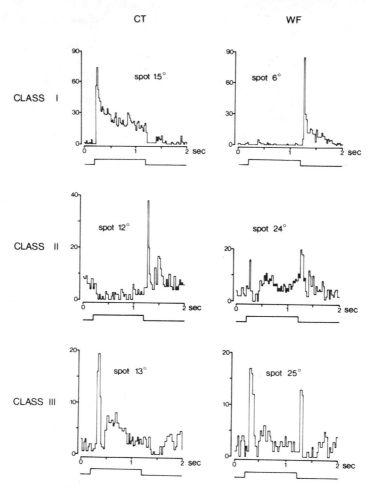

Fig. 3. Surround responses obtained by suprathreshold whole-field (WF) stimulation. Whole-field stimulation of class I cells elicits a response to the offset of light. In class II and class III cells, ON-OFF responses were obtained by whole-field stimulation.

II is an OFF center cell. For the class I unit shown in Fig. 3, the onset of the whole-field illumination produces a decrease of firing to spontaneous levels and a high-frequency burst to the offset of light. For the class II and III cells, whole-field stimulation evokes an ON-OFF response. This mixed response might be the result of a combined contribution from the center and the surround of the receptive field. We have detected surround-type responses to whole-field stimulation in two out of five class I, nine out of 20 class II, and seven out of 18 class III units. Therefore, it is evident that most of the responses elicited under full-

field stimulation are ON-OFF mixed responses. Relatively few cells be-
haved in a fashion to show purely antagonistic reponses.

SURROUND STIMULATION

If no surround response could be obtained by whole-field stimulation, the procedure was then to apply a flashing annulus confined to
the periphery of the field. This procedure was effective in driving the
surround in 8 cells out of 25 analyzed. In Fig. 4, the responses of an
OFF center cell to center (CT), whole-field (WF), and annulus stimulation (AN) are compared. The OFF discharges of the cell to center and
to whole-field stimulation are quite similar (class III cell); on the other
hand, the onset of the 20-deg spot does not evoke a clear surround-
type response. However, flashing an annulus in the periphery of the
field provokes a response to both the onset and offset of light.

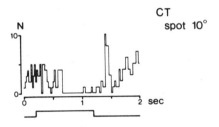

CT
spot 10°

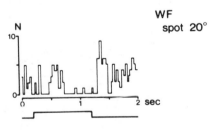

WF
spot 20°

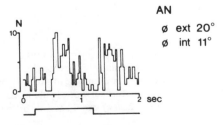

AN
Ø ext 20°
Ø int 11°

Fig. 4. Responses from an off center cell
obtained by center (CT), whole-field (WF),
and annulus stimulation (AN). The center
field was stimulated by a 10-deg spot and
the entire field by a 20-deg spot. Annulus
inner diameter (Ø int) was 11 deg; annulus
outer diameter (Ø ext) was 20 deg. There is
a slight reduction in the OFF activation to
WF stimulation as compared to that obtained by CT stimulation. Surround stimulation by annulus evokes ON-OFF responses.

In six units, the surround response could be demonstrated only by indirect ways as, for example, by first illuminating the center and then using a flashing annulus to drive the surround discharge. Figure 5 shows an example for a class II ON center cell. Center stimulation (CT) by a 3-deg spot provokes a response to the onset of light; after a burst, the firing remains significantly higher than the spontaneous activity. Both the burst and the sustained activity are decreased by whole-field stimulation (WF). Flashing an annulus in the surround is without effect (AN). If the annulus is presented in conjunction with a central steady spot which evokes a high level of spike activity, there is tonic inhibition at the onset of the annulus followed by a slight excitation at the offset. This technique was not effective for the remaining 11 units studied. Since we did not try to change the size or the intensity of the adapting

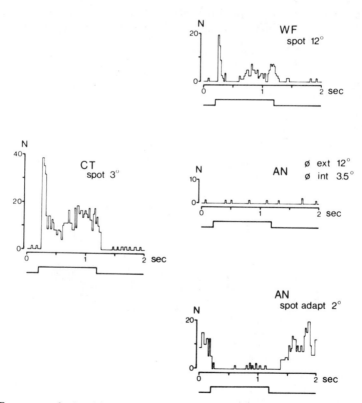

Fig. 5. Responses obtained from an ON center cell by flashing an annulus on the surround during continuous illumination of the center. An annulus of 3.5 deg inner diameter (∅ int) and 12 deg outer diameter (∅ ext) does not drive the surround response. Flashing the same annulus in the surround during continuous illumination of the center (annulus spot adaptation 2 deg) provokes inhibition to light onset and excitation to light offset.

spot, the existence of a surround response cannot be absolutely excluded.

The results of the foregoing experiments indicate that the proportion of cells which yield a surround response increases when the appropriate stimulus is applied. Furthermore, similar to the results of whole-field stimulation, most of the cells give ON-OFF responses to isolated stimulation of the surround of the field.

MAPPING OF THE CENTER AND THE SURROUND OF THE RECEPTIVE FIELD WITH STATIONARY SPOTS OF LIGHT

This series of experiments was performed to analyze the distribution of the center and the surround responses in the receptive fields. Fourteen cells were analyzed in the following way. For each cell, we first tried to find the smallest stimulus able to evoke a detectable response at suprathreshold intensity. Afterward, the field was mapped with the selected spot in the horizontal and vertica directions; PSTHs were recorded for each position. All but two of the receptive fields analyzed have almost concentrically organized center and surround regions.

Concentrically Organized Fields

The PSTHs in Fig. 6 show the responses of an OFF center cell to small light stimuli within and at variable distances from the receptive field center. PSTHs 1 and 2 are responses obtained from the center region. When the light was turned on, there was a partial suppression of the maintained activity; when the light was turned off, there was a sharp rise in firing followed by a slow decay to a maintained firing level. At stimulus positions 3 and 4, the OFF activation was reduced and a small response appeared to the onset of light (PSTHs 3 and 4). Locating the stimulating spot farther away from the center produced an increase in the amplitude of the ON discharge and a further decrease of the OFF discharge (PSTHs 5 and 6). Near the outer limit of the field, both responses almost disappeared (PSTH 7). Thus this cell has a field composed of an OFF center region surrounded by a broad area giving ON-OFF responses.

The variations in amplitude along the whole horizontal diameter of the field of the cell are shown in Fig. 7. The measure of amplitude used is the number of spikes of the unit during the first 100 msec after

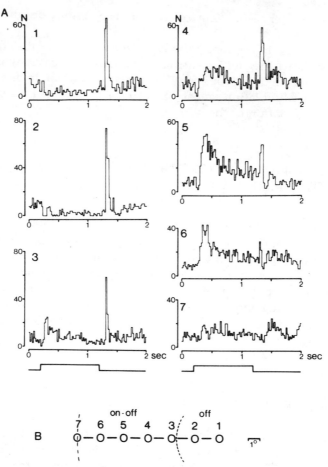

Fig. 6. A: Responses of an OFF center neuron with a concentric field to stimuli in different parts of its receptive field. Stimuli have 0.5 deg diameters. The numbers refer to the stimulus map in B at the bottom of the figure. OFF responses were obtained from stimulus positions 1 and 2, which were placed in the center of the field. Stimuli placed in the receptive field surround (PSTHs 3–7) evoke ON-OFF responses. The ON-OFF surround response can be elicited from a wider area than the OFF center response.

the beginning of the response. It is evident from this figure that (1) the amplitude of the OFF discharge is markedly reduced at positions in the field where the ON response increases (see positions 3–5 and 8–9), and (2) the ON discharge is smaller on the right side of the field than on the left side of the field. It is also interesting to note that the receptive field of this cell was radially asymmetrical, with the center region situated away from the geometric center of the field. The response sequence to

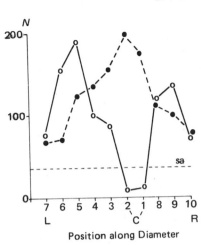

ON   o——o
OFF   ●– –●

Fig. 7. Amplitude of the responses of the same cell as in Fig. 6 to a spot of light (0.5 deg diameter) as a function of the position of the stimulus. Measurements were taken along the whole horizontal diameter of the field. The ordinate shows the number of spikes (N) during a 100-msec period just after the response begins. The numbers on the abscissa refer to the stimulus map shown in Fig. 6B. Positions 1 and 2 correspond to the center (C) of the field. Positions 3–7 and 8–10 correspond, respectively, to the left side (L) and the right side (R) of the surround. Spontaneous activity (sa) = 36 spikes/sec.

spot positions in the field, shown in Figs. 6 and 7, corresponds roughly to the response sequence of most of the concentric fields we studied. However, in two units near the outer limits of the surround region, the center-type response disappeared while the antagonistic surround response could still be evoked.

Figure 8 shows a cell which possessed a more complex receptive field. PSTH 1 represents the ON response obtained by stimulating the center of the field. When the stimulus was located 1 deg from the center, the ON response was followed by an OFF activation (PSTH 2). At a stimulus position 2 deg from the center, the center-type response was greatly reduced (PSTH 3), and it disappeared at position 3 deg (PSTH 4) while the activation to the OFF was still rather significant. Thus the ON center region is surrounded by an ON-OFF region, which in turn is then surrounded by an area of pure OFF responses. However, when the spot is located at positions 4 and 5 deg from the center, a high-amplitude ON response develops again, while the OFF discharge first diminishes and afterward disappears (PSTHs 5–7).

Nonconcentrically Organized Fields

Two cells were included in the category of nonconcentrically organized fields. They had receptive fields that could be subdivided into two parallel regions on the basis of their responses to flashed bars of light. Figure 9 shows PSTHs obtained from one of the cells. The map

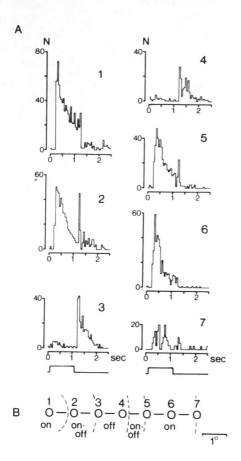

Fig. 8. A: PSTHs from a concentric field with a complex surround. Stimulus diameter 0.7 deg. Numbers on the abscissa refer to the stimulus map in B. PSTH 1 shows the ON response obtained from the center of the field. The surround is formed by four concentric regions that are, from inward to outward: (1) ON-OFF (PSTH 2); (2) OFF (PSTHs 3 and 4); (3) ON-OFF (PSTH 5); (4) ON (PSTHs 6 and 7).

stimuli are shown in Fig. 10B. Flashing a 0.5 × 8 deg bar in the left part of the field evokes an ON discharge that increases in amplitude from position 1 to 4 (PSTHS 1-4). Light offset is without effect in positions 1–3 and evokes a barely detectable activation in position 4. On the right side of the field, the ON response decreases and the OFF discharge markedly increases (PSTHs 5 and 6). At more extreme positions to the right of the field, both discharges decrease continuously and simultaneously (PSTHs 7-9). Thus the receptive field of this cell has an ON region paralleled by an ON-OFF region. The variations in amplitude of the responses along the field are represented in Fig. 10. The measure of amplitude used is the same as that in Fig. 7. It is clear from Fig. 10 that in the right side of the field, simultaneous with the rise of the amplitude of the OFF discharge, a marked decrease in the amplitude of the ON response occurs (see positions 5 and 6).

DISCUSSION

Experimental evidence in avian retinal ganglion neurons (Maturana, 1962; Maturana and Frenk, 1963; Miles, 1972; Pearlman and Hughes, 1976) suggests that the surround region of the receptive field has an inhibitory effect on the center discharge which is not paired by surround firing. However, a more recent work (Holden, 1977) shows that in the pigeon the retinal fields are concentrically organized; i.e.,

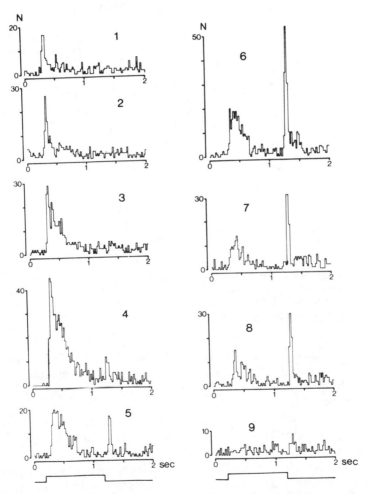

Fig. 9. PSTHs from a nonconcentrically organized field. Stimulus 0.5 × 8 deg bar of light. The numbers refer to stimulus position shown in Fig. 10B. PSTHs 1-3 from the left part of the field show ON responses. The ON activation is maximal at PSTH 4; a small activation is also seen at OFF. PSTHs 5-8 show ON-OFF responses obtained from the left part of the field.

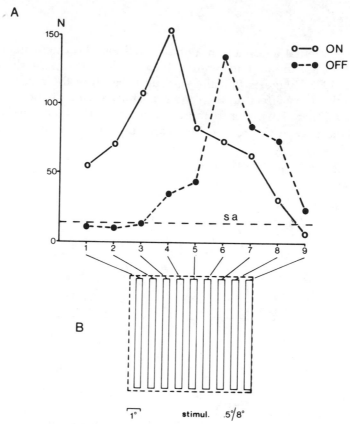

Fig. 10. A: Amplitude of the response of the cell shown in Fig. 9 to a bar of light (0.5 × 8 deg) as a function of stimulus position. On the ordinate is the number of spikes during a 100-msec period just after the response begins. The numbers on the abscissa refer to the stimulus map in B. Spontaneous activity (sa) = about 12 spikes/sec.

an annulus flashed in the surround evokes discharge at offset in ON center cells and at onset in OFF center cells. Similarly, most of the DLA units in the pigeon we have reported here have receptive fields made up of two concentric regions: center and surround. The surround region of the ON center and OFF center DLA neurons has, as does the surround of the pigeon retinal cells, the ability to generate a response when appropriately stimulated. In this regard, the DLA receptive fields are similar to those which have been described in the retina. Nevertheless, it is evident from our results that the majority of the DLA receptive fields differ from ganglion cell receptive fields in a particular way. Indeed, light stimulation of the surround of ganglion cell receptive fields leads to a change in firing rate in the opposite direction to that elicited by center stimulation. In contrast, as we have shown here, most DLA neurons give ON-OFF responses to whole-field or to annular stimulation. Furthermore, stimulation with small spots of light elicits ON-OFF responses in every part of the surround of the majority of the DLA fields. Only in two cells does the surround show a narrow area of responses of opposite sign to those recorded from the center area.

A Scheme for the Elaboration of Surround Responses of DLA Receptive Fields

Our results suggest that considerable modification of the visual message must occur at the DLA level. It is natural to ask what this means in terms of input. At present, we do not have direct evidence on how the DLA transforms the incoming visual information. However, the properties of both the ON center and OFF center DLA cells can be better accounted for by supposing that the afferents to the cells' surround originate from the center of the field of retinal cells situated in the appropriate retinal regions. For example, the cell shown in Fig. 6 gives ON-OFF responses throughout its surround region. One may imagine that the surround is formed by the projection of a group of ON center retinal cells, largely superimposed on the OFF center retinal cells projecting to the center of the DLA field. Such a system would account for the reduction in the amplitude of the center-type response in the surround part of the field that we observed. Another possibility is that the surround receives afferents from a group of ON-OFF center retinal cells. Such a projection system, shown in Fig. 11A, would appear consistent with the observation that most of the ganglion cell receptive fields in the bird retina have ON-OFF centers (Maturana, 1962; Maturana and Frenk, 1963; Miles, 1972; Pearlman and Hughes, 1976). In a similar way, the nonconcentric DLA field shown in Fig. 9 may be constructed by supposing that retinal cells with ON center fields project to the left side of the field and that retinal cells with ON-OFF center fields project to the right side of the field.

The properties of the cell represented in Fig. 8 are not easily accounted for by supposing that ON-OFF center retinal cells project to the surround area. Its field is formed by an ON center region surrounded by a broad area of ON-OFF responses, which is encircled by a region of pure OFF responses. Farther out, there is another region of ON-OFF discharges and an outermost area of ON responses. One may speculate, as is shown in Fig. 11B, that the center of this DLA field is formed by projections from retinal ganglion cells having ON center fields. The innermost part (which gives OFF responses) and the outermost part (which gives ON responses) of the surround might be formed, respectively, by the projection of OFF center and ON center retinal cells. The superposition of both, the ON center and the OFF center retinal fields,

A   B

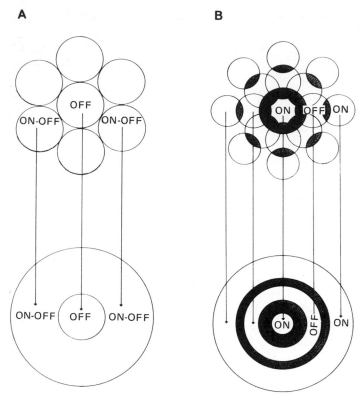

Fig. 11. Retina-DLA connections. In each schema, a DLA receptive field is represented at the bottom of the figure, together with some retinal receptive fields projecting on it at the top. To simplify the schemata, only one center retinal neuron projecting to the center of DLA fields is shown. A: One OFF center retinal neuron projects to the center of the DLA field and six ON-OFF center retinal neurons project to the surround. B: One ON center retinal neuron projects to the center of the DLA field. Eight OFF center retinal neurons project to the surround. The ON and OFF retinal neurons are largely superimposed. Another eight ON center retinal cells project to the outermost region of the surround and overlap with the OFF center retinal cells. The hatched regions show the area of superposition of ON center and OFF center retinal fields and the ON-OFF region on the DLA receptive field.

might account for the two ON-OFF areas of the surround. A further possibility is that both ON-OFF regions are made up by the superposition of the surrounds of the ON center and the OFF center retinal cells.

These propositions are obviously tentative and should not be interpreted literally. However, it does seem probable, regardless of the details of the process, that the surround of the DLA receptive fields is built up from the centers of retinal receptive fields. A similar model has been proposed for the cat lateral geniculate fields (Hubel and Wiesel, 1961; Maffei and Fiorentini, 1972; Singer and Creutzfeldt, 1970).

Functional Implication

The thalamic relay of the retina–hyperstriatum pathway in birds, the DLA, is thought to be homologous to the lateral geniculate body of mammals (Karten et al., 1973; Karten and Nauta, 1968). Therefore, it is interesting to compare our present results in the DLA with those obtained by other authors on geniculate fields. Following the work of Hubel and Wiesel (1961), other investigators (Maffei and Fiorentini, 1972; Singer and Creutzfeldt, 1970) have provided evidence that the surround of the cat lateral geniculate receptive fields is more powerful in antagonizing the center response than the surround of the ganglion cells. Within this line of thought, it seems worthwhile to ask what our results imply in terms of function. That is, is there an increase in the strength of the surround in DLA receptive fields? If, as we have proposed above, retinal centers project onto DLA surrounds, the surrounds of both peripheral and central neurons should be largely superimposed. Thus the peripheral surrounds should reduce the inhibitory effects arising from the surrounds of the central neurons. At first glance, our results show that this interpretation might apply at least to some of the DLA fields. In fact, we have found that, in spite of the great variation in spatial antagonism between center and surround observed in the DLA cells, a large number yield responses to whole-field stimulation that are nearly as large as those elicited by stimuli confined to the center region. There is not a direct correlation between the ease of generating a surround response and the degree to which stimulation of the surround decreases the response from the center. These results, however, are not conclusive. To answer the question, a more systematic investigation of center and surround interactions at the pigeon retinal level would be highly desirable.

REFERENCES

Cowan, W. M., Adamson, L., and Powell, T. P. S.: An experimental study of the avian visual system. *J. Anat.* **95:**545–563 (1961).

Holden, A. L.: Concentric receptive fields of pigeon ganglion cells. *Vision Res.* **17:**545–554 (1977).

Hubel, D. H., and Wiesel, T. N.: Integrative activity in the cat's lateral geniculate body. *J. Physiol. (London)* **155:**385–398 (1961).

Hughes, C. P., and Pearlman, A. L.: Single unit receptive fields and the cellular layers of the pigeon optic tectum. *Brain Res.* **80:**365–377 (1974).

Hunt, S. P., and Webster, K. E.: Thalamo-hyperstriate interrelations in the pigeon. *Brain Res.* **44:**647–651 (1972).

Jacobs, G. H., and Yolton, R. L.: Center-surround balance in receptive fields of cells in the lateral geniculate nucleus. *Vision Res.* **10:**1127–1144 (1970).

Jassik-Gerschenfeld, D., and Guichard, J.: Visual receptive fields of single cells in the pigeon's optic tectum. *Brain Res.* **40**:303–317 (1972).

Jassik-Gerschenfeld, D., Minois, F., and Conde-Courtine, F.: Receptive field properties of directionally selective units in the pigeon's optic tectum. *Brain Res.* **24**:407–421 (1970).

Jassik-Gerschenfeld, D., Teulon, J., and Ropert, N.: Visual receptive field types in the nucleus dorsolateralis anterior of the pigeon's thalamus. *Brain Res.* **108**:295–306 (1976).

Karten, H. J., and Hodos, W.: *A Stereotaxic Atlas of the Brain of the Pigeon (Columba livia).* Johns Hopkins Press, Baltimore (1967).

Karten, H. J., and Hodos, W.: Telencephalic projections of the nucleus rotundus in the pigeon *(Columba livia). J. Comp. Neurol.* **140**:35–52 (1970).

Karten, H. J., and Nauta, W. J. H.: Organization of the retino-thalamic projections in the pigeon and owl. *Anat. Rec.* **160**:373, Abstr. (1968).

Karten, H. J., and Revzin, A. M.: The afferent connections of the nucleus rotundus in the pigeon. *Brain Res.* **2**:368–377 (1966).

Karten, H. J., Hodos, W., Nauta, W. J. H., and Revzin, A. M.: Neural connections of the "visual Wulst" of the avian telencephalon. Experimental studies in the pigeon *(Columba livia)* and owl *(Speotyto cunicularia). J. Comp. Neurol.* **150**:253–278 (1973).

Maffei, L., and Fiorentini, A.: Retinogeniculate convergence and analysis of contrast. *J. Neurophysiol.* **35**:65–72 (1972).

Maturana, H. R.: Functional organization of the pigeon retina. In *22nd Int. Congr. Physiol. Sci. Leyden* (1962). Pp. 170–178.

Maturana, H. R., and Frenk, S.: Directional movement and horizontal edge detectors in the pigeon retina. *Science* **150**:977–979 (1963).

Meier, R. E., Mihailovic, J., and Cuenod, M.: Thalamic organization of the retino-thalamo-hyperstriatal pathway in the pigeon *(Columba livia). Exp. Brain Res.* **19**:351–364 (1974).

Michael, C. R.: Visual receptive fields of single neurons in superior colliculus of the ground squirrel. *J. Neurophysiol.* **35**:815–832 (1972).

Michael, C. R.: Opponent-color and opponent-contrast cells in lateral geniculate nucleus of the ground squirrel. *J. Neurophysiol.* **36**:536–550 (1973).

Miles, F. A.: Centrifugal control of the avian retina. I. Receptive field properties of retinal ganglion cells. *Brain Res.* **48**:65–92 (1972).

O'Flaherty, J. J., and Invernizzi, G.: Organizzazione funzionale dei campi recettivi di singole unita visive del "Wulst" nel piccione. *Boll. Soc. Ital. Biol. Sper.* **48**:137–138 (1971).

Pearlman, A. L., and Hughes, C. P.: Functional role of efferents to the avian retina. I. Analysis of retinal ganglion cell receptive fields. *J. Comp. Neurol.* **166**:111–122 (1976).

Pettigrew, J. D., and Konishi, M: Neurons selective for orientation and binocular disparity in the visual Wulst of the Barn Owl *(Tyto alba). Science* **193**:675–677 (1976).

Repérant, J., Raffin, J. P., and Miceli, D.: La voie retino-thalamo-hyperstriatale chez le Poussin *(Gallus domesticus L). C.R.Acad.Sci.* **279**:279–282 (1974).

Revzin, A. M.: A specific visual projection area in the hyperstriatum of the pigeon *(Columba livia). Brain Res.* **15**:246–249 (1969).

Singer, W., and Creutzfeldt, O.: Reciprocal lateral inhibition of on- and off-center neurones in the lateral geniculate body of the cat. *Exp. Brain Res.* **10**:311–330 (1970).

Thomas, R. C., and Wilson, V. J.: Marking single neurons by staining with intracellular recording microelectrodes. *Science* **151**:1538–1539 (1966).

Wiesel, T. H., and Hubel, D. H.: Spatial and chromatic interactions in the lateral geniculate body of the rhesus monkey. *J. Neurophysiol.* **29**:1115–1156 (1966).

10

Functional Localization in the Nucleus Rotundus

A. M. REVZIN

INTRODUCTION

Recent work of Benowitz and Karten (1976) has shown that the projections from the optic tectum to the nucleus rotundus in the pigeon are spatially organized, with specific regions of layers of the optic tectum projecting to specific, anatomically defined areas of rotundus. The present study, in part a reexamination of previous data, was initiated to see whether regional differences in rotundal functions could be correlated with the anatomical areas defined by Benowitz and Karten (1976).

METHODS

Extracellular unit recordings were taken from rotundal neurons in urethane-anesthetized White Carneaux pigeons (*Columba livia*). Projected spots of light or black cardboard targets were moved against a light-gray tangent screen to elicit visual responses in spontaneously active cells. The tangent screen was mounted vertically, parallel to the parasagittal plane, at a distance of 1.5 m from the pigeon's left eye. Absolute room illumination levels varied but were usually in the low

A. M. REVZIN • Neuropharmacology Research Unit, Aviation Toxicology Laboratory, Civil Aeromedical Institute, Federal Aviation Administration, Oklahoma City, Oklahoma 73125.

photopic range. Although more elaborate data reduction techniques such as poststimulus-time histograms were used, most data were taken as subjective evaluations of the unit firing frequency heard on the audiomonitor (Lettvin et al., 1959; Bishop, 1967). A 5 point intensity scale was used: strong, moderate, and weak excitation, no effect, and inhibition. Recording techniques and equipment and electrode localization procedures were conventional (Karten and Hodos, 1967).

The sampling procedures were such that only spontaneously active neurons or clusters of neurons were selected for detailed study because the general procedure was to advance the electrode until a spontaneously active unit was found and then examine its characteristics. In 20 tracks, we simply advanced the electrodes in 50-μm increments and tested at each point to see if unit activity was evokable. The data suggested that only one in three of the visually driven neurons was spontaneously active. For the most part, the evoked responses of "active" and "quiet" neurons were similar, although it is quite possible that "active" and "quiet" neurons represent functionally distinct populations. More than 600 units or small clusters of units were examined in 62 electrode penetrations. The tracks sampled activity in the rotundus throughout its rostrocaudal and dorsoventral extent. However, some bias was present: the central, lateral, and dorsal areas of the nucleus were sampled more extensively than medial and ventral zones.

For each isolated unit or cluster of units, we determined field size, directional responses for each of a wide range of target configurations, responses to changes in ambient illumination, and responses to stationary diffuse or discrete light flashes.

RESULTS

Qualitative Description of Response Characteristics

Much of this material has previously been reported (Revzin, 1966, 1967, 1970) and what follows is, for the most part, a review and summary. About 80% of the rotundal units had very large visual fields, ranging from 100 deg to 175 deg (Revzin, 1966; Revzin and Karten, 1967). Most of the units with smaller fields were seen in the ventral quarter of the rotundus or as occasional units with large, long-duration spikes mixed with other units in the posterior rotundus (see below).

Figure 1 diagrams the most common types of responses seen in the nucleus rotundus. In each diagram, the length of the vector indicates response magnitude and the direction of the vector indicates the direction of movement of the target on the tangent screen, 0 deg being

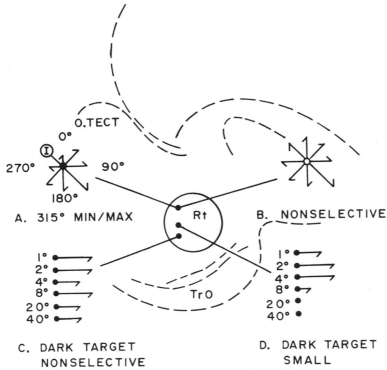

Fig. 1. Some neuron response patterns found in the nucleus rotundus. For each diagram, the length of the arrow represents response magnitude, the direction of the arrow indicates the direction of stimulus movement. A circled I signifies an inhibition of spontaneous activity. The uppermost neuron was interrogated with two stimuli: a small dark cardboard target (A) and a projected spot of light of the same size (B). In A a movement along the 315-deg axis produces an inhibition of ongoing activity, while the opposite movement, in the 135-deg direction, produces a maximum response. This defines a "315-deg min/max" axis for this neuron. However, little directional sensitivity was apparent when this unit was tested with a projected spot of light (B). This unit was also tested with dark targets of various sizes (C). As shown, there is little variation in response correlated with stimulus size. Responses to horizontal (90 deg) movement are shown for simplicity, although this class of cells simply does not discriminate target size, whatever other selectivity characteristics the cell may demonstrate. In D are shown response characteristics of a cell that responds only to relatively small targets. Abbreviations for Figs. 1 and 2: O.Tect., optic tectum; Rt, nucleus rotundus; TrO, optic tract; GLV, lateral geniculate nucleus, pars ventralis.

vertical and 90 deg being anterior. Figure 1A shows the variations in response seen as a target is moved in various directions. Clearly, the maximum response is seen at 135 deg. The circled I at 315 deg indicates that movement in this direction caused an inhibition of spontaneous activity of the neuron. Thus a "315-deg min/max" axis is defined. This pattern was elicited by a 2-deg-diameter, 3-mm-thick, black cardboard target. Such targets were commonly the most "efficient" visual stimuli in that they usually elicited the largest-amplitude and most parametrically selective responses seen in any given rotundal unit. Figure 1B shows the response elicited in the same cell by a projected white spot of light, also of 2 deg diameter. Clearly, the response to the moving light spot is not so directionally selective as the dark-target response. Figure 1C shows amplitudes of the responses of the same neuron to horizontal movements of targets of the indicated sizes. This unit is nonselective for size; that is, the response intensity is independent of target size. The response pattern of Fig. 1D shows a "size-selective" unit, so called because the response intensity is clearly a function of target size.

The smallest targets used subtended 4 min of arc. About 10% of the units tested responded, weakly or moderately, to this stimulus; this response suggests an ultimate angular threshold for this system of less than 2 min of arc. The two most common rotundal response patterns were the combinations of the configurations in Fig. 1A, D (directionally selective for small dark targets) and those in Fig. 1B,C (nonselective for anything but movement).

About 40% of the directionally sensitive cells also show a dead zone in their response pattern; that is, a unit will respond to an appropriate stimulus only if the stimulus moved in a straight line through a distance of more than 2–10 deg of arc. This is not a latency phenomenon because the size of the dead zone is not a function of stimulus velocity, and the simulus may be moved within the dead zone in any manner and for any length of time without affecting the firing of the unit. The diameter of the dead zone was, as indicated, always in the range of 2–10 deg and, for any given unit, of constant size. Surprisingly, dead zones were seen in units selective for large targets as well as in those selective for small stimuli.

The neurons selected for examination in these studies showed little adaptation to repeated presentation of a stimulus. However, about 10% of all rotundal units encountered do show some kind of adaptation phenomena. About a third of these are directionally selective cells requiring priming; that is, after a rest period of more than 5 min during which there is no movement in the visual field, the initial 1–3 sec of stimulation evokes only generalized, nonselective response patterns. The selective reponse patterns develop rapidly after this initial lethargy and remain stable and consistent throughout the remainder of the examination. The other units show complex patterns of adaptation, usually a function of the stimulus parameters, that have not been examined in detail (Revzin, 1970) but are generally similar to those described for tectal units by Woods and Frost (1977).

Although rotundal responses have been categorized to some extent in the preceding paragraphs, these categories are neither complete nor mutually exclusive. Indeed, it seems as if every possible combination of size, directional, and brightness response preferences has been seen. Figure 2 shows some of the various response patterns that can be seen during one electrode penetration. Figure 2A shows a cluster of three units that have the "common" pattern. Figure 2B is similar but the min/max axis is rotated 45 deg; there is no inhibitory response to movement, and there are equal responses to small dark and small light targets. Figure 2C shows a very sharply tuned response to an 8 × 1 deg dark bar. Figure 2D is similar, but the response is only to targets greater than 20 deg, while Fig. 2E is a common variant on the Fig. 1A response. More complex response patterns are also seen. One type, the "left turn" neuron, responds only if something the size and shape of a human stands more than 1 m from the bird and pivots or turns

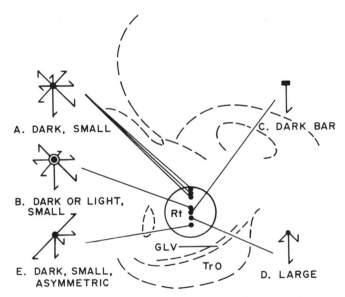

Fig. 2. Typical response patterns seen in the course of single electrode penetration. The first three units in sequence responded only to small dark targets with some directional sensitivity (A). The next unit (B) was similar but with different directional preferences, and it responded to either dark or light spots. Neuron C responded only to a dark bar (8 × 1 deg) moved downward. Cell D responded only to a very large dark target, greater than 30 deg, moving downward. Unit E is similar, again, to A and B.

sharply to the left (five units) or right (two units). These and other equally whimsical cells occur chiefly in the most lateral and anterior part of the rotundus. Furthermore, some of our very first unit studies suggested that excitability as well as size and directional preferences could be affected by substantial changes in ambient illumination (Bisti et al., 1977) or by electrical stimulation in brain stem areas traditionally associated with the "reticular activating system" concept (unpublished observations). Because, say, directional selectivity can also be affected by such things as dark vs. light stimuli (Fig. 1), it is apparent that the response characteristics of rotundal neurons depend, to an uncomfortable extent, on the minutiae of the experimental arrangements.

Regional Distribution of Responses

Perhaps the simplest categorization of rotundal cells is directionally selective vs. not selective. In Fig. 3 we have plotted, for each cell in each of ten tracks, whether it was directionally selective. The two different classes of directionally sensitive cells were plotted because they differ pharmacologically, but they should be considered as one

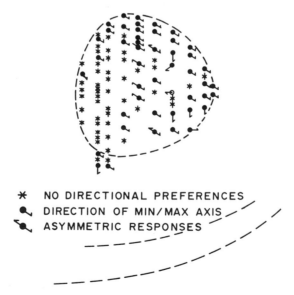

Fig. 3. Visual response patterns seen in ten selected electrode tracks are plotted against a diagram of a sagittal section through the center of the nucleus rotundus. The neurons were classified according to their responses to different directions of stimulus movement as described in Figs. 1 and 2. There is a clear tendency for units without directional selectivity or preferences to cluster in the posterior third of the rotundus.

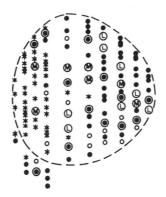

* ANYTHING EXCITES   ◉ LIGHT OR DARK
● SMALL DARK   Ⓜ MIDDLE SIZE
○ SMALL LIGHT SPOT   Ⓛ LARGE

Fig. 4. Responses from another set of ten tracks plotted as before. The responses are categorized according to size preferences (Fig. 1C, D). The units nonselective for size seem to cluster in the posterior third of the rotundus.

group here. Clearly, the cells showing no directional preferences tend to cluster in the posterior third of the nucleus.

There is a good deal of overlap between categories, but the distribution does suggest that the posterior third of the rotundus differs from the remainder. In six tracts in the dorsal anterior rotundus, the min/max axis of successive directionally selective units rotated clockwise as the electrode was advanced along the usual dorsoventral axis. This rotation of response axis, taken together with the "left turn" cells, for example, suggests a high degree of functional localization in the rotundus, although the complexity of the responses, the limited number of test patterns used, and the paucity of data on any given neuron response pattern make verification impossible now.

Rotundal units also differ with respect to the size of their preferred stimulus. In Fig. 4, we have plotted size preferences seen in rotundal units. We used a ten track subset of the total for simplicity but sampled ten tracks different from those used in Fig. 3. Again, as in Fig. 3, the nonselective units, the ones fired by anything moving, tend to be grouped in the posterior third of the rotundus. There is a sampling error here, though. Were all tracks plotted, the separation, although still clear, would not be so sharp as it appears in this figure. In eight tracts, preferred stimulus size increased as the electrode advanced through the dorsal half of the anterior rotundus. This increase suggests, again, that there may be a much higher degree of functional organization within the rotundus than that suggested in Figs. 3 and 4, based, as they are, on quite simple categorizations.

Although posterior rotundal responses have been described in terms of single-unit responses, what occurs is, in fact, rather complex. Spontaneously active single units are fairly easy to isolate in this area, at least in deeply anesthetized animals. In the "posterior rotundus," the probability of finding spontaneously active neurons increases with depth of anesthesia, although the rate for any given unit does not increase with an increase in anesthesia depth. The presence of a moving stimulus induces a characteristic 30–100 Hz rhythmic high-frequency activity in the local EEG and also causes virtually every neuron in the area of the electrode to fire at rates of up to 250 spikes/sec. There is some tendency for the neuron firing to cluster on the positive-going slope of the EEG waves. This evoked multiunit activity usually makes it difficult to discern whether the spontaneously active unit shares its neighbor's excitement over the stimulus, although this is usually the case. This pattern of activity is unique to the posterior rotundus.

There are also pharmacological differences between anterior and posterior rotundal neurons. For example, ethanol inhibits anterior rotundal spontaneous activities at very low doses, while posterior rotundal cells show a complex, dose-dependent inhibitory-exitatory-inhibitory sequence of changes (Revzin, unpublished data). Nonvisual dorsal thalamic neurons are usually inhibited by ethanol, but the threshold doses are 3–5 times those for the rotundal effects. Thus it again appears that the posterior third of the rotundus is not concerned with the same matters as is the rest of the nucleus.

Some rotundal units do respond to nonmoving light flashes (Revzin, 1966, 1970). In Fig. 5, we have plotted the distribution of these. Twenty tracks were plotted, including some of the ones used above. The separation of areas is less clear then above, but it does

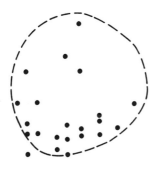

Fig. 5. Responses to single, nonmoving flashes of light, spots or whole field, seldom seen in the rotundus. In this diagram, we have condensed results from 20 electrode tracks. Units responding to flash tend to cluster in the ventral third of the nucleus.

appear that the probability of finding a flash response increases sharply as the microelectrode reaches the ventral quarter of the rotundus.

The preceding data suggest that the nucleus rotundus is divided into at least three parts. The neurons in the posterior one-third of the nucleus seem to respond to anything that moves. The anterior two-thirds contain cells that respond best to certain abstract characteristics of the stimulus. A less certainly differentiable ventral quarter seems more concerned with luminance-related phenomena than do the other areas. These cells also tend to have smaller fields than do those located more dorsally, and they usually respond only to small stimuli. These subareas of the rotundus, functionally differentiated, resemble the parcellation of the rotundus proposed by Benowitz and Karten (1976), which was based on patterns of connections determined anatomically. Our posterior and ventral areas correspond roughly to their posterior and ventral subdivisions, while our anterior area is roughly equal to their anteromedial plus dorsal anterior plus medial subdivisions. This rough correspondence between anatomical and physiological data reinforces the idea that the rotundus is subdivided into functionally distinct subareas.

DISCUSSION

As we have seen, the available data suggest that the nucleus rotundus is functionally differentiated. Neurons in the posterior rotundus tend to respond to any image movement on the retina, whereas anterior rotundal responses tend to be selective for such abstract qualities of the moving stimulus as size, direction, contrast, and velocity. Ventral rotundal responses are similar to anterior response patterns, but these cells seem more concerned about brightness than the others. These are broad, even crude, distinctions. There is evidence that suggests far more precise and complex localizations. In some penetrations, a series of "315-deg min/max" units would be followed by a series of units that are not directionally selective but, say, size selective. Further, in some penetrations a systematic variation in size or directional selectivity of the units was seen as the micropipette moved ventrally. Lastly, Benowitz and Karten (1976) reported an anatomical parcellation that was rather more complex than the functional parcellations seen here.

The characteristic response properties of rotundal units seem to be determined in the tectum (Cotter, 1976; Hughes and Pearlman, 1974; Jassik-Gerschenfeld and Guichard, 1972; Jassik-Gerschenfeld et al., 1970; Pearlman and Hughes, 1976; Revzin, 1970) or retina (Pearlman and Hughes, 1976). This determination, taken together with the functional localization discussed above and the characteristic wide visual field of rotundal neurons (De Britto et al., 1975; Revzin, 1970), suggests that the responses of all tectal neurons having some unique set of response properties are summed and sent to a specific and unique subarea of the rotundus. That is, localization in the tectum is a function of the spatial localization of the stimulus; in the rotundus, it is a function of the responses to some set of abstractions about the stimulus.

A good deal of recent research in mammalian visual function has suggested that form perception depends on a kind of parallel processing (Dow, 1976) in which the identification of the stimulus depends on an integration of the outputs of numbers of neurons or neuronal systems, each responding to a different subset of abstract stimulus qualities (Sprague et al., 1977). In the rotundus, each subset of neurons seems to respond preferentially in the presence of some defined set of stimulus qualities; that is, the firing of any given group of rotundal neurons signifies that a stimulus of defined properties exists somewhere in the visual field. This information is relayed to the ectostriatal "core" (Karten and Hodos, 1970), where the response patterns are very similar to those in the rotundus (Kimberly et al., 1971). This ectostriatal core, in turn, projects to the ectostriatal "belt," as does the hyperstriatal visual area, the functional homologue, perhaps, of the striatal cortex (Karten and Hodos, 1970). Thus the major area of integration of information from two major avian visual projection pathways may be the ectostriatal belt, which thus may also be a major center controlling form and motion perception in the bird.

REFERENCES

Benowitz, L. I., and Karten, H. J.: Organization of the tectofugal visual pathway in the pigeon. *J. Comp. Neurol.* **167**:503–520 (1976).

Bishop, P. O.: Central nervous system: Afferent mechanisms and perception. *Annu. Rev. Physiol.* **29**:427–484 (1967).

Bisti, S., Clement, R., Maffei, L., and Mecacci, L.: Spatial frequency and orientation tuning curves of visual neurones in the cat: Effects of mean luminance. *Exp. Brain Res.* **27**:335–345 (1977).

Cotter, J. R.: Visual and nonvisual units recorded from the optic tectum of *Gallus domesticus. Brain Behav. Evol.* **13**:1–21 (1976).

De Britto, L. R. G., Brunelli, M., Francesconi, W., and Magni, F.: Visual response pattern of thalamic neurons in the pigeon. *Brain Res.* **97**:337–343 (1975).

Dow, B. M.: Central mechanisms of vision: Parallel processing. *Fed. Proc.* **35(1)**:54–59 (1976).

Hughes, C. P., and Pearlman, A. L.: Single unit receptive fields and the cellular layers of the pigeon optic tectum. *Brain Res.* **80**:365–377 (1974).

Jassik-Gerschenfeld, D., and Guichard, J.: Visual receptive fields of single cells in the pigeon's optic tectum. *Brain Res.* **40**:303–317 (1972).

Jassik-Gerschenfeld, D., Minois, F., and Conde-Courtine, F.: Receptive field properties of directionally selective units in the pigeon's optic tectum. *Brain Res.* **24**:407–421 (1970).

Karten, H. J., and Hodos, W.: *A Stereotactic Atlas of the Brain of the Pigeon (Columba livia)*. Johns Hopkins University Press, Baltimore (1967).

Karten, H. J., and Hodos, W.: Telencephalic projections of the nucleus rotundus in the pigeon (*Columba livia*). *J. Comp. Neurol.* **140**:35–52 (1970).

Kimberly, R. P., Holden, A. L., and Bamborough, P.: Response characteristics of pigeon forebrain cells to visual stimulation. *Vision Res.* **11**:475–478 (1971).

Lettvin, J. Y., Maturana, H. R., McCulloch, W. S., and Pitts, W. H.: What the frog's eye tells the frog's brain. *Proc. IRE* **47**:1940–1951 (1959).

Pearlman, A. L., and Hughes, C. P.: Functional role of efferents to the avian retina. I. *J. Comp. Neurol.* **166**:111–122 (1976).

Revzin, A. M.: Flash evoked unit response patterns in the diencephalon of the pigeon. *Fed. Proc.* **25(1)**:395 (1966).

Revzin, A. M.: Unit responses to visual stimuli in the nucleus rotundus of the pigeon. *Fed. Proc.* **26**:2238 (1967).

Revzin, A. M.: Some characteristics of wide-field units in the brain of the pigeon. *Brain Behav. Evol.* **3**:195–204 (1970).

Revzin, A. M., and Karten, H. J.: Rostral projections of the optic tectum and the nucleus rotundus in the pigeon. *Brain Res.* **3**:264–276 (1967).

Sprague, J. M., Levy, J., Di Berardino, A., and Berlucchi, G.: Visual cortical areas mediating form discrimination in the cat. *J. Comp. Neurol.* **172**:441–488 (1977).

Woods, E. J., and Frost, B. J.: Adaptation and habituation characteristics of tectal neurons in the pigeon. *Exp. Brain Res.* **27**:347–354 (1977).

11

Receptive Fields of Movement-Sensitive Cells in the Pigeon Thalamus

J. H. MAXWELL and A. M. GRANDA

INTRODUCTION

Pigeons have adapted to an environmental niche that requires visually controlled behavior as diverse as swiftly executed flying maneuvers and the detection of minute particles of food. Because they depend on vision as a primary source of sensory information, their visual system has been studied extensively. The anatomy is known in some detail: the synaptically complex retina (Yazulla, 1974) transmits visual information to well-developed central visual structures (Karten et al., 1973) over pathways constructed parallel to the mammalian plan (Webster, 1974). Behaviorally, the pigeon's ability to discriminate wavelengths (Wright, 1972) and its visual acuity (Hodos et al., 1976) are well documented. Less well understood than either anatomy or behavior is the physiology of the pigeon visual system.

Visual information to forebrain structures flows along two main routes. The tectofugal pathway can be traced from the retina to the optic tectum, OT; from OT to the nucleus rotundus of the thalamus, Rt; from Rt to the ectostriatum (Benowitz and Karten, 1976). The thalamofugal pathway projects to the hyperstriatum by way of the dorsal

J. H. MAXWELL and A. M. GRANDA • Institute for Neuroscience and Behavior, University of Delaware, Newark, Delaware 19711. This work was supported by Grant No. 01540 from the National Eye Institute, National Institutes of Health.

thalamic nuclear complex (Karten et al., 1973). The thalamus, then, provides an opportunity to compare the functioning of the two pathways since they lie in close proximity there.

Cells isolated in Rt are generally responsive to moving stimuli over large receptive fields, RFs (Revzin, 1967, 1970, this volume). Dorsal thalamic units also respond to moving stimuli but over much smaller RFs (De Britto et al., 1975; Jassik-Gerschenfeld et al., this volume). Contradictions exist concerning the directional selectivity of cells in the two regions. Jassik-Gerschenfeld et al. (1976) found no directionally selective units in the dorsal thalamus, while such cells were observed by Revzin in Rt. De Britto et al. reported opposite results for both regions. In terms of color processing, even fewer comparative data are available. Granda and Yazulla (1971) and Yazulla and Granda (1973) reported the action spectra for units in both the dorsal thalamic area and Rt. Units in both areas displayed narrow-band spectral sensitivities indicative of input from single receptor types: either rods with sensitivity peaks near 500 nm or cones with multiple peaks near 540 nm and 600–620 nm. Opponent-color units were observed only in Rt. The anatomical distribution of unit types in Rt was uneven, with the ventral portion favoring the existence of opponent cells.

The experiments reported here were designed to examine the RF properties of units in both the dorsal thalamus and Rt in order to determine the functional differences between the two major visual pathways.

METHODS

Subjects

The experiments were conducted on mature White Carneaux pigeons (*Columba livia*) obtained from the Palmetto Pigeon Plant, Sumter, South Carolina. The subjects ranged in weight from 400 to 500 g and were of undetermined age and sex.

Surgery

Each pigeon was anesthetized with methoxyflurane and an endotracheal cannula was inserted with the aid of local anesthetics. The bird was cradled in a rigid styrofoam holder for insulation and support and placed in a stereotaxic head holder (Lab-Tronics, Inc., Chicago, IL) that afforded a clear field of view for the left eye. The head was oriented in the same stereotaxic plane employed by Karten and Hodos

(1967). An opening was made in the skull and dura overlying the right posteromedial portion of the cerebrum and the exposed brain surface was protected with a warmed agar–saline solution. The eyelids of the left eye were sutured open and a protective drop of methylcellulose (Isopto Tears, Alcon Laboratories, Fort Worth, TX) was applied to the cornea. Following the initial preparation, general anesthesia was discontinued and paralysis was initiated with an injection of Flaxedil (20 mg/kg body weight) and tubocurarine chloride (5 mg/kg body weight) in normal saline into the right pectoralis muscle. The pigeon was respirated using a one-way air flow technique. Air from a small animal respirator (Phipps and Bird, Inc., Richmond, VA) flowed to the lungs through the endotracheal cannula and the expirate escaped from the left sacral air sac through a hole drilled in the synsacrum. The bird was maintained in good condition for 12–15 hr.

Stimulus System

In the stereotaxic head holder, the pigeon was held with its left eye at the center of a 1-m-radius hemispherical screen, the surface of which was painted flat white. Light for the optical system was provided by a 450-W xenon arc lamp (Osram, Berlin, West Germany). Two optical channels were used, one for a stimulus disk and one for background illumination. In both channels, intensity was controlled by Kodak Wratten neutral density filters. In the stimulus channel, wavelength was controlled by a 0.25-m Ebert monochromator (Jarrell-Ash, Waltham, MA) whose entrance and exit ports were selected to provide a bandwidth down 3 dB, 5.1 nm either side of the nominal wavelength. Wavelength in the background channel was controlled by Kodak Wratten color filters. The unattenuated white stimulus disk measured 3.0×10^{-5} W/cm^2/ster. The chromatic stimulus disks were equated at a maximum of 1.9×10^{12} quanta/sec/cm^2/ster. The unattenuated white background measured 1.17×10^{-7} W/cm^2/ster, and the chromatic backgrounds were equated for maximum energy at 2.4×10^{-8} W/cm^2/ster.

Scanning System

Receptive fields (RFs) were mapped using an automated scanning system. The stimulus used to map the RFs consisted of a 1-deg disk of light projected onto the hemispherical surface. Light for the stimulus disk was projected off a circular first-surface mirror driven on two axes by powerful, single-turn, d.c. motors governed by a servocontrol mechanism (Behavior Technics, Lemont, PA). The control mechanism could be operated in a free-run mode where the stimulus disk's position on the screen was controlled by a joystick or in an automatic scanning mode in which the stimulus disk traced a horizontal or vertical raster pattern. For each RF map, the disk made 60 sweeps (30 in one direction and 30 in the return direction), with equally spaced steps between sweeps. Each sweep was 90 deg in length and each step was 1.5 deg, so that an area 90 × 90 deg was mapped. Smaller maps of 45 × 45 deg could also be produced. A delay of 2.5 sec, where the stimulus was motionless, occurred between sweeps. Stimulus velocity could be controlled between the limits of 0.5 and 1000 deg/sec. Outputs from the control mechanism allowed the position of the stimulus disk to be monitored by a PDP-12 computer.

Recording System

Extracellular recordings were made with stainless steel microelectrodes. The microelectrodes were etched electrolytically to tip diameters of 1–2 μm. The electrodes were double insulated with Insl-x (Insl-x Products Corp., Yonkers, NY) and had resistances at 1000 Hz ranging from 10 to 40 MΩ.

The output of the microelectrode, measured with respect to an indifferent platinum electrode inserted into a neck muscle, was led to a Bak electrometer (Electronics for Life Sciences, Rockville, MD) and then to a Tektronix 122 preamplifier (Tektronix, Inc., Beaverton, OR) set at a bandpass of 80 Hz to 10 kHz. The signal, amplified a thousandfold, was sent to a window discriminator (R. Adler, Department of Electrical Engineering, University of Delaware) with a parallel signal going to an audiomonitor (Grass Instruments, Quincy, MA). The output of the window discriminator was monitored by a 502 Tektronix oscilloscope and the PDP-12 computer.

Mapping Procedure

The search for visual cells along the electrode track began at the most dorsal aspect of the thalamus and continued downward to the most ventral portion of Rt. Micrometer settings on the microelectrode drive were recorded for each isolated unit. After a visual thalamic unit was isolated and its RF located by moving the stimulus disk around with the joystick, the RF was mapped by scanning it automatically. The computer simultaneously monitored the disk's position and the cell's electrical activity. When an action potential occurred, the computer stored the current position of the disk on the raster pattern. Several stimulus and background parameters were manipulated, including wavelength, velocity, intensity, and direction. Since each complete scan took several minutes to complete, it was necessary to hold a unit several hours in order to complete the examination.

At the termination of each electrode track, a final reading was made of the microdrive position, and an electrolytic lesion was produced in the tissue by passing an anodal current of 100 μA for 10 sec through the electrode. The electrode was then raised and a second lesion was placed 2–3 mm above the first so that tissue shrinkage might be estimated after fixation. This procedure established a calibrated reference distance against which the entire track could be reconstructed.

Histology

At the termination of an experimental session, the pigeon was sacrificed and the brain was blocked and removed. After fixation and staining, the brain was sectioned serially at 70 μm for comparison with the Karten and Hodos (1967) atlas for the pigeon brain. Using the lesions as calibrated bench marks in conjunction with the microdrive readings from the experimental log, the entire electrode track was plotted. A summary set of schematic frontal brain sections showing the locations of all mapped units is shown in Fig. 1.

RESULTS

The results described here are based on data collected for 53 visual thalamic units responsive to the moving stimulus disk. The anatomical nomenclature used here for the thalamic nuclei generally follows that of Karten and Hodos (1967). The major exception is the partitioning of the nucleus dorsolateralis anterior thalami pars lateralis, DLL, which more recent studies (e.g., Miceli et al., 1975) divide into subunits: pars ventralis, DLLv, and pars dorsalis, DLLd. The present study further divided DLLd into anterior, DLLd(A), and posterior, DLLd(P), regions on the basis of RF area.

Receptive-field maps for each scan were reconstructed by the computer. Although data were collected during a scan for two opposite directions, the maps generated by the computer were for sweeps in a single direction only. A complete scan, then, provided the data for two maps, one each for opposite directions of movement. Responses along the sweep length, either 90 or 45 deg, were collected into 60 equal-length bins. For map displays, the data were shown as an array: 30 rows of 60 bins. The computer was programmed to display a dot on an oscilloscope for each bin in the array that contained some spike activity

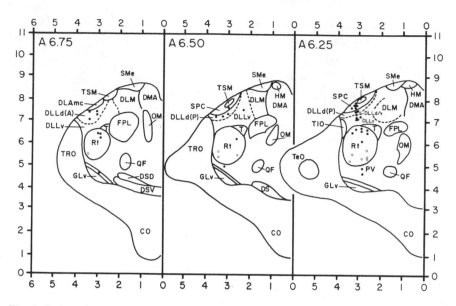

Fig. 1. Series of schematics showing the location of isolated units. Sections were taken from the atlas of Karten and Hodos (1967) and represent anterior planes 6.25, 6.50, and 6.75. The division of DLL into dorsal and ventral subdivisions and certain other modifications are after Miceli et al. (1975). The anterior and posterior portions of DLLd are indicated by the notations (A) and (P). The arrow in section A6.25 indicates a group of units designated DLLd/v all with approximately the same anatomical position on the border between DLLd(P) and DLLv (see text). The open symbols designate ventral Rt units. Abbreviations: DLLd, nucleus dorsolateralis anterior thalami pars lateralis pars dorsalis, (A) anterior and (P) posterior regions; DLAmc, nucleus dorsolateralis anterior thalami pars magnocellularis; DLLv, nucleus dorsolateralis anterior thalami pars lateralis pars ventralis; DLM, nucleus dorsolateralis anterior thalami pars medialis; DMA, nucleus dorsomedialis anterior thalami; DS, decussatio supraoptica; DSD, decussatio supraoptica dorsalis; DSV, decussatio supraoptica ventralis; FPL, fasciculus prosencephali lateralis; GLv, nucleus geniculatus lateralis ventralis; HM, nucleus habenularis medialis; OM, tractus occipitomesencephalicus; PV, nucleus posteroventralis thalami; QF, tractus quintofrontalis; Rt, nucleus rotundus; SMe, stria medullaris; SPC, nucleus superficialis parvocellularis; T, nucleus triangularis; TRO, tractus opticus; TSM, tractus septomesencephalicus.

so that the region in the scanning area that was excited by the passage of the stimulus disk appeared as a group of dots defining the RF. For most spontaneously active units, it was necessary to set a criterion level for spike activity in each bin so that only the more active regions were displayed.

Receptive Field Properties

The RFs of all visual units could be altered, sometimes significantly, by the manipulation of the stimulus parameters of velocity, intensity, wavelength, and direction of motion, as well as background intensity, contrast, and the pigeon's state of light adaptation. In other words, the RF for any visual cell is a retinal region, variable in size, shape, and sensitivity, from which information is drawn.

Effect of Stimulus Velocity. Units were examined with single sweeps through their RFs at a variety of velocities from 4.5 to 60 deg/sec. The majority of units responded most actively to slow-moving stimuli. Velocity preferences varied slightly between individual units, but there were no systematic differences between anatomical regions.

No unit ever responded well to velocities exceeding 40–50 deg/sec, and most units preferred stimulus speeds below 10 deg/sec. As an example, the RF maps for a DLLd(P) unit scanned at 4.5, 9, and 15 deg/sec are shown in column a of Fig. 2. At 9 deg/sec, the unit responded uniformly over a circular RF approximately 45 deg in diameter. At 15 deg/sec, the unit was unresponsive, while at 4.5 deg/sec the unit fired but with an irregular bursting pattern over a diffuse and irregularly shaped RF. The firing pattern of the unit, as the stimulus disk passed through the RF at the different velocities, is shown in column b.

Effect of Stimulus Intensity. Units were examined using a white or monochromatic stimulus which was reduced in intensity for a series of scans. The RF maps of a DDLd/v unit scanned at 9.4, 0.5, and 0.2 × 10^{11} quanta/sec/cm^2/ster against a dark background are shown in Fig. 3. For this unit, there was a decrease in RF size as stimulus intensity was reduced. A similar trend was observed for all units tested in this way: larger RFs were associated with more intense targets.

The number of dots displayed on a map of a RF was directly related to the total RF area. Thus it was possible to quantify the relative RF areas for different cells as a function of stimulus intensity. The relationship between displayed dot count and stimulus intensity for six units mapped with white light is graphed in Fig. 4. The relationship was uniform for all units, with the highest intensity values always favoring highest displayed dot counts. The same correlation between intensity and area held for cells isolated in all anatomical regions and for monochromatic as well as white stimuli.

Effect of Background Intensity. The DLLd(P) unit whose RF maps are shown in Fig. 5 was scanned with a white stimulus disk having a radiance of 3.0 × 10^{-5} W/cm^2/ster under two background conditions. The unit was first mapped with the disk projected against a dark background and then, after the white background of 1.17 × 10^{-7} W/cm^2/ster had been on for 5 min, the unit was mapped again at the same stimulus radiance. The effect of the background was to reduce the RF from a diameter of approximately 45 deg to one of approximately 30 deg. A reduction in RF size was observed for most units, both dorsal thalamic and Rt, when they were scanned against a lighted back-

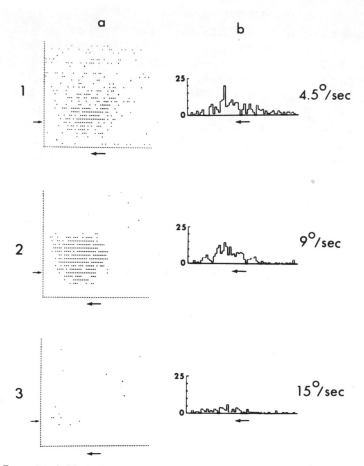

Fig. 2. Receptive fields and single-sweep histograms for a unit in DLLd (P) mapped at
4.5 deg/sec in 1a, 9 deg/sec in 2a, and 15 deg/sec in 3a with white light. Histograms
(column b) are for sweeps indicated by small arrows next to the maps. Map size 90 × 90
deg; scan direction left; radiance 3.0 × 10⁻⁵ W/cm²/ster; criterion level 5. Scale on each
histogram is in numbers of spikes per bin.

ground. Such effects have been recognized to be the result of an antagonistic balance between an inhibitory surround and an excitatory
center (Kuffler, 1953; Barlow et al., 1957). The implication here is that
many pigeon visual thalamic units are of the center-surround type, as
recent evidence suggests is the case for pigeon ganglion cells (Pearlman
and Hughes, 1976a).

Effects of Scanning Direction. The majority of units were scanned
in four directions: up, down, left, and right. Directional effects were
grouped into four categories. For each category, the feature of directionality appeared to have different degrees of relevance. The group-

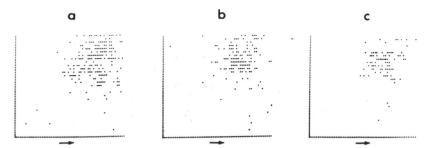

Fig. 3. Receptive fields for a unit in DLLd/v mapped with radiances of 9.4, 0.5, and 0.2 × 10^{11} quanta/sec/cm²/ster in a, b, and c, respectively. Map size 90 × 90 deg; scan direction right; wavelength 540 nm; sweep speed 9 deg/sec; criterion level 3.

ings were as follows: no directional effect, where the RF was unaffected by scan direction; directional differences, where the RF changed in shape but was generally equally responsive to all scan directions; directional preferences, where there was a greater response to one direction or set of directions; directional specificity, where a definite "null" as well as a preferred direction was evident. The RF maps for a directionally selective unit isolated in DLLd(P) are shown in Fig. 6.

Only the last of the aforementioned groups can be considered "directional units" in the classically defined sense (Maturana and Frenk, 1963; Barlow and Levick, 1965), since a "null" or inhibitory

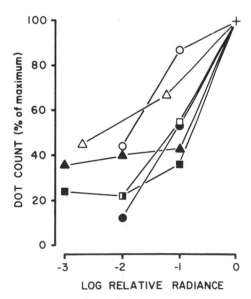

Fig. 4. Radiance response curves for six units. Response values were determined by counting the number of displayed dots in each RF map for each unit at various stimulus radiances. Dot counts were normalized at the peak of each curve.

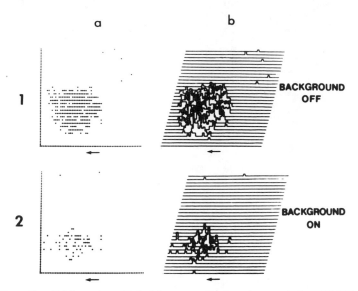

Fig. 5. Receptive fields and multiple-histogram displays for a unit in DLLd(P) mapped with a white disk at 3.0×10^{-5} W/cm²/ster against a dark background in row 1 and against a white background measuring 1.17×10^{-7} W/cm²/ster in row 2. Map size 90 × 90 deg; scan direction right; sweep speed 9 deg/sec; criterion level 5.

response eliminates the possibility of directional ambiguity and is therefore a more reliable indicator of movement direction. Only eight out of the 53 units sampled were classified as directionally selective. Of these eight, seven were located anatomically in dorsal thalamic regions and only one was found in Rt. Directional classifications within anatomical subdivisions are presented in Table 1.

Surround Responses. In some of the directionally selective units, a

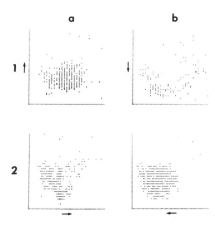

Fig. 6. Receptive fields for a directionally selective unit in DLLd(P) with white light in four different scan directions indicated with the arrows next to each map. Note the burst of activity which accompanies the exit of the stimulus disk from the inhibitory center in the downward, "null" direction (1b). Map size 90 × 90 deg; radiance 3.0×10^{-5} W/cm²/ster; sweep speed 9 deg/sec; criterion level 5.

Table 1. Directional Classification of Units Grouped into Anatomical Subdivisions[a]

Anatomical site	Directional classification (number of units)			
	No effect	Differences	Preferences	Specific
SPC	1	1	4	1
DLLd(A)	1		2	1
DLLd(P)	1	1	2	2
DLLd/v		2		3
DLLv	1	2	3	
Rt(dorsal)	2	1	7	1
Rt(ventral)[b]	3	3	4	
PV	1		2	
GLv			1	
Totals	10	10	25	8
Percent of total sample	19	19	47	15

[a] Subdivisions of thalamus are shown in Fig. 1.
[b] Shown as open symbols in Fig. 1.

burst of firing accompanied the exit of the stimulus disk from the RF center (see Fig. 6). These units were reminiscent of Spinelli's (1967) "out-surround" cat ganglion cell units and the "out-responses" of OFF cells in the cat lateral geniculate described by Lee et al. (1977). The out-responses seen here for pigeon thalamic units appeared to be the result of disinhibition; i.e., responses occurred only after the stimulus disk passed through the inhibitory RF center and not as the disk passed through the surround prior to entering the center region or when the disk passed by the center laterally.

Responses to direct surround stimulation were observed only rarely. This is very much in keeping with previous observations in pigeons that surrounds usually are inactive when stimulated alone (Hughes and Pearlman, 1974; Pearlman and Hughes, 1976a). For two dorsal thalamic units, maps were generated that demonstrated responses to stimulus movement in the surround portion of the RF, i.e., responses that did not depend on the stimulus disk moving through the center for activation. Two different sorts of active-surround responses were observed. The first unit was inhibited while the target traversed the surround, while the second unit could be either excited or inhibited by movement through the surround. Both types of surround responses were dependent on the direction of scan. Figure 7 illustrates the RF maps for the first unit, which had an excitatory center and an inhibitory surround. A curious feature of this unit, which was isolated in DLLd/v, was the fact that both the center and surround mechanisms became active only when stimulated with vertical move-

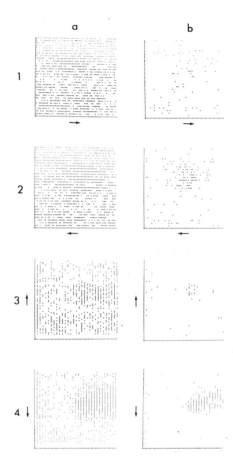

Fig. 7. Receptive fields for an active-surround unit in DLLd/v mapped with white light in four different scan directions indicated with the arrows next to each map. A criterion level of 1 in column a shows both excitatory and inhibitory regions, while the higher criterion level of 5 in column b permits a clearer comparison of the excitatory regions. The map in 1a, shows mainly spontaneous activity, which can be compared to the activity level in the inhibitory surround seen in 4a. Both the excitatory center and the inhibitory surround are visible but reduced in size in 3a. Map size 90 × 90 deg; radiance 1.5 × 10⁻⁵ W/cm²/ster; sweep speed 9 deg/sec.

ment. Both regions, in fact, had a preferred down direction. A most unusual series of maps is shown in Fig. 8 for the second unit, isolated in the nucleus superficialis parvocellularis (SPC), a dorsal thalamic nucleus. This unit demonstrated a center-surround RF organization that was associated with scan direction in an opponent fashion. When scanned horizontally, this unit reacted vigorously in a well-defined center region but was inactive or slightly inhibited over a large surround region. When scanned vertically, the unit was inhibited over the center area but was excited by movement through the surround region.

Effects of Wavelength. Monochromatic stimuli were used to map 33 out of the total 53 units studied. Often it was possible to hold a unit long enough to map a unit with a series of monochromatic stimuli distributed across the visible spectrum. One such series is shown in Fig. 9. The DLLd(A) unit shown here was tested with 450-nm (1a), 580-nm (1b), and 620-nm (2a) stimuli equated for quanta. This unit was

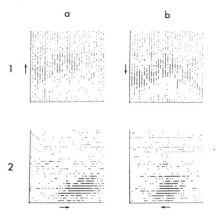

a   b

Fig. 8. Receptive fields for an active-surround unit in SPC mapped with white light in four different scan directions indicated with the arrows next to each map. The unit was manually scanned with the joystick control below the region mapped here, and the surround response to vertical movement seen in row 1 was easily detected below the horizontal-movement-sensitive center. Map size 90 × 90 deg; radiance 3.0 × 10⁻⁶ W/cm²/ster; sweep speed 9 deg/sec; criterion level 1.

typical of most units tested in this way: there was a positive correlation between RF size and the wavelength to which the unit responded most strongly. The RF for 620-nm light was clearly reduced in size in comparison to the RFs for either 580- or 450-nm light. It is unlikely, however, that the RF differences in this case indicate a color-processing function for this cell since it was possible to make good matches to the 620 nm map by reducing the intensity of either the 580-nm or the 450-nm stimulus. As an example, a RF map obtained with the 450-nm stimulus reduced in intensity by 2 logarithmic units is shown in 2b of Fig. 9.

The type of spectral response described above was typical of the nine dorsal thalamic units tested with a series of wavelengths. Spectral response curves were obtained for these nine units by plotting displayed dot counts vs. wavelength. All units had curves resembling those shown in Fig. 10 for a DLLd unit scanned horizontally. Response

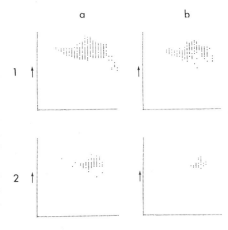

a   b

Fig. 9. Receptive fields for a unit in DLLd(A) mapped with a series of monochromatic stimuli. The unit was mapped with stimuli of 450 nm in 1a, 580 nm in 1b, and 620 nm in 2a, all equated at 1.9 × 10¹² quanta/sec/cm²/ster. In 2b is shown the RF for the 450-nm stimulus at 1.9 × 10¹⁰ quanta/sec/cm²/ster. The receptive field for the dim blue stimulus makes a good match to the RF for the bright red one. Map size 45 × 45 deg; sweep speed 9 deg/sec; criterion level 1.

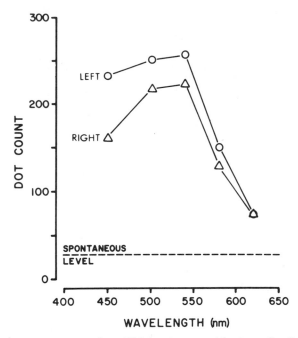

Fig. 10. Spectral response curves for a DLLd unit scanned horizontally. Total displayed dots are plotted as a function of stimulus wavelength. The unit showed a peak response at 540 nm with a slight preference for movement to the left. Spontaneous level was determined by scanning with the stimulus channel blocked.

peaks were at 540 nm. Spontaneous levels were determined by counting the dots on maps made by "scanning" with the stimulus light channel blocked.

Among those Rt units tested with monochromatic stimuli were some whose spectral responses peaked at 540 nm, much like the curves plotted in Fig. 10. It is likely that a similar spectral mechanism is responsible for the spectral curves of those Rt units and the previously described dorsal thalamic units. The remainder of Rt units tested with monochromatic light responded with combinations of excitation and inhibition or unique spatial distributions of spectral responsiveness suggestive of a process of wavelength comparison. Two examples are given below.

One ventral Rt unit was tested with 450- and 580-nm light in four scan directions. The displayed dot counts for each map are shown in Fig. 11. The unit was excited by movement in all directions when scanned with 450-nm light but was inhibited by movement in all directions when scanned with 580-nm light. In terms of opponent-color processing, this unit should be classified as a (+ blue − yellow) type.

The data points here fit the curve shown by Yazulla and Granda (1973; cf. their Fig. 2) for a $(+ B - Y)$ unit also isolated in ventral Rt.

Receptive-field maps for a dorsal Rt unit that possessed a unique blue-yellow center–surround organization are shown in Fig. 12. In 1a, a RF map is shown for a 450-nm stimulus disk scanned against a dark background. The unit was uniformly excited over a compact, oblong region. The RF map for a 580-nm stimulus, also on a dark background, is shown in 1b. For 580-nm light, the only excitatory region was the surround of the blue-selective center; i.e., the unit appeared to be inhibited in the center when scanned with yellow light. The inhibitory nature of the center's response to 580-nm light was further revealed when the RF was mapped with the 580-nm disk against a blue background. The flood of blue background light adapted out, i.e., made less sensitive, the mechanism inhibiting responses to 580-nm stimuli in the center. Chromatic adaptation revealed a yellow-sensitive region extending over the whole RF. When the RF was scanned with 450-nm light against a yellow background equated in energy with the blue background, the effect was to shift the RF downward by about 20 deg.

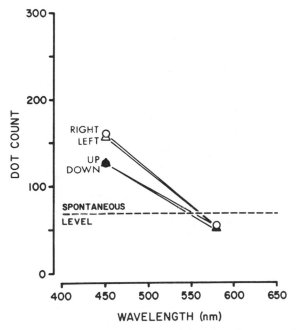

Fig. 11. Spectral response points for four scanning directions for a ventral Rt unit. This unit was tested at 450 and 580 nm at 1.9×10^{12} quanta/sec/cm²/ster. The displayed dot counts for all receptive fields mapped with 580-nm stimuli were below the spontaneous level determined by scanning with the stimulus channel blocked.

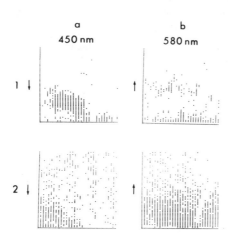

Fig. 12. Receptive fields for a dorsal Rt unit mapped with a 450-nm and a 580-nm stimulus. Stimuli were equated at 1.9 × 10¹² quanta/sec/cm²/ster. In row 1, the stimuli were presented against a dark background. In 2a the 450-nm stimulus was presented against the yellow background, and in 2b the 580-nm stimulus was presented against the blue background. Both backgrounds were equated at 2.4 × 10⁻⁸ W/cm²/ster. The preferred direction for each condition is shown next to each map, although there were no strong directional preferences with this unit and the main points could be seen for all directions. Map size 90 × 90 deg; sweep speed 9 deg/sec; criterion level 3.

This shift reflects a delay in the response latency of about 2 sec since the unit was scanned at 9 deg/sec. The increased latency is presumably due to an increase in relative sensitivity to 450-nm light as a result of yellow chromatic adaptation. A similar increase in response latency was reported by Granda and Yazulla (1971) for some inhibitory Rt units when short-wavelength stimulus intensity increased.

RF Size and Shape Correlated with Anatomical Area. The fullest extent of each unit's RF was estimated from maps obtained with an intense stimulus disk (usually white at 3.0 × 10⁻⁵ W/cm²/ster) scanned at 9 deg/sec over a dark background. Each RF was designated as having either a generally oblong or a circular shape, although no RF was perfectly regular in form. The area of each oblong RF was estimated by multiplying together the measurements for the long and short axes. Table 2 presents each anatomical region in which units were isolated (see Fig. 1), along with the number of units within each region either oblong or circular in shape and the mean area for all units in each region.

Table 2 shows that the RFs of dorsal thalamic units are about equally divided between oblong and circular shapes. In Rt, the distribution is uneven, with the dorsal portion containing only units with oblong RFs and the ventral portion favoring circular RFs at a ratio of 9:1.

In terms of area, the RFs mapped in DLLd(A) were the smallest. They were a little more than one-half the RF areas of units in SPC, DLLd(P), or DLLd/v, regions with nearly equal average areas. The RFs in DLLd(P) and DLLd/v were so nearly equal in size that most probably those units designated DLLd/v could properly be considered part of

Table 2. *Shape and Size of RFs Grouped into Anatomical Subdivisions* [a]

Anatomical site	Shape (number of units)		Area (deg^2) [b]
	Oblong	Circular	
SPC	2	5	1500
DLLd(A)	3	1	800
DLLd(P)	4	2	1200
DLLd/v	3	2	1300
DLLv	3	3	5100
Rt(dorsal)	11	0	5300
Rt(ventral) [c]	1	9	8900
PV	2	1	900
GLv	1	0	2200

[a] Subdivisions of thalamus are shown in Fig. 1.
[b] Rounded to nearest 100 deg^2.
[c] Shown as open symbols in Fig. 1.

DLLd(P). More ventral units in DLLv had RFs averaging 3 or 4 times larger than any DLLd group.

The well-known distinction between relatively compact dorsal thalamic RFs and much larger Rt RFs (Revzin, 1967, 1970; Webster, 1974) is supported here, although RFs in DLLv were close in size, if not in shape, to RFs in dorsal Rt. Ventral Rt RFs were the largest of all, with a mean diameter of about 100 deg. Ventral Rt RFs were nearly twice the average area of dorsal Rt RFs and were 8 times the area of all DLLd RFs.

DISCUSSION

Several differences were found between the RF characteristics of dorsal thalamic and Rt units.

1. All dorsal thalamic units scanned with monochromatic stimuli showed maximal responses to 540-nm light. Some Rt units also had a 540 nm spectral response peak; however, other Rt units demonstrated an opponent-color response.
2. Seven of the eight units classified as directionally selective were evenly distributed throughout the dorsal thalamic nuclei. Only one directionally selective unit was located in Rt.
3. The mean RF area of dorsal thalamic units was approximately one-third the mean RF area of Rt units.

4. In each of the dorsal thalamic nuclei, the RFs were about equally divided between oblong and circular shapes; however, there was an uneven distribution of shape classifications within Rt. All 11 dorsal Rt units were oblong in shape, while nine out of ten ventral Rt units had circular RFs.

There were also some RF characteristics shared by all units studied.

1. Receptive fields increased in size for more intense stimuli up to some upper limit of stimulus intensity.
2. Backgrounds had an effect complementary to the effect of stimulus intensity: more intense backgrounds produced smaller RFs.
3. A few units responded to direct stimulation of their RF surrounds, but most were unresponsive to surround stimulation.
4. Most units responded best to a stimulus velocity of 9 deg/sec.

Functional Comparisons of the Two Visual Pathways

Tectofugal Pathway. Multiple topographical maps of the retina are arranged in layers of the tectum (McGill et al., 1966; Crossland et al., 1975). Different functions are apparently assumed by different layers: the smallest, most stimulus-selective RFs are found in superficial tectal layers, and progressively larger RFs, less selective to stimulus qualities, are associated with units of the deeper layers (Holden, 1969; Jassik-Gerschenfeld et al., 1970; Hughes and Pearlman, 1974; Frost and Di-Franco, 1976). The segregation of particular functions to particular layers may be quite exact. For instance, Jassik-Gerschenfeld et al. (1975) found virtually all directional units to be restricted to the stratum griseum et fibrosum superficiale.

The wide-field units of the tectum may be part of a system that orients the pigeon's attention to the vicinity of possibly significant stimuli. This system might also initiate those reflexive reactions which seem to dominate much of avian visual behavior. In any case, the relatively enormous size of the pigeon's optic tectum suggests that it plays a major role in controlling visual behavior.

The present work and other findings (Granda and Yazulla, 1971; Yazulla and Granda, 1973; Benowitz and Karten, 1976; Revzin, this volume) show that functionally similar units from individual tectal layers project to specific portions of Rt. The still larger size of RFs in Rt indicates a further generalization of spatial information. Units of Rt may be "wired" to respond to general stimulus types, e.g., horizontal bars or edges, or stimuli of specific wavelengths, moving across large portions of the visual field or even over the whole monocular viewing area. Wavelength processing is largely but not entirely restricted to ventral Rt units.

Thalamofugal Pathway. Units in the dorsal thalamic nuclear complex receive input from the retina and feedback from the Wulst (De Britto et al., 1975; Miceli et al., 1975). Most of the feedback projects to ventral DLLd and ventral DLLv. These subdivisions of the dorsal thalamus, especially DLLv, were found here to have the largest RFs. The correspondence between Wulst projections and large RF size suggests a possible disinhibitory role for Wulst feedback similar to the disinhibitory isthmooptic nucleus relationship to the retina. The reversible cooling experiments which so successfully revealed the nature of centrifugal feedback to the retina (Miles, 1972; Pearlman and Hughes, 1976b) should be repeated in the Wulst–dorsal thalamus circuit.

The results here and elsewhere (De Britto et al., 1975; Jassik-Gerschenfeld et al., this volume) indicate that many dorsal thalamic units have small, frequently directionally selective RFs with antagonistic surrounds. The impression gained is one of good spatial localization and contrast analysis. The thalamofugal system may direct fine head or eye movements to hold images on the central retina for examination. Interconnections with the Wulst suggest that the dorsal thalamus serves as more than a simple relay and that its transmission characteristics may be influenced by the activity of more central processing centers.

Higher-Order Visual Processing

Higher-order perceptual events probably occur where the thalamofugal and tectofugal pathways rejoin. As Revzin (this volume) suggests, the periectostriatal belt (Ep) is likely to be one site of recombination. Signals encoding such stimulus dimensions as wavelength and orientation may be carried by wide-field tectofugal units to Ep cells, where signals from narrow-field thalamofugal units encoding location, contrast, direction of movement, or size also project. Stimulus dimensions such as wavelength and directionality, which seem to be encoded by inhibition, may act on Ep cells in a gating fashion. For example, an Ep cell might receive *inhibitory* input from a tectofugal ($-B$ $+Y$) opponent-color fiber whose RF covers nearly the entire visual field. The same Ep cell might also receive *excitatory* input from a thalamofugal fiber with a small, oblong RF. The result could be a detector-type Ep cell maximally responsive to small blue bar-shaped objects imaged on the retina in a precise location. This type of visual processing allows the growth of specificity to particular dimensions as well as the generalization to other dimensions. It is also efficient since it permits individual wide-field units to service many spatially specific units. The parallel transport of visual information along anatomically separate pathways may be simply a way to preclude interfering crosstalk between stimulus dimensions.

REFERENCES

Barlow, H. B., and Levick, W. R.: The mechanism of directionally selective units in rabbit retina. *J. Physiol. (London)* **178**:477-504 (1965).

Barlow, H. B., FitzHugh, R., and Kuffler, S. W.: Change of organization in the receptive fields of the cat's retina during dark adaptation. *J. Physiol. (London)* **137**:338-354 (1957).

Benowitz, L. I., and Karten, H. J.: Organization of the tectofugal visual pathway in the pigeon. *J. Comp. Neurol.* **167**:503-520 (1976).

Crossland, W. J., Cowan, W. M., and Rogers, L. A.: Studies in the development of the chick optic tectum. IV. An autoradiographic study of the development of retinotectal connections. *Brain Res.* **91**:1-23 (1975).

De Britto, L. R. G., Brunelli, M., Francesconi, W., and Magni, F.: Visual response pattern of thalamic neurons in the pigeon. *Brain Res.* **97**:337-343 (1975).

Frost, B. J., and DiFranco, D. E.: Motion characteristics of simple units in the pigeon optic tectum. *Vision Res.* **16**:1129-1234 (1976).

Granda, A. M., and Yazulla, S.: The spectral sensitivity of single units in the nucleus rotundus of pigeon, *Columba livia. J. Gen. Physiol.* **57**:363-384 (1971).

Hodos, W., Leibowitz, R. W., and Bonbright, J. C., Jr.: Near-field visual acuity of pigeons: Effects of head location and stimulus luminance. *J. Exp. Anal. Behav.* **25**:129-141 (1976).

Holden, A. L.: Receptive properties of retinal cells and tectal cells in the pigeon. *J. Physiol. (London)* **201**:56P-57P (1969).

Hughes, C. P., and Pearlman, A. L.: Single unit receptive fields and the cellular layers of the pigeon optic tectum. *Brain Res.* **80**:365-377 (1974).

Jassik-Gerschenfeld, D., Minois, F., and Condé-Courtine, F.: Receptive field properties of directionally selective units in the pigeon's optic tectum. *Brain Res.* **24**:407-421 (1970).

Jassik-Gerschenfeld, D., Guichard, J., and Tessier, Y.: Localization of directionally selective and movement sensitive cells in the optic tectum of the pigeon. *Vision Res.* **15**:1037-1038 (1975).

Jassik-Gerschenfeld, D., Teulon, J., and Ropert, N.: Visual receptive field types in the nucleus dorsolateralis anterior of the pigeon's thalamus. *Brain Res.* **108**:295-306 (1976).

Karten, H. J., and Hodos, W.: *A Stereotaxic Atlas of the Brain of the Pigeon (Columba livia).* The Johns Hopkins Press, Baltimore (1967). Pp. 193.

Karten, H. J., Hodos, W., Nauta, W. J. H., and Revzin, A. M.: Neural connections of the "visual Wulst" of the avian telencephalon: Experimental studies in the pigeon (*Columba livia*) and owl (*Speotyto cunicularia*). *J. Comp. Neurol.* **150**:253-278 (1973).

Kuffler, S. W.: Discharge patterns and functional organization of mammalian retina. *J. Neurophysiol.* **16**:37-69 (1953).

Lee, B. B., Virsu, V., and Creutzfeldt, O. D.: Responses of cells in the cat lateral geniculate nucleus to moving stimuli at various levels of light and dark adaptation. *Exp. Brain Res.* **27**:51-59 (1977).

Maturana, H. R., and Frenk, S.: Directional movement and horizontal edge detectors in the pigeon retina. *Science* **142**:977–979 (1963).

McGill, J. I., Powell, T. P. S., and Cowan, W. M.: The retinal representation upon the optic tectum and isthmooptic nucleus in the pigeon. *J. Anat.* **100**:5–33 (1966).

Miceli, D., Peyrichoux, S., and Repérant, J.: The retino-thalamo-hyperstriatal pathway in the pigeon (*Columba livia*). *Brain Res.* **100**:125–131 (1975).

Miles, F. A.: Centrifugal control of the avian retina. IV. Effects of reversible cold block of the isthmo-optic tract on the receptive field properties of cells in the retina and isthmo-optic nucleus. *Brain Res.* **48**:131–145 (1972).

Pearlman, A. L., and Hughes, C. P.: Functional role of efferents to the avian retina. I. Analysis of retinal ganglion cell receptive fields. *J. Comp. Neurol.* **166**:111–122 (1976a).

Pearlman, A. L., and Hughes, C. P.: Functional role of efferents to the avian retina. II. Effects of reversible cooling of the isthmo-optic nucleus. *J. Comp. Neurol.* **166**:123–132 (1976b).

Revzin, A. M.: Unit responses to visual stimuli in the nucleus rotundus of the pigeon. *Fed. Proc.* **26**:656 (1967).

Revzin, A. M.: Some characteristics of wide-field units in the brain of the pigeon. *Brain Behav. Evol.* **3**:195–204 (1970).

Spinelli, D. N.: Receptive field organization of ganglion cells in the cat's retina. *Exp. Neurol.* **19**:291–315 (1967).

Webster, K. E.: Changing concepts of the organization of the central visual pathways in birds. In Bellairs, R., and Gray, E. G. (eds.): *Essays on the Nervous System*. Clarendon Press, Oxford. (1974). Pp. 258–298.

Wright, A. A.: Psychometric and psychophysical hue discrimination functions for the pigeon. *Vision Res.* **12**:1447–1464 (1972).

Yazulla, S.: Intraretinal differentiation in the synaptic organization of the inner plexiform layer of the pigeon retina. *J. Comp. Neurol.* **153**:309–324 (1974).

Yazulla, S., and Granda, A. M.: Opponent-color units in the thalamus of the pigeon (*Columba livia*). *Vision Res.* **13**:1555–1563 (1973).

12

Discrimination of Line Orientation by Pigeons after Lesions of Thalamic Visual Nuclei

PATRICK MULVANNY

INTRODUCTION

Two pathways are known to carry visual information to the avian telencephalon. The more highly developed tectofugal pathway proceeds from the retina to the optic tectum (Cowan et al., 1961), to the nucleus rotundus thalami (Karten and Revzin, 1966), and to the ectostriatum of the telencephalon (Karten and Hodos, 1970). The smaller thalamofugal pathway proceeds from the retina to a nuclear complex in the dorso-lateral thalamus designated the nucleus opticus principalis thalami (OPT) (Karten and Nauta, 1968). Component nuclei of this complex are the nucleus lateralis anterior (LA), the nucleus dorsolateralis anterior pars magnocellularis (DLAmc), and the nucleus dorsolateralis anterior pars lateralis (DLL). The OPT complex has been shown to project on distinct groups of cells in the telencephalon called, collectively, the visual Wulst (Hunt and Webster, 1972; Karten et al., 1973). The origin of this projection, which consists of both ipsilateral and contralateral components, has been identified as DLL (Meier et al., 1974).

Receptive fields of neurons along the two visual pathways show

PATRICK MULVANNY • Department of Psychology, University of Maryland, College Park, Maryland 20742. Present address: Department of Psychology, Ursinus College, Collegeville, Pennsylvania 19426. This work was supported by NIH Fellowship MH-05165 to Patrick Mulvanny and NIH Grant EY-00735 to William Hodos.

differences which suggest that the information reaching the telence-phalon by the tectofugal route differs from that ascending by the thal-amofugal route. The tectofugal pathway is characterized by expansion of receptive field size within the tectal strata (Jassik-Gerschenfeld and Guichard, 1972) and in both the nucleus rotundus and the ectostriatum (Revzin, 1970). The receptive fields of neurons along the thalamofugal pathway remain small by comparison, both in the OPT complex (Cross-land, 1972) and in the visual Wulst (Revzin, 1969; O'Flaherty and Invernizzi, 1972). At the thalamic level, several investigators have re-corded from both tectofugal and thalamofugal relay nuclei using the same methods; they invariably report larger receptive fields for rotun-dal than for OPT neurons (Crossland, 1972; Jassik-Gerschenfeld and Guichard, 1972; Jassik-Gerschenfeld et al., 1976; De Britto et al., 1975; Maxwell and Granda, this volume).

These differences in response characteristics of cells in the two pathways suggest hypotheses about the respective roles of the path-ways in the analysis of visual information, for example, that the thal-amofugal pathway contributes more to the processing of spatial infor-mation than does the tectofugal pathway. This view is supported by the identification of a few units in the dorsolateral thalamus sensitive to stimulus orientation (De Britto et al., 1975), and predicts impairment of form discrimination following lesions of the OPT complex.

The effects of lesions of the nucleus rotundus and of OPT seem at first to be inconsistent with this hypothesis. Hodos and Karten (1966) placed lesions in the nucleus rotundus after training pigeons to perform one intensity and three form-discrimination problems. They found severe initial decrements in performance on all four problems, with eventual return to preoperative levels of accuracy following extensive retraining. Lesions of the OPT complex, however, produced little or no impairment on these same discrimination problems. However, as these authors point out, the differences between stimuli used in their exper-iment may have been too great to reveal sensory losses resulting from lesions of the thalamofugal pathway: even a small postoperative visual capability may have been sufficient for highly accurate discrimination between the elements of their stimulus pairs.

Hodos and Bonbright (1974) examined this possibility by testing pigeons with a psychophysical procedure that required discrimination between stimuli differing in luminance by as little as 0.05 log unit. Postoperative difference thresholds for subjects with lesions of the nucleus rotundus showed the pattern seen in the Hodos and Karten (1966) experiment: thresholds rose following surgery, then returned to their preoperative levels following many sessions of retraining. OPT cases, on the other hand, showed smaller elevations of threshold postoperatively, but these did not return to preoperative levels despite extensive retraining.

The present experiment was a psychophysical assessment of the role of visual thalamic nuclei in performance of a discrimination based on a spatial stimulus property. Line orientation was chosen as the stimulus continuum because it is nonintensive and because its discrimination would seem to require neurons with small receptive fields or highly selective response properties. Care was taken to exclude intensity as a basis for response, both by controlling the physical stimulus and by considering stimulus effects that might resemble intensity. For example, since contours are highly effective stimuli at the retinal level, stimuli varying in the amount of contour present might differ in their "intensive" effect on central structures (Weiskrantz, 1963). For the same reason, horizontal and vertical lines were not included in the stimulus set for which data are reported (although they serve as training stimuli) because lines with these orientations may receive special processing at the retina (Maturana, 1962) and thus be discriminated on the basis of their intensive central effect.

METHOD

Subjects

Subjects were ten White Carneaux pigeons (Columba livia) of both sexes obtained from the Hillside Pigeon Farm of Hyattstown, Maryland. They were 1-2 years old at the start of the experiment and weighed 450-600 g before food deprivation sufficient to reduce them to 70-80% of free-fed weight, levels that were maintained throughout the course of the experiment.

Apparatus

Sessions took place in a Lehigh Valley, Inc., pigeon chamber equipped with a blower for ventilation and a speaker supplying white noise to mask external sounds. The chamber's front panel supported a standard grain feeder and feeder light for reinforcement of key pecking, and a houselight that maintained panel luminance at 145 cd/m^2 in the region of the pecking keys. Three keys were arranged on a horizontal line 240 mm from the floor of the chamber. Keys were 25 mm in diameter and centered 31 mm apart. The left and right keys were made from translucent plexiglas and could be transilluminated by bulbs set behind them to a level of 216 cd/m^2. The center key was made from pyrex glass to avoid scratches in the area of the stimulus; its rear surface was ground to serve as a projection screen for the optical system described below. All keys operated attached microswitches with application of 30 g pressure, measured at the center.

The optical system condensed the light from a Sylvania CEW 150-W lamp powered at 1.3 A through a voltage regulator set to 100 VAC, and sent it through a 9.0 by 0.8-mm slit in a sheet of thin brass. Light then passed through a Kodak Wratten filter of 1.0 nominal neutral density and a lens that formed an image of the source at the entrance of a Dove prism in a ball-bearing mount. A final lens focused the light leaving the prism to form an image of the slit on the rear surface of the center pecking key. The projected line was in sharp focus, was precisely centered, and measured 16.0 by 1.4 mm. Luminance of the line was 785 cd/m^2. Line orientation was controlled by rotation of the Dove prism through a belt-and-pulley arrangement from a DC stepping motor (Superior Electric Co.). Effects of lash in the drive system were minimized by ensuring that a given prism setting was always approached from the same direction and that the prism always returned to its resting position between trials, and by discarding the data from the very few sessions after which the position of the prism differed from its resting position.

All experimental events, including moving the stepping motor and recording data, were controlled by solid-state logic modules.

Procedure

Preoperative Training and Testing. The behavioral procedure was based on the method of Heinemann et al. (1969), with modifications developed by Hodos and Bonbright (1972) for behavioral tests of brain-lesioned subjects.

After pigeons learned to eat grain from the upraised feeder, they were trained, using 2.0-sec operation of the feeder as reinforcement, to peck whichever of the two side keys was illuminated. After 20 reinforced responses had been made to each side key, pretraining trials began. Each pretraining trial began with presentation of a vertical or a horizontal line on the center key. The order of vertical-line and horizontal-line trials was determined by a pseudorandom discrimination sequence. Pecks to the center key darkened it and illuminated the correct side key, which was the right key on vertical-line trials and the left on horizontal-line trials. The number of pecks required on the center key was raised gradually from one to ten. Pecks to the correct side key were followed by reinforcement with probability 1.0 at first, decreasing gradually to 0.4. Unreinforced side-key pecks operated the feeder light but not the feeder itself. Pecks to the incorrect side key turned off the houselight for 2.0 sec and caused a correction trial to be programmed for the next trial. Correction trials were identical to the trials they followed, except that no data were recorded and correct side-key responses led only to operation of the feeder light, not the feeder. Their purpose was to discourage subjects from pecking only one of the side keys. All trials were separated by a 3.0-sec pause, and were grouped into daily sessions of 324 trials each.

Following one full session with center-key requirement and rein-forcement probability at their final values, discrimination training began. Discrimination training sessions were identical to pretraining sessions except that completion of the center-key requirement illumi-nated both correct and incorrect side keys. Thus the subject was re-quired to respond to one side key or the other on the basis of the line's orientation rather than the luminance of the side keys.

When a subject chose the correct key on more than 90% of all trials for three consecutive discrimination training sessions, psychophysical testing began. In the psychophysical testing condition, the 324-trial session was divided into nine 36-trial blocks, with a single pair of stimuli presented during each block. The first block served as a warmup and consisted of discrimination training trials as described above. The second block was an assessment to determine whether the animal's performance warranted psychophysical testing. Its primary purpose was to prevent cessation of response during presentation of difficult discrimination problems by subjects incapable of discriminating reli-ably even between horizontal and vertical lines. If a subject responded to the incorrect side key on more than three trials during the assessment block, the entire session consisted of discrimination training with ver-tical and horizontal lines. If a subject made fewer than three errors, the horizontal and vertical lines were replaced in subsequent blocks by the test stimuli. Stimulus orientation was measured and stimuli were class-ified according to their direction and degree of rotation relative to a "zero" position 45 deg clockwise of vertical. Each pair of stimuli con-sisted of one member rotated clockwise (−) and one rotated counter-clockwise (+) of the zero position. Stimuli in the "−" class were treated as horizontal lines, i.e., they signaled reinforcement for pecking the left key. Stimuli in the "+" class were treated as vertical lines and signaled reinforcement for pecking the key on the right. The degrees of rotation from zero for stimuli in each of the seven test blocks were 17, 11, 5, 20, 14, 8, and 2 deg, in order of presentation. Stimulus magnitude descended in two interlocking series to permit an evaluation of within-session stability of performance. With this arrangement, im-provement or deterioration of performance would show up in the data as large differences in accuracy of response to adjacent values of orientation. The sequence of trial events for both classes of stimuli is summarized in Fig. 1.

Data Treatment. The rationale underlying analysis of the data is based on the theory of signal detection (see Treisman and Watts, 1966, for a discussion of this type of data treatment), and is illustrated in Fig. 2. The internal events evoked by presentation of a line with a given orientation are assumed to be normally distributed along a decision axis, with considerable overlap between the distributions of events evoked by lines differing little in orientation. A subject responds according to a criterion which partitions the decision axis into regions for which events will lead to left- and right-key responses. Thus the subject responds "left" to the stimulus generating internal event *a* in Fig. 2, even though it may well have been evoked by a stimulus for which a "right" response was correct. The probability of a right-key response to a stimulus is given by the area of its event distribution falling to the right of the criterion line. If the distributions generated by the stimuli are equally spaced along the decision axis, probability of response should grow with orientation according to a cumulative normal curve. That the spacing of these distributions is in fact equal when pigeons and equal orientation differences are used has been demonstrated by Blough (1972).

The slope of a line fitted to the psychometric function when response probabilities are expressed as their normal deviates gives the change in response probability occurring with changes in orientation, expressed as z scores per degree. Since this unit is inconvenient for discussion, its reciprocal will be used here. This unit is the SD and represents the number of degrees of orientation change needed to move response probability through one standard deviation. It is analogous to the difference-threshold measure of classical psychophysics.

The SD was computed from a line fitted to each subject's normalized response probabilities by the method of least squares following

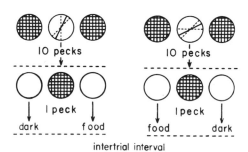

Fig. 1. Sequence of events during training and psychophysical testing trials. Ten pecks to a line projected on the center key illuminated two side keys. A single peck to a side key produced either food reinforcement or a brief period of darkness. The assignment of outcomes to side keys depended on whether the orientation of the line on the center key had been positive (left panel) or negative (right panel).

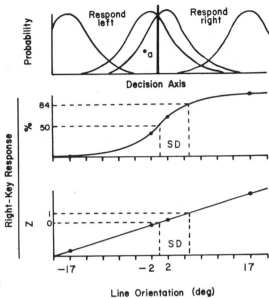

Fig. 2. Theoretical basis for analysis of the behavioral data. Refer to the text for details.

every session. Subjects were run until data from a ten-session series met criteria for variability and trend. The variability criterion specified that the standard deviation of the ten SDs be less than 0.15 times their mean. The trend criterion specified that monotonicity of SDs over the same ten-session period not be significant according to a two-tailed Mann–Kendall nonparametric test for trend (Bradley, 1968), using a significance level of 0.20. Note that this criterion specifies that the extent of monotonicity be limited; it does not mean that subjects neither improved nor deteriorated in their performance over a 10-day period.

Data from the ten sessions satisfying these criteria were pooled to form a single psychometric function reflecting preoperative performance.

Surgery. Within 24 hr of the final preoperative session, subjects were anesthetized with methoxyflurane carried in a mixture of 95% oxygen and 5% carbon dioxide and given subcutaneous injections of xylocaine at the intended incision site. Bilateral, anodal electrolytic lesions were made in the area of the dorsolateral thalamus or in the nucleus rotundus, using stereotaxic coordinates from the Karten and Hodos (1967) atlas of the pigeon brain.

Postoperative Testing. After a 5–7 day recovery period, subjects resumed psychophysical testing. Procedures, treatment of data, and criteria for termination were as they had been for preoperative testing.

Histology. At the completion of postoperative testing, each subject was deeply anesthetized by intravenous injection of sodium pentobarbitol and perfused through the left ventricle with normal saline followed by Heidenhain's solution without mercuric chloride. The head was then severed from the body and the calvarium removed to expose the brain. The head was submerged in Heidenhain's solution overnight, then transferred to 10% formol-saline for 1–5 days of additional fixation. The head was then placed in the stereotaxic instrument and blocked in the stereotaxic plane with a scalpel blade mounted on an electrode carrier. The brain was removed from the skull and stored in formol-saline for several days. Following this, the brain was dehydrated in an ethanol series, cleared in cedarwood oil, embedded in paraffin, and sectioned on a rotary microtome at 10 μm. Every tenth section was mounted and stained according to a modification of the Klüver and Barrera (1953) method for cells and myelinated axons. Brain sections were examined under a microscope and the lesions were reconstructed on standard drawings of the pigeon brain adapted from the Karten and Hodos (1967) atlas. In addition to necrotic areas, indications of gliosis, retrograde chromatolysis, cell loss, and demyelination were recorded.

RESULTS

Anatomical

The ten cases in this experiment were assigned to three groups, depending on the location of the lesion. Because of the proximity of OPT and the nucleus rotundus, lesions intended for one usually involve some direct damage to the other. In addition, since the efferent fibers of the nucleus rotundus pass through the area of OPT en route to the telencephalon, OPT lesions often produce some retrograde degeneration in the nucleus rotundus. Classification of lesions into OPT and rotundus groups is therefore not absolute, but is based to some extent on the degree and bilaterality of damage to the structures involved.

Four cases in the anterior OPT group sustained lesions confined to the anterior portion of the OPT complex, involving LA, DLAmc, and the anterior pole of DLL, but sparing DLL posterior to the A 6.75 plane of the Karten and Hodos (1967) atlas. Posterior OPT cases included substantial damage to DLL, including the area posterior to the A 6.75 plane. Subjects were assigned to this group on the basis of involvement of DLL, regardless of the amount of damage to more anterior components of the OPT complex. In each of the OPT groups, bilateral damage to the nucleus rotundus was slight. Cases were assigned to the nucleus rotundus group on the basis of varying degrees of bilateral direct or retrograde damage to the nucleus rotundus with little or no bilateral involvement of any nucleus of the OPT complex.

Figure 3 presents a series of transverse sections through the pigeon brain stem, with nuclei and tracts identified by abbreviations. The number beside each section indicates the plate in the Karten and Hodos (1967) atlas from which the drawing was derived.

Anterior OPT. Figure 4 shows the reconstructions of lesions in the anterior OPT group. Bilateral damage to elements of the OPT complex was slight in birds 302 and 309. Bird 302 showed bilateral destruction of dorsal LA and of the lateral tip of DLAmc, but in each of the nuclei of OPT the majority of cells were spared. The OPT complex of bird 309 was completely destroyed on the right, but damage on the left resembled that seen in the case of bird 302: ventral LA, medial DLAmc, and virtually all of DLL were spared.

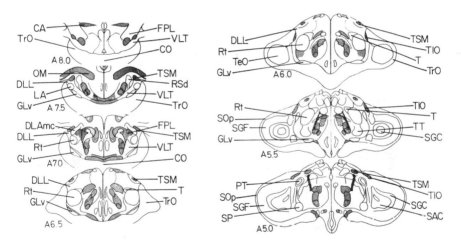

Fig. 3. Key for the identification of structures in Figs. 4–6. The number next to each transverse section of the pigeon brain stem indicates that plate in the Karten and Hodos (1967) atlas from which the drawing was derived. Abbreviations: CA, commissura anterior; CO, chiasma opticum; DLAmc, nucleus dorsolateralis anterior pars lateralis; FPL, fasciculus prosencephali lateralis; GLv, nucleus geniculatus lateralis pars ventralis; LA, nucleus lateralis anterior; OM, tractus occipitomesencephalicus; PT, nucleus pretectalis; RSd, nucleus reticularis superior pars dorsalis; Rt, nucleus rotundus; SAC, stratum album centrale; SGC, stratum griseum centrale; SGF, stratum griseum et fibrosum superficiale; SOp, stratum opticum; SP, nucleus subpretectalis; T, nucleus triangularis; TeO, tectum opticum; TIO, tractus isthmoopticus; TrO, tractus opticus; TSM, tractus septomesencephalicus; TT, tractus tectothalamicus; VLT, nucleus ventrolateralis thalami.

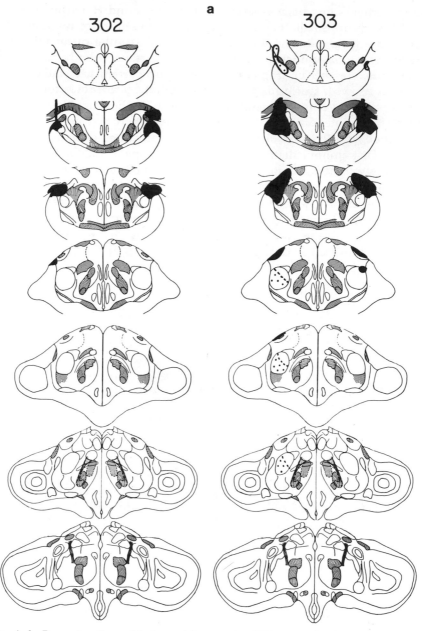

Fig. 4a,b. Reconstructions of lesions of the anterior OPT group. See Fig. 3 for identification of structures. In this and the following two figures, black areas indicate zones of necrosis; stippling indicates gliosis or demyelination in fiber bundles and retrograde degeneration or cell loss in cell groups. The density of stippling corresponds to the severity of damage.

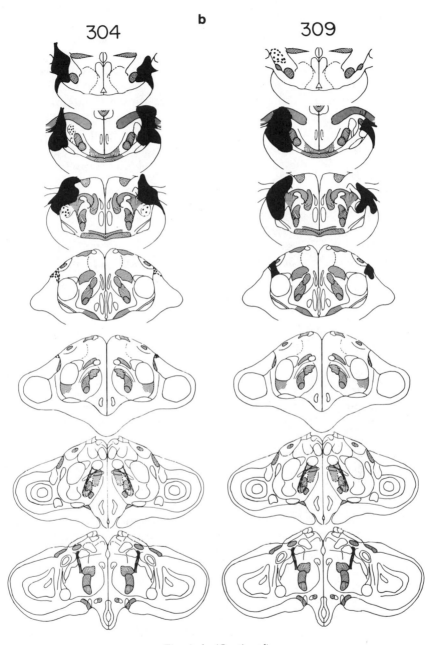

Fig. 4a,b. (*Continued*)

Damage to anterior OPT was more nearly complete in the cases of birds 303 and 304. Bird 303 showed complete destruction of LA and near-total involvement of DLAmc bilaterally, with sparing of all but the anterior pole of DLL. In addition, the right nucleus rotundus showed a moderate amount of retrograde degeneration, as evidenced by the presence of chromatolytic cells in its ventrolateral two-thirds. The left nucleus rotundus remained virtually intact. Bird 304 sustained a large lesion that completely destroyed LA bilaterally and spared only the medial tip of DLAmc on the left. Damage to DLL was again confined to its anterior pole, as was retrograde degeneration in the nucleus rotundus. This subject also showed extensive cell loss in the right nucleus reticularis superior pars dorsalis (RSd), as well as extensive direct damage to the fasciculus prosencephali lateralis (FPL) bilaterally.

Posterior OPT. Figure 5 shows the reconstructions of the lesions in the posterior OPT group. For both subjects, most of DLL lay in the necrotic area produced directly by the passage of current. Bird 307 showed complete bilateral destruction of all elements of the OPT complex; only the extreme medial pole of left DLAmc was spared. In addition to damage in OPT, some bilateral invasion of the nucleus geniculatus lateralis pars ventralis (GLv) was evident. Retrograde degeneration in the right nucleus rotundus was moderate to extensive in its anterior two-thirds, as evidenced by some loss of cells and chromatolytic changes among many of those remaining. Damage to the left nucleus rotundus, however, was slight, and was confined entirely to its anterior pole. Bird 311 sustained a lesion largely restricted to DLL. LA was spared bilaterally, as was the medial half of DLAmc. Direct invasion of the nucleus rotundus was limited to its anterior and dorsal aspects bilaterally; retrograde changes were evident only in the right nucleus rotundus and took the form of a few scattered chromatolytic cells.

Nucleus Rotundus. Figure 6 displays the lesion reconstructions from the four cases in the nucleus rotundus group. Bird 362 sustained a small lesion of the dorsal portion of the nucleus rotundus bilaterally; damage was slightly more extensive on the left. Retrograde degeneration was confined to the area immediately surrounding the necrotic area. Damage to OPT was limited to the extreme posterolateral tip of left DLL. Bird 360 showed a slightly asymmetrical but extensive pattern of damage confined almost entirely to the nucleus rotundus, with some involvement of right posterolateral DLL. Both the nucleus triangularis and all but the rostral pole of nucleus rotundus were destroyed on the right. Direct and retrograde damage on the left extended throughout the anterior two-thirds of the nucleus rotundus but spared its posterior pole as well as the nucleus triangularis.

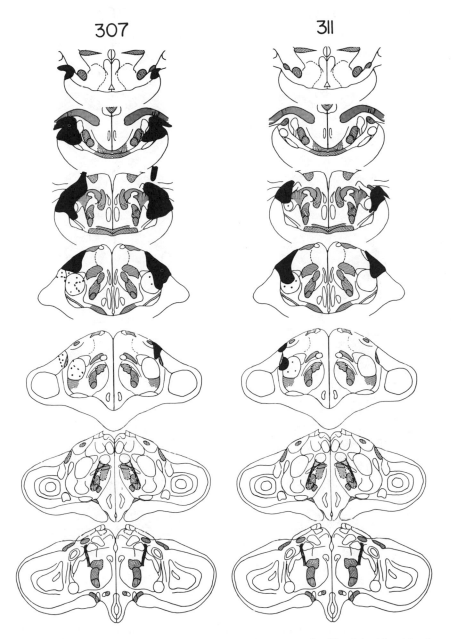

Fig. 5. Reconstructions of lesions of the posterior OPT group. See Fig. 3 for identification of structures.

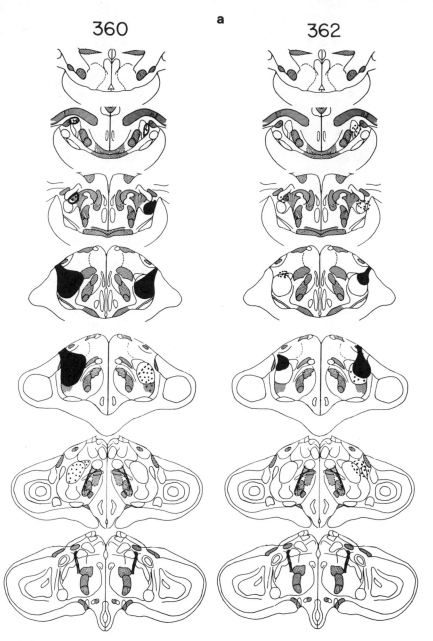

Fig. 6a,b. Reconstruction of lesions of the nucleus rotundus group. See Fig. 3 for identification of structures.

b

364 367

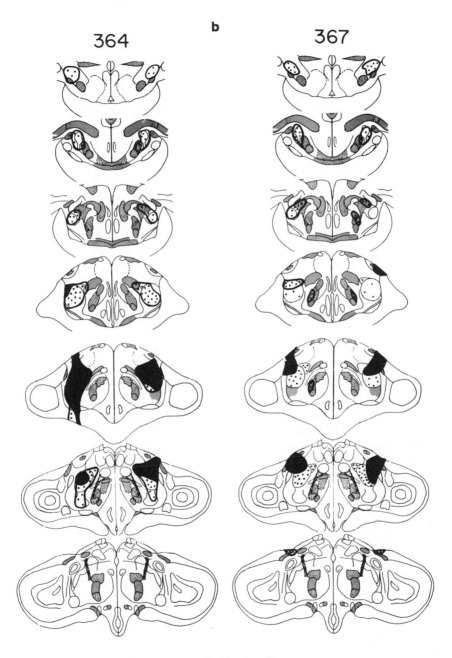

Fig. 6a,b. (Continued)

The remaining two cases, birds 364 and 367, sustained bilateral damage throughout the nucleus rotundus, with consequent demyelination of FPL, which contains the projection fibers of the nucleus rotundus on the ectostriatum. In addition, both birds suffered retrograde degeneration in RSd. In neither case did examination of OPT reveal any significant damage. In the case of bird 364, bilateral direct and retrograde destruction of the nucleus rotundus was virtually complete, with only a few cells on the left spared. The lesion also included posterior right GLv and the tectothalamic tract bilaterally. Damage to the nucleus rotundus of the final case, bird 367, consisted mainly of retrograde degeneration, which was severe in the posterior half bilaterally and slight to moderate elsewhere. Many chromatolytic cells were also identified bilaterally in the nucleus triangularis.

Behavioral

Behavioral data from the three groups of cases are presented in two ways. Figures 7, 9, and 11 show the SDs calculated from daily preoperative and postoperative sessions, with the average SD over the 10-day periods of stable performance represented by dashed horizontal lines. Data from these 10-day periods were pooled to produce the psychometric functions of Figs. 8, 10, and 12. In these figures, response probabilities are plotted as their normal deviates, and each point represents 180 presentations of a stimulus. Lines fitted to the points by the method of least squares are also displayed; slope and intercept constants of these lines are given in Table 1, as is the SD for each subject based on the pooled data. The slope constant indicates sensitivity to changes in orientation, i.e., the change in response probability generated by a change in line orientation. The intercept constant represents response bias, i.e., a subject's propensity to respond to the right (+) or left (−) key regardless of line orientation.

Several features of the psychometric functions are apparent. First, the data are well fitted by straight lines, lending further support to the idea that equal differences in orientation yield equal differences in discriminability over the range of orientations presented. Second, adjacent orientation values generated similar probabilities of response despite the fact that these values were presented half a session apart. This demonstrates the freedom from progressive improvement or deterioration in data from rather lengthy sessions. This fact, taken with the stringent criteria for stability and lack of trend met by the data, reflects the overall stability and homogeneity of performance during the sessions from which pre- and postoperative performance data were collected.

Table 1. Regression Constants and SDs Calculated from the Preoperative and
Postoperative Psychometric Functions of Each Subject[a]

Group, subject	Preoperative			Postoperative		
	a	b	SD (deg)	a	b	SD (deg)
Anterior OPT						
302	0.0575	0.0779	17.38	0.1013	−0.0021	9.88
303	0.1192	−0.0971	8.39	0.1225	−0.1750	8.16
304	0.1077	−0.0271	9.29	0.1044	0.0129	9.58
309	0.1016	−0.1114	9.84	0.1185	−0.4164	8.44
Posterior OPT						
307	0.0803	0.0786	12.45	0.0651	−0.0793	15.36
311	0.1088	0.5050	9.19	0.0871	−0.2885	11.48
Nucleus rotundus						
360	0.0741	−0.2979	13.50	0.0775	−0.0029	12.90
362	0.1120	0.0750	8.93	0.1154	−0.0600	8.67
364	0.1239	−0.2007	8.07	0.0919	−0.1879	10.88
367	0.0720	0.1393	13.89	0.0929	0.0800	10.76

[a] Constants a and b are taken from the regression equation $Y = aX + b$, where Y is the normal deviate of response probability and X is line orientation in degrees. SD gives the number of degrees of orientation change needed to move response probability through 1 standard deviation; it is equal to $1/a$.

Figures 7 and 8 show the performance of the anterior OPT cases. Preoperative SDs ranged from 8.39 deg to 17.38 deg. Postoperative SDs of birds 303 and 304 stabilized rapidly within a fraction of a degree of their preoperative values. Some initial loss of sensitivity, reflected in a rise in SD immediately following surgery, was seen in the data of bird 309. But for this subject, and more dramatically for bird 302, postoperative stabilization was delayed primarily by a trend toward decreasing SDs to below preoperative levels. These improvements in performance are seen as postoperative increases in slope of the psychometric functions of Fig. 8, and are probably due to continued training on the discrimination task rather than to any effect of the lesion.

Data from the posterior OPT group are presented in Figs. 9 and 10. Preoperative thresholds for birds 307 and 311 were 12.45 deg and 9.19 deg, respectively. In contrast to the anterior OPT group, SDs of these cases showed an immediate and stable elevation above the preoperative level to final values of 15.36 deg and 11.48 deg, respectively. In addition to the loss of sensitivity seen in the performance of both subjects, Fig. 10 reveals the only substantial change in response bias seen in the experiment, a switch by bird 311 from a right-key to a left-key preference.

The behavioral data for the nucleus rotundus group, shown in Figs. 11 and 12, reveal a range of effects. The SDs of bird 362, the subject with least damage to the rotundus, stabilized almost immedi-

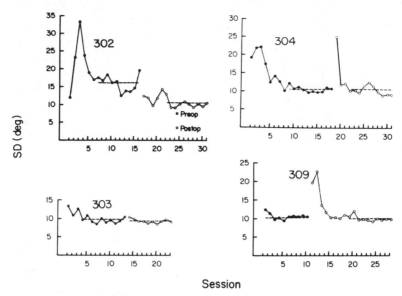

Fig. 7. Daily performance of subjects in the anterior OPT group. The dashed horizontal lines indicate the average of the final ten preoperative or postoperative SDs.

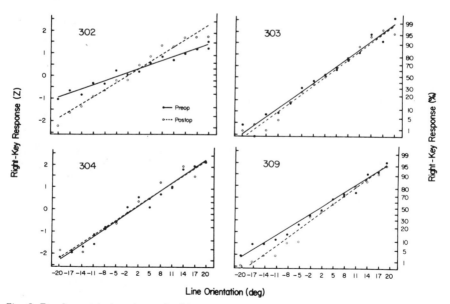

Fig. 8. Psychometric functions of subjects in the anterior OPT group taken from the final ten preoperative and postoperative sessions. Lines were fitted to the data points by the method of least squares.

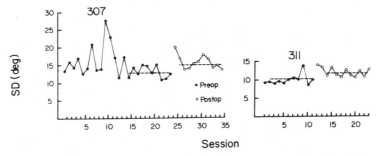

Fig. 9. Daily performance of subjects in the posterior OPT group. See Fig. 7 for details.

ately at the preoperative level, with no significant change in either sensitivity or bias apparent from the psychometric function. Birds 360 and 367, both with considerable involvement of the rotundus, showed severe performance losses immediately following surgery, coupled with increased session-to-session variability. With continued training, SDs stabilized below preoperative levels: the final pooled SD of bird 360 dropped from 13.50 deg to 12.90 deg; that of bird 367 from 13.89 deg to 10.76 deg. Paradoxically, bird 364, with the greatest damage to nucleus rotundus and no involvement of OPT, showed a behavioral effect resembling that seen in cases from the posterior OPT group. Data from individual sessions show an immediate and sustained rise in SD following surgery. Pooled data show a flattening of the psychometric function, and a rise in SD from 8.07 deg to 10.88 deg.

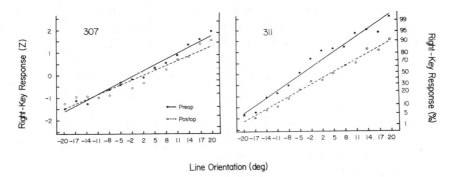

Fig. 10. Psychometric functions of subjects in the posterior OPT group. See Fig. 8 for details.

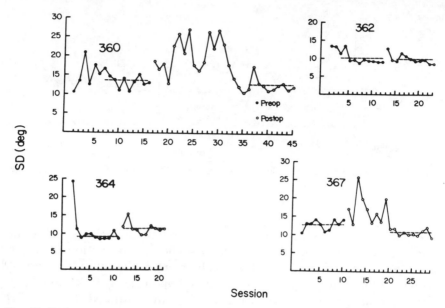

Fig. 11. Daily performance of subjects in the nucleus rotundus group. See Fig. 7 for details.

DISCUSSION

The results presented above extend the quantitative psychophysical analysis of lesions in the avian visual thalamus to include effects on processing of a spatial stimulus feature. Results from the nucleus rotundus and posterior OPT groups clearly demonstrate the influence of thalamic components of both tectofugal and thalamofugal visual pathways on the discrimination of stimulus orientation.

Similarities and differences between the present results and those obtained for intensity discrimination by Hodos and Bonbright (1974) are instructive.

In three of four cases, lesions of the nucleus rotundus affected orientation discrimination in the same way that such lesions affect intensity discrimination. When little tissue is involved, as in the case of bird 362, no deficit is seen. When bilateral damage to the rotundus is extensive, as in the cases of birds 360 and 367, discriminative performance deteriorates and becomes variable, but losses are ameliorated with continued testing.

The fourth case, bird 364, sustained the most complete damage to the nucleus rotundus, yet it did not show the postoperative deficit typical of other nucleus rotundus cases both in this experiment and in that of Hodos and Bonbright (1974). Rather, elevation of the SD after surgery was moderate and stable, resembling losses seen in perform-ance of the posterior OPT group. This paradoxical result suggests a more complex role for the nucleus rotundus than has been suspected. It is especially intriguing in light of Revzin's (this volume) report of receptive-field differences among neurons in several zones within the nucleus rotundus and bears investigation with additional subjects.

Pigeons in the posterior OPT group, like OPT cases in the intensity study, showed moderate but stable losses in the amount of stimulus change needed to bring about a fixed change in response probability. As Hodos and Bonbright (1974) emphasize, even apparently small elevations of threshold (or SD) actually represent considerable loss of the total resolving power of the visual system for differences along the tested stimulus dimension. Nevertheless, losses experienced by these subjects would not be revealed by most behavioral tests of vision, such as the vertical vs. horizontal line discrimination used by Hodos et al. (1973). The survival of considerable orientation-processing capacity after interruption of the thalamofugal pathway demonstrates that this is not the only pathway involved in analyzing spatial properties of stimuli.

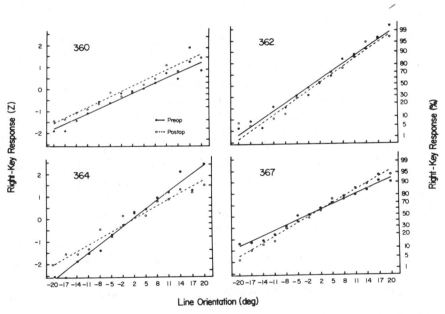

Fig. 12. Psychometric functions of subjects in the nucleus rotundus group. See Fig. 8 for details.

The most significant finding of the present study is the functional specialization revealed among the cell groups that compose OPT. Subjects in the anterior OPT group, with lesions confined primarily to LA and DLAmc, failed to show any postoperative deficits of orientation discrimination. This contrasts with the effects of similar lesions on intensity discrimination: two of the subjects in the Hodos and Bonbright (1974) study (birds C-431 and C-158) sustained lesions that would have placed them in the anterior OPT group of the present experiment, yet they showed clear postoperative losses of intensity discrimination. In view of the similarities between the methods used in the two studies, it is reasonable to look for the difference of results in the organization of visual processing in the thalamus.

One possible explanation rests on putative differences between the neural codes for intensity and for orientation. There is support for the view that intensity is coded as response frequency throughout the visual system, but that discrimination of strictly spatial features depends on the response of neurons "tuned'" for those features (Uttal, 1973, Chapters 6 and 8). According to this view, lesions anywhere in the OPT complex would lower the precision of intensity judgments by restricting the range of total visual system response to intensity. Orientation discrimination, on the other hand, would remain at preoperative levels of precision as long as specific groups of neurons, some presumably in posterior OPT, survived the lesion. The question of whether any such group of neurons exists in posterior and not anterior OPT requires electrophysiological investigaton.

A related explanation places the orientation-sensitive neurons in the projection field of OPT rather than in OPT itself. The area of OPT in which lesions produce orientation discrimination deficits is approximately coextensive with DLL, which projects to the visual Wulst (Meier et al., 1974). The Wulst contains neurons with oval receptive fields that may be especially sensitive to stimulus orientation (Revzin, 1969; O'Flaherty and Invernizzi, 1972). Thus lesions of posterior OPT may affect orientation discrimination by removing visual input from the Wulst. Parker (1971) has demonstrated that pigeons with Wulst ablations are capable of responding differentially to orientation. But neither the behavioral method (generalization testing) nor the stimulus spacing (10 deg) used in that study was intended to reveal sensory losses of the magnitude reported here. A replication of that study seems appropriate, using a psychophysical procedure and closely spaced stimuli.

The present results support comparison of the avian thalamofugal pathway to the mammalian geniculostriate pathway. A recent study by Pasik and Pasik (1976) demonstrated that monkeys exhibit modest orientation discrimination deficits after removal of striate cortex. That moderate and sustained losses of performance of this task follow interruption of the thalamofugal pathway in a bird and of the geniculo-striate pathway in a primate adds to the growing body of evidence that the structural similarities between these pathways (Nauta and Karten, 1970) are reflected in their contribution to visual behavior.

ACKNOWLEDGMENTS. The author thanks Dr. William Hodos for much useful discussion and assistance, and Eddie Penland and Beverly West for their help with processing of the histological materials.

REFERENCES

Blough, D. S.: Recognition by the pigeon of stimuli varying in two dimensions. *J. Exp. Anal. Behav.* **18**:345–367 (1972).

Bradley, J. V.: *Distribution-Free Statistical Tests*. Prentice-Hall, Englewood Cliffs, N.J. (1968).

Cowan, W. M., Adamson, L., and Powell, T. P. S.: An experimental study of the avian visual system. *J. Anat.* **95**:545–563 (1961).

Crossland, W. J.: Receptive field characteristics of some thalamic visual nuclei of the pigeon *Columba livia* (Abstr.). Ph.D. dissertation, University of Illinois at Urbana-Champaign (1972).

De Britto, L. R. G., Brunelli, M., Francesconi, W., and Magni, F.: Visual response pattern of thalamic neurons in the pigeon. *Brain Res.* **97**:337–343 (1975).

Heinemann, E. G., Avin, E., Sullivan, M. A., and Chase, S.: Analysis of stimulus generalization with a psychophysical method. *J. Exp. Psychol.* **80**:215–224 (1969).

Hodos, W., and Bonbright, J. C., Jr.: The detection of visual intensity differences by pigeons. *J. Exp. Anal. Behav.* **18**:471–479 (1972).

Hodos, W., and Bonbright, J. C., Jr.: Intensity difference thresholds in pigeons after lesions of the tectofugal and thalamofugal visual pathways. *J. Comp. Physiol. Psychol.* **87**:1013–1031 (1974).

Hodos, W., and Karten, H. J.: Brightness and pattern discrimination deficits in the pigeon after lesions of nucleus rotundus. *Exp. Brain Res.* **2**:151–167 (1966).

Hodos, W., Karten, H. J., and Bonbright, J. C., Jr.: Visual intensity and pattern discrimination deficits after lesions of the thalamofugal visual pathway in pigeons. *J. Comp. Neurol.* **148**:447–468 (1973).

Hunt, S. P., and Webster, K. E.: Thalamo-hyperstriate interrelations in the pigeon. *Brain Res.* **44**:647–651 (1972).

Jassik-Gerschenfeld, D., and Guichard, J.: Visual receptive fields of single cells in the pigeon's optic tectum. *Brain Res.* **40**:303–317 (1972).

Jassik-Gerschenfeld, D., Teulon, J., and Ropert, N.: Visual receptive field types in the nucleus dorsolateralis anterior of the pigeon's thalamus. *Brain Res.* **108**:295–306 (1976).

Karten, H. J., and Hodos, W.: *A Stereotaxic Atlas of the Brain of the Pigeon (Columba livia)*. Johns Hopkins Press, Baltimore (1967).

Karten, H. J., and Hodos, W.: Telencephalic projections of the nucleus rotundus in the pigeon *(Columba livia)*. *J. Comp. Neurol.* **140**:35–52 (1970).

Karten, H. J., and Nauta, W. J. H.: Organization of retino-thalamic projections in the pigeon and owl. *Anat. Rec.* **160**:373 (1968).

Karten, H. J., and Revzin, A. M.: The afferent connections of the nucleus rotundus in the pigeon. *Brain Res.* **2**:368–377 (1966).

Karten, H. J., Hodos, W., Nauta, W. J. H., and Revzin, A. M.: Neural connections of the "visual Wulst" of the avian telencephalon: Experimental studies in the pigeon (*Columba livia*) and owl (*Speotyto cunicularia*). *J. Comp. Neurol.* **150**:253–278 (1973).

Klüver, H., and Barrera, E.: A method for the combined staining of cells and fibers in the nervous sytem. *J. Neuropathol. Exp. Neurol.* **12**:400–403 (1953).

Maturana, H. R.: Functional organization of the pigeon retina. *22nd Int. Congr. Physiol. Soc., Leyden* (1962). Pp. 170–178.

Meier, R. E., Mihailović, J., and Cuénod, M: Thalamic organization of the retino-thalamo-hyperstriatal pathway in the pigeon (*Columba livia*). *Exp. Brain Res.* **19**:351–364 . (1974).

Nauta, W. J. H., and Karten, H. J.: A general profile of the vertebrate brain with sidelights on the ancestry of cerebral cortex. In Schmitt, F. O. (ed.): *The Neurosciences: Second Study Program*. Rockefeller University Press, New York (1970). Pp. 7–26.

O'Flaherty, J. J., and Invernizzi, G.: Functional organization of receptive fields of single visual units in the Wulst of the pigeon. *Boll. Soc. Biol. Sper.* **48**:137–139 (1972).

Parker, D. M.: Electrophysiological and behavioral studies of vision in the pigeon. Ph.D. dissertation, Durham (1971).

Pasik, P., and Pasik, T.: Discrimination of orientation in monkeys after removal of striate cortex. *Conf. Soc. Neurosci., Montreal* (1976).

Revzin, A. M.: A specific visual projection area in the hyperstriatum of the pigeon (*Columba livia*). *Brain Res.* **15**:246–249 (1969).

Revzin, A. M.: Some characteristics of wide-field units in the brain of the pigeon. *Brain Behav. Evol.* **3**:195–204 (1970).

Treisman, M., and Watts, T.R.: Relation between signal detectability theory and the traditional procedures for measuring sensory thresholds: Estimating d' from results given by the method of constant stimuli. *Psychol. Bull.* **66**:438–454 (1966).

Uttal, W. R.: *The Psychobiology of Sensory Coding*. Harper and Row, New York (1973).

Weiskrantz, L.: Contour discrimination in a young monkey with striate cortex ablation. *Neuropsychologia* **1**:145–164 (1963).

13

The Avian Visual Wulst:
I. An Anatomical Study of Afferent and Efferent Pathways.
II. An Electrophysiological Study of the Functional Properties of Single Neurons

D. MICELI, H. GIOANNI, J. REPÉRANT,
and J. PEYRICHOUX

INTRODUCTION

A number of anatomical studies using orthograde and retrograde degeneration techniques have provided data regarding the afferent and
efferent projections of the visual Wulst in the pigeon and the owl (Hunt
and Webster, 1972; Karten et al., 1973; Meier et al., 1974). The thalamo-
Wulst visual projection has also been investigated in the pigeon using
the method of retrograde labeling with horseradish peroxidase (HRP)
(Miceli et al., 1975). This chapter compares earlier findings related to
the organization of the retinothalamohyperstriatal pathway in the pi-

D. MICELI, H. GIOANNI, J. REPÉRANT, and J. PEYRICHOUX • Laboratoire de Psy-
chophysiologie Sensorielle, Université Pierre et Marie Curie, 75230 Paris Cédex 05, France.
This work was supported by INSERM Grants No. 76.1.042.6, No. 76.5.043.6, and C.N.
R.S. Grant (ERA No. 333).

geon with further observations made in the chick (*Gallus domesticus*) and herring gull (*Larus argentatus*) using the HRP method. It also reexamines the descending hyperstriatal projections in these species using the Fink–Heimer and autoradiographic techniques.

Another line of investigation has involved extracellular microelectrode recording of single-unit responses in the pigeon's Wulst to visual stimulation. Initial data derived from studies of the receptive-field properties of single neurons in the Wulst of the pigeon (Revzin, 1969; O'Flaherty and Invernizzi, 1971) have indicated movement to be a very effective stimulus parameter in driving units. However, the findings reported varied concerning the topographical location of visual units, the size and organization of receptive fields (RFs), and the existence of units with specific requirements for stimulus size, direction, and velocity of movement. We believe that the present study of the pigeon's Wulst is of interest not only because it attempts to elucidate some of the physiological properties characterizing Wulst neurons, but also in view of the recent reports of Pettigrew and Konishi (1976), who have described units in the owl's Wulst with functional properties similar to those of cells in the mammalian visual cortex. They have suggested, as has Revzin (1969), an analogous function between these structures.

ANATOMICAL STUDY

Material and Methods

The different anatomical procedures were undertaken jointly in the three species. Besides examining retinal projections with the Fink–Heimer and autoradiographic techniques (27 specimens), thalamohyperstriatal projections were investigated (38 specimens) using the HRP method after unilateral injection of 0.1–0.3 μl of HRP into different regions of the hyperstriatum, with survival periods ranging from 24 to 48 hr. Hyperstriatal projections were examined using the Fink–Heimer method after lesions of the Wulst produced by thermocoagulation (12 specimens, survival periods ranging from 2 to 10 days), and also using the autoradiographic technique following unilateral injections of 0.3–0.5 μl [^{3}H]proline (diluted to 15 μCi/μl) in the hyperstriatum (11 specimens, survival periods ranging from 2 to 8 days).

The nomenclature used in this chapter is essentially that of Karten and Hodos (1967).

Table 1. Abbreviations Used in this Chapter

AL	Ansa lenticularis	OM	Tractus occipitomesencephalicus
AP	Area pretectalis		
DLA	Nucleus dorsolateralis anterior thalami	Ov	Nucleus ovoidalis
		PPC	Nucleus principalis precommissuralis
DLAlr	Nucleus dorsolateralis anterior thalami pars lateralis rostralis	PT	Nucleus pretectalis
		PTM	Nucleus pretectalis medialis
DLAmc	Nucleus dorsolateralis anterior thalami pars magnocellularis	QF	Tractus quintofrontalis
		R	Nucleus rotundus
DLL	Nucleus dorsolateralis anterior thalami pars lateralis	RS	Nucleus reticularis superior
		SAC	Stratum album centrale
DLLd	Nucleus dorsolateralis anterior thalami pars lateralis pars dorsalis	SCE	Stratum cellulare externum
		SCI	Stratum cellulare internum
DLLv	Nucleus dorsolateralis anterior thalami pars lateralis pars ventralis	SGC	Stratum griseum centrale
DLM	Nucleus dorsolateralis anterior thalami pars medialis	SGF	Stratum griseum et fibrosum superficiale
		SMe	Stria medullaris
DLP	Nucleus dorsolateralis posterior thalami	SOp	Stratum opticum
		SP	Nucleus subpretectalis
DMA	Nucleus dorsomedialis anterior thalami	SPC	Nucleus superficialis parvocellularis
DSO	Decussatio supraoptica	SpL	Nucleus spiriformis lateralis
EM	Nucleus ectomammillaris	SpM	Nucleus spiriformis medialis
FPL	Fasciculus prosencephali lateralis	SR	Nucleus subrotundus
GLP	Nucleus geniculatus lateralis pretectalis	SS	Nucleus superficialis synencephali
GLv	Nucleus geniculatus lateralis pars ventralis	T	Nucleus triangularis
		TIO	Tractus isthmoopticus
GT	Nucleus griseus tectalis	TO	Tectum opticum
HA	Hyperstriatum accessorium	TR	Tractus opticus
		TSM	Tractus septomesencephalicus
HD	Hyperstriatum dorsale	TSMd	Tractus septomesencephalicus pars dorsalis
HIS	Hyperstriatum intercalatus superior	TSMv	Tractus septomesencephalicus pars ventralis
HM	Nucleus habenularis medialis	VLT	Nucleus ventrolateralis thalami
HV	Hyperstriatum ventrale	4,5,6,7,8,9,10	tectal layers 4–10 of Ramón y Cajal
ICT	Nucleus intercalatus thalami		
LA	Nucleus lateralis anterior thalami		

Results

The Retinothalamic Projection (Fig. 1). Similar results were produced with the Fink–Heimer and autoradiographic methods. Aside from contralateral retinal projections to the hypothalamus (zones 1, 2, and 3 of Meier, 1973), ventral thalamus (GLv), pretectum (AP, SS, GLP, GT), tectum (layers 1–7 of Ramón y Cajal), and tegmentum (EM), terminal arborization was observed in the dorsothalamic complex (LA, DLA). In DLA, the highest densities of optic fiber terminals were found in the ventral portion of DLLd, and lower densities were observed in ventrolateral regions of DLLv, as well as in DLAlr and DLAmc. On a number of Fink–Heimer preparations, some degenerating fibers were observed in the dorsal portion of DLLd and in SPC. Retinal projections were not detected in DLM and DLP.

Areas of the dorsal thalamus receiving retinal input were found to be more extensive and to contain higher densities of terminals in the gull compared to the pigeon and the chicken, respectively. In contrast to the thalamic projection, the GLv in *Larus* is much reduced, and in this species, as in *Columba*, the pretectal nuclei SS and GLP cannot be distinguished on the bases of cytoarchitectonic criteria. Conversely, in *Gallus*, the latter two nuclei are well differentiated and the GLv is well developed.

The Thalamohyperstriatal Pathway (Figs. 1A and 2). Following unilateral injection of HRP into the Wulst (HA, HIS, HD), peroxidase product was identified bilaterally in the dorsal thalamus; a similar pattern of labeling was observed in the three species examined. On the side ipsilateral to the injection, HRP-positive neurons were located in DLLv, in the ventral portion of DLLd, and more rostrally in DLAmc and DLAlr. The most prominent density of labeled neurons was observed in the ventral portion of DLLv overlying the nucleus rotundus. On the contralateral side, neurons containing HRP product were contained within a narrow region running along the dorsolateral edge of the DLA complex (DLLd, and in restricted regions of DLAlr and DLAmc). In the experimental cases where HRP injections were confined to superficial regions of the Wulst (HA and lateral, more superficial HIS), retrograde labeling was localized almost exclusively in the ipsilateral thalamus. No peroxidase product was ever observed in the nuclei LA, DLM, DLP, or DMA, and in SPC, contralateral to the injection, a small number of positive neurons were identified in only one case.

The retrograde HRP reaction was generally stronger in the chick material; this was particularly evident in the labeling observed in the

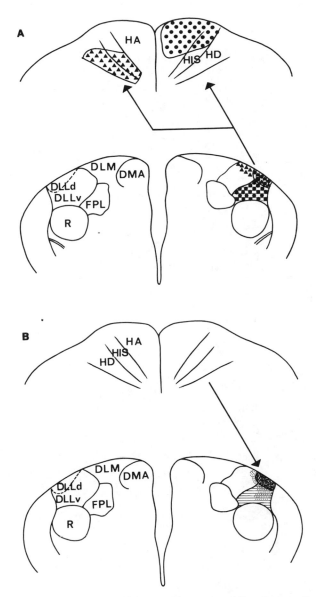

Fig. 1. Retinal projection to DLL. Vertical and horizontal lines, respectively, designate areas of high and low terminal density. Shown are areas of the DLL with ipsilateral (●), contralateral (▲), and bilateral projections to the Wulst (A) and the distribution of the Wulst projection onto DLL as indicated by fine dots (B). The highest density of Wulst fiber terminals is found in the ventral portion of DLLd, an area which is both a major target of retinal fibers attaining the DLL and at the origin of bilateral projections to the Wulst.

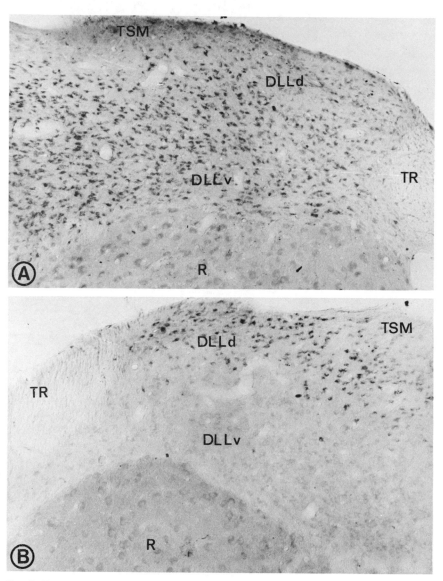

Fig. 2. Transverse sections through the thalamus of the chick showing the location of peroxidase-positive neurons in the ipsilateral DLLv and DLLd (A) and contralaterally in DLLd (B) following the injection of HRP into the Wulst. ×200, reproduced at 65%.

contralateral thalamus. Nevertheless, in all species, labeling was always heavier and more widespread in the ipsilateral thalamus than on the contralateral side. Labeled regions of the dorsal thalamus appeared to be more extensive in the gull than in the other species.

Efferent Pathways of the Wulst (Figs. 1B and 3–7). Aside from differences linked to the survival period and age of the animals, the pattern of fiber projections and terminals as determined with the Fink–Heimer and autoradiographic methods was consistent in all of the three species examined. From the Wulst, a very prominent system of fibers passed in the TSM, coursing medially to the ventricle in the telencephalon, and could be traced to the extreme dorsolateral edge of the rostral diencephalon. At this level, the main body of fibers (TSMd) continued caudally toward the mesencephalon by way of DLAlr, DLLd, and SPC, whereas a smaller fiber bundle coursed ventromedially, bypassing LA medially, and radiated through VLT to attain the GLv. From VLT, some fibers progressed medially and could be followed posteriorly as far as the level of EM, where they aggregated (TSMv) just dorsomedially to the latter nucleus. The destination of these fibers could not be determined on our material.

Fiber terminals were identified rostrally in the GLv, VLT, and ICT, and caudally the latter nuclei were innervated by fibers emerging between the nucleus rotundus and the marginal optic tract. Terminals were also observed in DLAlr and DLAmc. A very high terminal density was seen in the ventral portion of DLLd just above the optic tract, and relatively fewer terminals were observed in a restricted ventral region of DLLv and in SPC. From the latter nucleus, fibers passed ventrally to the visual AP, where some terminal arborizations were observed. These continued passing immediately lateral to PT, then passed ventrally to innervate other pretectal structures (SS, GLP, GT, PPC). Other fibers coursed laterally from AP in the direction of the tectum. In the latter, fibers terminated in the deeper layers (SGC, SAC), and more sparsely in the superficial layers. In the superficial layers, lower terminal densities were noted in the dorsal and lateral regions of the rostral tectum, and caudally fiber terminals were more difficult to detect. No projections were observed either to LA or to contralateral diencephalic and mesencephalic structures.

Evidence of another system of Wulst projections was suggested through the Fink–Heimer preparations, where some degenerating fibers of passage were seen to extend from the lesion site to subadjacent regions of HV. However, no degenerating boutons were detected in the latter or in any other areas of the telencephalon. On autoradiographic material, no silver grain concentrations were observed above

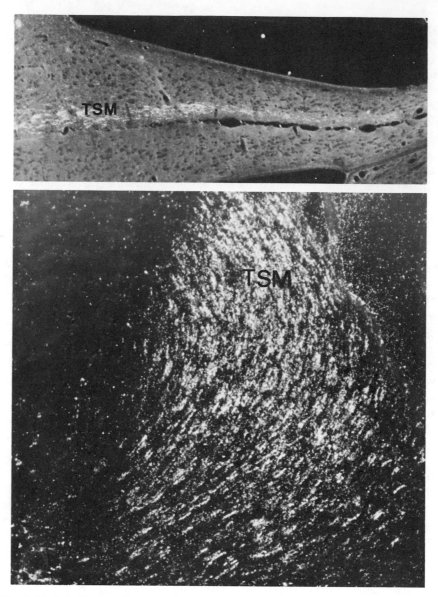

Fig. 3. Dark-field autoradiograms showing labeling of the ipsilateral TSM in the telece-phalon (top, ×50) and in the dorsolateral region of the rostral diecephalon (bottom, ×200) following the injection of [³H]proline into the Wulst.

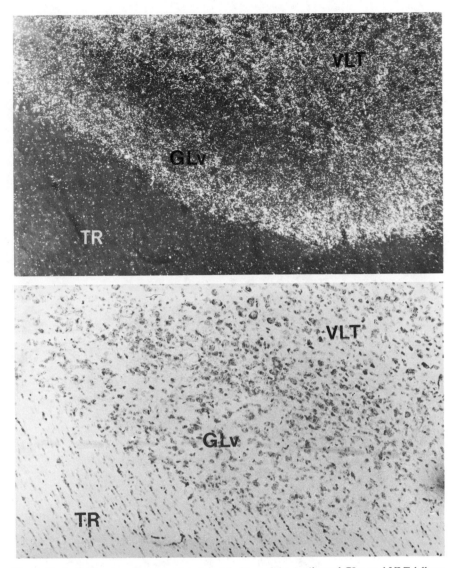

Fig. 4. Dark-field autoradiogram showing labeling of the ipsilateral GLv and VLT following the injection of [³H]proline into the Wulst (top) and the same region photographed under light-field conditions showing the cytoarchitecture of GLv and VLT (bottom). ×200, reproduced at 65%.

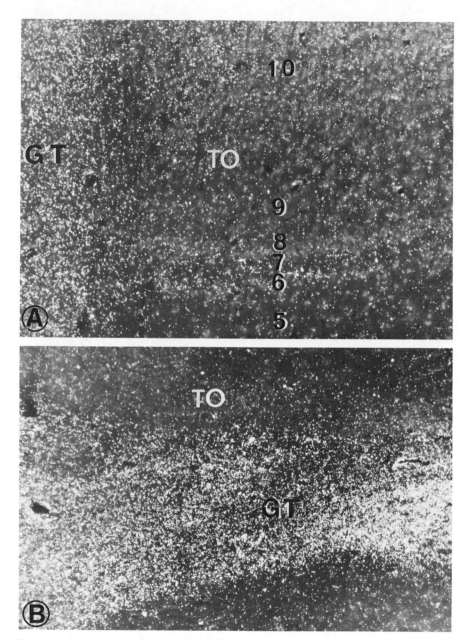

Fig. 5. Dark-field autoradiograms of labeling in ipsilateral tectopretectal regions after the injection of [³H]proline into the Wulst. A: Layers 5–10 of the ventral tectum and GT. Higher silver grain concentrations are present in GT (anterior portion) and in the deeper tectal layers. B: Heavy labeling of GT (rotated 90 deg clockwise). ×200, reproduced at 85%.

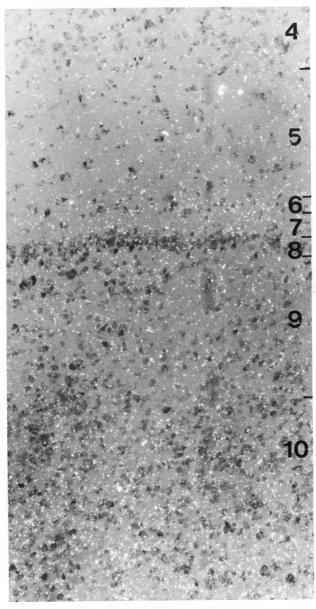

Fig. 6. Autoradiogram of the ipsilateral Wulst-tectal projection obtained 48 hr after the injection of [³H]proline into the Wulst. Higher silver grain concentrations are located in the deeper layers of the tectum. Photographed using a light-field–dark-field double exposure. ×200.

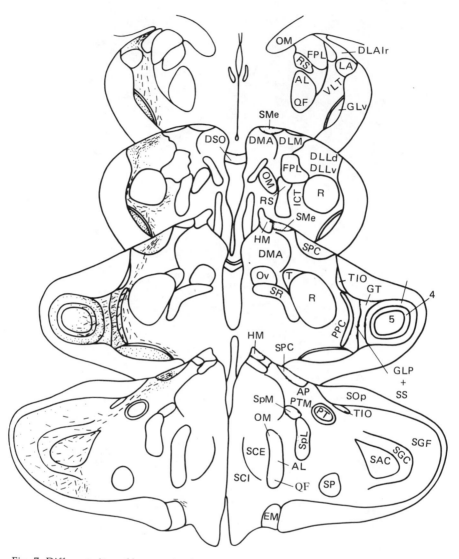

Fig. 7. Different sites of hyperstriatal projections in the diecephalon and mesencephalon of the pigeon. Fine dots indicate terminal arborizations, and thin dashes indicate fibers of passage.

the relatively high background levels present over large areas of the telencephalon.

Discussion

The thalamic nuclei which receive retinal fibers and in turn project to the Wulst are DLAlr, DLAmc, and DLL. Comparison of the ipsilateral and contralateral thalamic regions containing HRP product, after injections of the enzyme into the Wulst, revealed a partial overlap indicating the existence of three distinct areas with differential projections to the Wulst. In DLL, there exists a major area located in DLLv which projects to the ipsilateral Wulst, an area located in the dorsal portion of DLLd which projects to the contralateral Wulst, and an area situated in the ventral portion of DLLd which projects bilaterally to the Wulst. Differential projections to the Wulst were also apparent rostrally in DLAmc and DLAlr. The data obtained in the chick and the gull were consistent with the general pattern of organization of the thalamo-Wulst pathway previously described in the pigeon (Miceli et al., 1975).

A comparison of the thalamic labeling obtained with superficial and deep injections of HRP into the Wulst indicated that the ipsilateral and contralateral distributions of thalamic projections onto the Wulst were not homotopic (Fig. 1A). The visual thalamus projects ipsilaterally to HA and/or to lateral, more superficial regions of HIS and contralaterally to deeper, more medial regions of HIS and/or HD. Because of the extent of HRP spread at the injection site, we were unable to isolate HIS from HA, or HD from HIS and HA, which could account for the fact that exclusive labeling of the contralateral thalamus was never observed. These findings are compatible with data reported by Hunt and Webster (1972) and Webster (1974).

Descending projections from the Wulst were seen to terminate in the ipsilateral dorsal thalamus, ventral thalamus, pretectum, and tectum. This is in accord with the Wulst efferent system previously described in the owl and the pigeon (Karten et al., 1973). However, a projection to contralateral diencephalic and mesencephalic nuclei reported in the latter study was not observed in our material, or in Hunt and Webster's (1972) study, where only ipsilateral projections to the dorsal thalamus, tectum, and pretectum were noted. For all injections of tritiated proline, and even with very extensive lesions of the Wulst, labeling and orthograde degeneration were confined to ipsilateral structures. If there is indeed a contralateral projection, it is, in the species here examined, probably particularly reduced and difficult to detect with light microscopic techniques. Conclusive evidence could depend on demonstration at the electron microscopic level of either labeling or terminal degeneration.

The sites of termination of LA efferents are subject to controversy. For certain authors, this nucleus is part of the ventral thalamus (Rendahl, 1924; Powell and Cowan, 1961); for others, it has direct projections to the telencephalon and is part of the dorsal thalamus (Kuhlenbeck, 1937; Minelli, 1964; Meier et al., 1974) or, more precisely, projects to the Wulst (Edinger et al., 1903; Karten et al., 1973). Our results provided no indication that LA either contributes to the thalamo-Wulst pathway or receives a projection from the Wulst.

ELECTROPHYSIOLOGICAL STUDY

Material and Methods

Extracellular recordings of single units were obtained in the visual Wulst of pigeons immobilized with gallamine triethiodide (Flaxedil). Surgical procedures were carried out under light ethane disulfonate clometiazole (Hemineurine) anesthesia supplemented with xylocaïne anesthesia locally applied to all pressure points and surgical areas. The electrodes (15-20 MΩ) were glass micropipettes filled with a solution containing KCO_2CH_3 (0.1 M) and methyl blue. Blue markers were deposited by passing a 5-μA negative current through the electrode for 10 min at the deepest point of each vertical penetration and near the Wulst surface for later histological examination and reconstruction of the electrode path and unit recording coordinates. The Wulst was explored between the stereotaxic coordinates A 13.5-10.5 mm and L 2.5-0.75 mm (Karten and Hodos, 1967), because preliminary field potential recordings to diffuse light stimulation had shown the highest-amplitude and shortest-latency responses to be located within these regions (Miceli and Gioanni, unpublished data).

Contralateral RFs were mapped and analyzed on either a hemispheric screen (with the eye of the pigeon at the center) or a tangent screen. The experiments were carried out under low mesopic conditions (0.5-1 cd/m^2) employing light stimuli of a luminance of about 15 cd/m^2. Although stationary stimuli were tested, moving stimuli were mainly used because these were found to be the most effective in driving units. Light spots and bars of different sizes were displaced across the RF at various speeds and directions. Bar stimuli were oriented perpendicular to their axis of movement. The action potentials were led into a loudspeaker for auditory monitoring, were displayed on a storage oscilloscope, and could be filmed on a display oscilloscope or recorded on magnetic tape for later processing of poststimulus-time histograms (PSTHs cumulated over 20 stimulus presentations) on a Didac 4000 Intertechnique computer.

Results

Among the 170 units encountered in the Wulst, 90 responded to the different visual stimuli employed and 62 units were monitored for a sufficient length of time to allow various visual tests to be performed. In addition, five units were recorded which responded either to tactile and visual stimuli or to tactile stimulation alone. A number of units showed a rapid adaptation to repeated presentation of the same stimulus, a property which made the compiling of PSTHs difficult. Such units were excluded from the analysis. Forty-three percent of the visual units presented a continuous spontaneous average discharge of > 1 spike/sec, in many cases showing bursts of action potentials. A lower spontaneous activity (< 1 spike/sec) was observed in 45% of the units, while 12% showed occasional spikes separated by relatively long silent periods.

Figure 8 shows the center of each RF mapped, plotted on an equidistant polar projection of the visual field. In accordance with earlier reports (Galifret, 1968), the fovea, in relation to the center of the hemisphere, was placed at 10 deg eccentricity on the 150 deg meridian. The majority of the RFs (34, 55%) were located in the anterior–superior

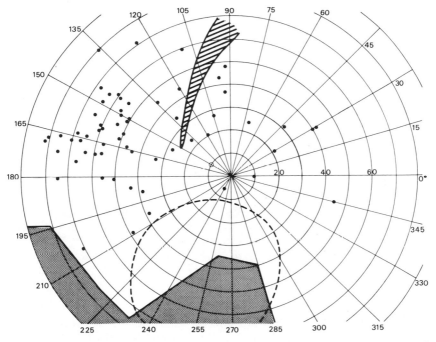

Fig. 8. Distribution of RF centers of the units studied shown on an equidistant polar projection of the visual field with the fovea (open circle) located on the 150-deg meridian at 10-deg eccentricity. The red-field projection area is bounded by the dashed line, and the segment of the visual field obscured by the containing apparatus is indicated by the shaded area.

quadrant between the meridians 135 and 180 deg and eccentricities 40 and 80 deg. RFs were not detected in either foveal or juxtafoveal areas of the visual field or in areas corresponding to the red-field projection of the retina.

As mentoned earlier, movement appeared to be the most potent stimulus parameter. Nevertheless, in the case of 22 units, audible ON and/or OFF discharges were detected with stationary stimuli. Moving light spots of small diameter (< 5 deg) were not very effective, and although the response increased with spot diameter, optimal responses were generated with straight edges or bars oriented perpendicular to their axis of movement. On the basis of their reponses to moving bar stimuli, the visual units studied were divided into two classes: non-orientation-selective cells (53%), which generated similar responses whatever the angular orientation or direction of movement of the stimulus, and orientation-selective cells (32%), which gave optimal responses to a particular orientation or range of orientations of the bar stimulus. In addition, for a given orientation of the bar, a number of units (15%) generated responses of higher magnitude for one direction of movement than for movement of the stimulus in the opposite direction, thus displaying direction selectivity.

RF Structure and Size. Most RFs of nonorientation units mapped were oval or approximately circular in shape. These cells gave either excitatory (increase in the cell's spontaneous discharge rate) or inhibitory (decrease in spontaneous discharge rate) responses to visual stimulation. Five units of this class had RFs composed of an excitatory central region and an inhibitory periphery, the latter either completely or only partially surrounding the center. RFs having inhibitory centers and excitatory surrounds were not observed. The RFs mapped for orientation-selective cells had rectangular or approximately rectangular shapes, and these units generated excitatory responses to visual stimulation. Inhibitory zones flanking two opposite margins of the excitatory region were detected in the case of four units and demonstrated by stimulating the RF with bars of different lengths.

The distribution of RF sizes for the visual units investigated is shown in the histogram of Fig. 9A. The dimensions ranged from 4.5 deg^2 to 2530 deg^2, with 75% of the units covering an area of the visual field between 20 deg^2 and 800 deg^2. The size distribution of RFs corresponding to orientation- and non-orientation-selective units are presented in the histograms of Fig. 9B. Nonorientation cells had RFs which were dominant in the 80–200 deg^2 size range (corresponding to a diameter of 10–16 deg). The RFs of orientation units showed a wider distribution extending toward the smaller size range, with 31% of these units having RFs smaller than 20 deg^2. The diversity of RF sizes with

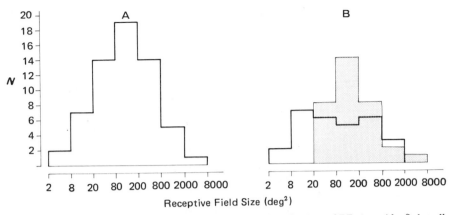

Fig. 9. Receptive field sizes. Histograms show the distribution of RF sizes (deg^2) for all of the units studied (A) and for non-orientation-selective (shaded area) and orientation-selective (thick line) units (B). The smallest and largest RFs were 4.5 deg^2 and 2530 deg^2.

respect to the location in the visual field for a sampling of 24 orientation-selective units is shown in Fig. 10.

Orientation, Movement Direction, and Velocity Selectivity. An example of the results obtained for an orientation-selective cell is shown in Fig. 11. The stimulus consisted of a light bar of 1.0 × 24.0 deg whose ends, for all angular orientations, extended well beyond the rectangular (4.0 × 9.0) excitatory region of the RF. The bar was displaced across the midpoint of the RF at constant velocity (1.8 deg/sec) and was always moved perpendicularly to its axis of orientation. PSTHs cumulated for opposite directions of movement to four angular orientations of the bar (radial intervals of 45 deg) are shown in Fig. 11A. The magnitude of the responses in terms of total number of spikes recorded for each direction of motion has been plotted using polar coordinates in Fig. 11C. The cell responded maximally for W-E and SW-NE orientations of the stimulus and hardly responded when the bar was oriented 90 deg to the latter, thus displaying orientation selectivity.

This same unit was subsequently tested using a shorter light bar which was displaced at the same velocity across the center of the RF perpendicular to the preferred and nonpreferred axes of orientation. The dimensions of the bar (1.0 × 2.0 deg) were such that, for all angular orientations, its extremities did not extend beyond the limits of the excitatory region. The PSTHs of the responses are shown in Fig. 11B, and the response magnitude for each direction of motion has been included in Fig. 11C. The previously observed orientation selectivity of the cell to the long bar stimulus was no longer apparent with the short bar. Responses of comparable amplitude were obtained for bar

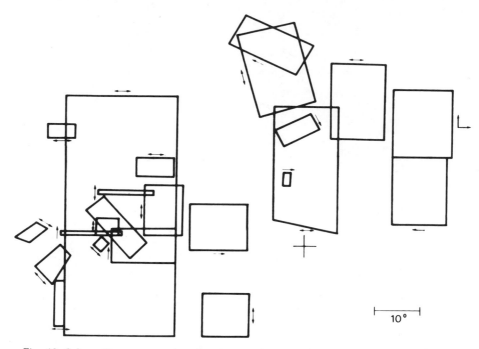

Fig. 10. Schematic representation showing the location and diversity of dimensions of the RFs for a sampling of 24 orientation-selective cells. The arrows indicate the direction of stimulus movement generating maximal responses. The anterior and superior visual fields are on the left and at the top of the diagram, respectively. The location of the fovea is indicated by the cross.

displacements in the SW, NE, and NW directions. Although all of the responses increased with the short bar, this stimulus provoked approximately a twofold increase in the response of the optimal axis of orientation and a more than tenfold average increase in the response of the nonpreferred axis of orientation. The changes in the response properties dependent on stimulus bar length can be explained by the presence of inhibitory regions flanking the longer axis of the rectangular excitatory center of the RF. Furthermore, these inhibitory regions appear to be a critical factor in determining the cell's orientation specificity.

The data obtained for another orientation-selective cell are shown in Fig. 12. The RF (1.5 × 3.0 deg) of this unit was stimulated with a light bar (0.5 × 5.0 deg) moving at constant speed (3.4 deg/sec). The responses to eight directions of movement (four orientations at 45-deg intervals) were recorded and processed as described for the preceding unit, and are shown in the illustration in the upper right-hand corner, using polar coordinates. The cell responded weakly to a SW-NE orientation, while more vigorous responses were obtained for a bar orientation 90 deg to the latter. Furthermore, the cell manifested a certain degree of directional selectivity; the responses obtained for movement in the NE and E directions were, respectively, 1.3 and 3.2 times larger than those recorded for motion in the corresponding opposite directions.

A velocity of 3.4 deg/sec was used in the orientation preference determination because an initial analysis, which consisted of adjusting bar orientation and displacement velocity until the loudest audible discharge was obtained, indicated that the optimal velocity fell within this range. The RF of this unit was stimulated by the same bar stimulus displaced in the optimal direction (toward E) and the responses to different velocities of movement were recorded (tested in ascending order: 0.85, 1.7, 3.4, 5.0, 10.0, and 20.0 deg/sec). The velocity preference curve of Fig. 12 was obtained by plotting the relative response at different velocities (total number of spikes cumulated in PSTHs) in relation to the optimal response (at 3.4 deg/sec). A fourfold decrease in the velocity (0.85 deg/sec) caused about a 45% decrease in the response. With a 1.5-fold increase in velocity, the response diminished by about 29%. For higher velocities tested, the response remained weak and relatively stable. The visual units showed varying degrees of selectivity for the velocity of stimulus movement. Depending on the unit, the preferred velocity ranged from about 1 to 50 deg/sec.

RFs with Complex Functional Structure. The data in Fig. 13A are the responses of a unit to the passage of a light bar of 0.5 × 26.0 deg across the RF and moving at a constant velocity of 5.6 deg/sec. This cell showed directional selectivity in that, for a NW-SE angular orientation of the bar, it was unresponsive to stimulus displacement in the NE direction and responded well for stimulus displacement in the opposite direction. In addition, the cell showed maximal firing for a N-S orientation of the bar and responded less vigorously for a bar orientation 90 deg to the latter, thus also exhibiting orientation selectivity.

An interesting feature of the response to the moving bar was seen when we compared the discharge patterns obtained with different axes of movement. In the axis of movement generating maximal responses (W-E), the discharge comprised two distinct components. This bimodal characteristic was also observed, although to a lesser degree, for the NW-SE axis of movement and was absent in the two remaining axes tested. The observed bimodality cannot be attributed to an ON-OFF type of effect produced by the stimulus entering and leaving the RF, as the intermodal interval was in the order of 1.2 sec, whereas the time taken by the stimulus to scan the RF was approximately 3 sec. It would

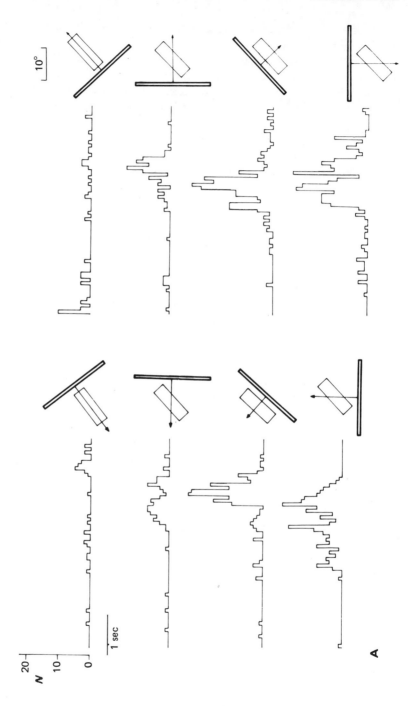

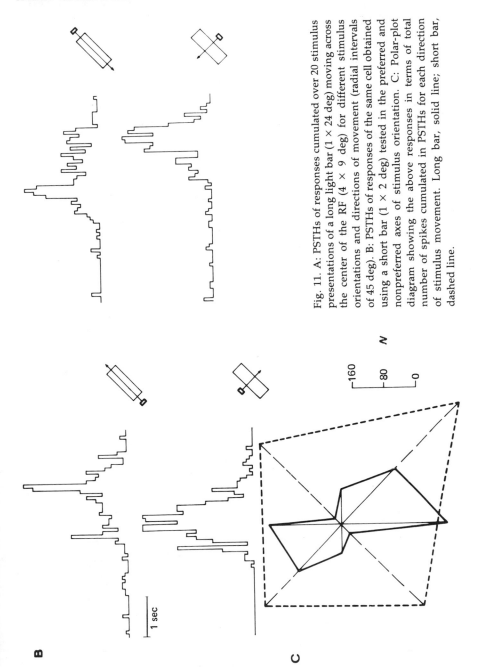

Fig. 11. A: PSTHs of responses cumulated over 20 stimulus presentations of a long light bar (1 × 24 deg) moving across the center of the RF (4 × 9 deg) for different stimulus orientations and directions of movement (radial intervals of 45 deg). B: PSTHs of responses of the same cell obtained using a short bar (1 × 2 deg) tested in the preferred and nonpreferred axes of stimulus orientation. C: Polar-plot diagram showing the above responses in terms of total number of spikes cumulated in PSTHs for each direction of stimulus movement. Long bar, solid line; short bar, dashed line.

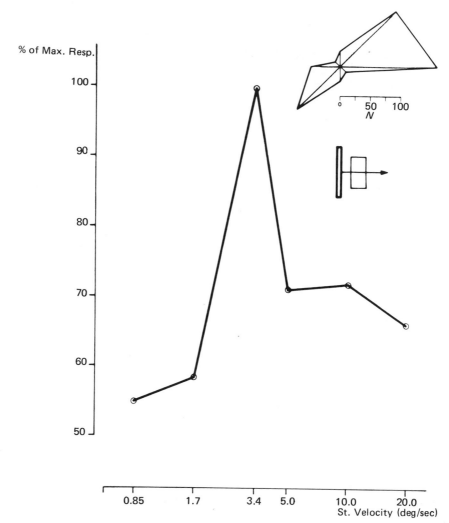

Fig. 12. Stimulus-velocity preference curve of an orientation-selective unit showing the response magnitude measured as a percentage of the optimal response obtained using a stimulus velocity of 3.4 deg/sec (total number of spikes in PSTHs cumulated over 20 stimulus presentations). The preliminary orientation-direction preference data for this unit are illustrated by the polar-plot diagram in the upper right-hand corner of the figure. The velocity preference determinations were performed under optimal stimulus-orientation (N-S) and displacement-direction (toward E) conditions.

appear that the excitatory region of the RF is not homogeneous but is made up of two distinct and highly excitable zones. Presumably, the bimodal response is most clearly manifest when these two zones are stimulated in succession (E-W axis).

The RF of this unit was also tested with stationary ON-OFF type stimuli; the PSTHs of responses to three different rectangular light stimuli of increasing size (1.6 × 8.0 deg, 6.0 × 12.0 deg, 8.5 × 17.0 deg) presented at the center of the RF (5-sec duration) are shown in Fig. 13B. The smallest stimulus evoked phasic ON and OFF responses accompanied by a sustained subtotal inhibition of the cell's spontaneous activity lasting throughout the period of stimulation. Increasing the stimulus size resulted in a depression of the ON response which was almost totally suppressed by a stimulus completely covering the area of the RF. This was also associated with a sustained inhibition during the stimulation period and a considerable increase in the OFF response. These modifications of the response produced by stimulation of ever-larger areas of the RF suggest the progressive involvement of inhibitory regions present in the field, in addition to the previously described excitatory regions.

Location of Visual Units in the Wulst. The data regarding the location of the visual units investigated are shown in Figure 14. The cells were situated in HA and HIS, and although HD was also explored no cell in this layer appeared to respond to any of our visual stimuli. In the Wulst, neither a particular topographical arrangement of orientation- and non-orientation-selective units nor a precise retinotopic organization in the rostrocaudal or mediolateral plane was observed. Some evidence of a relationship between the RF location and the depth of recording in the Wulst was apparent for electrode penetration at *A* 12.0 mm (comprising 45% of the visual units studied). The RFs of cells near the surface (0–100 μm) were situated in the posterior visual field. The RF location of deeper units (101–1000 μm) showed a sharp transition to anterior regions of the field and with increasing depth beyond about 1 mm, the mean RF position passed high in the superior field, then progressed in the direction of the fovea. A similar consistent displacement of the RF position was not detected at other anterior planes in the Wulst.

Although tactile stimulation was not performed systematically, three units were identified which generated either excitatory or inhibitory responses to stroking of the feathers on the animal's back. Furthermore, two units were found which responded to both tactile and visual stimulation by a sustained discharge in activity lasting the duration of the stimulation. In the latter cases, the tactile stimulation was

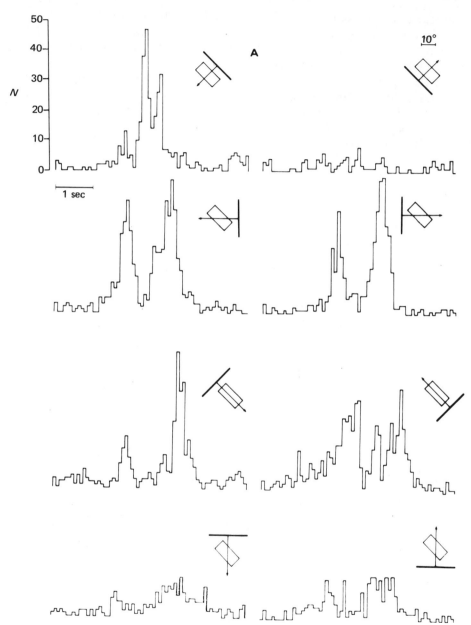

Fig. 13. A: PSTHs of responses of an orientation-direction-selective unit whose RF (7.5 × 16.0 deg) was stimulated with a moving light bar (0.5 × 26.0 deg) according to the same procedure described in Fig. 11A. B: PSTHs of responses of this same unit to stationary rectangular light stimuli of increasing size (1.6 × 8.0 deg, 6.0 × 12 deg, 8.5 × 17.0 deg) centered on the midpoint of the RF. Stimulus duration 5 sec.

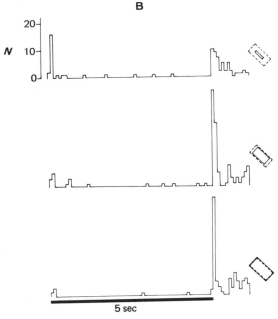

Fig. 13. (*Continued*)

restricted either to the back of the animal or to the leg extremities. The visual stimuli employed in driving these units were either diffuse light stimulation of relatively large areas of the visual field or randomly moving spots or bars of light. The visual RFs of these units could not be delineated. All effective stimuli were contralateral to the recording and these units were located in HA of the Wulst (A 12.5 and 12.0 mm) and in proximity to purely visual units (Fig. 15).

Discussion

Much of our data are in agreement with findings obtained in the owl Wulst (Pettigrew and Konishi, 1976), yet oddly enough striking differences appear among the findings derived from the Wulst of the pigeon, particularly concerning the topographical distribution of visual units, the size and complexity of organization of RFs, and the specific requirements for stimulus shape, orientation, direction, and velocity of movement. Visual units responding to contralateral eye stimulation were found throughout the superficial layers HA and HIS of the Wulst. A wide distribution of visual units in the pigeon Wulst, extending from 100 μm to 2700 μm beneath the surface, was also reported by O'Flaherty and Invernizzi (1971). By comparison, Revzin (1969), who

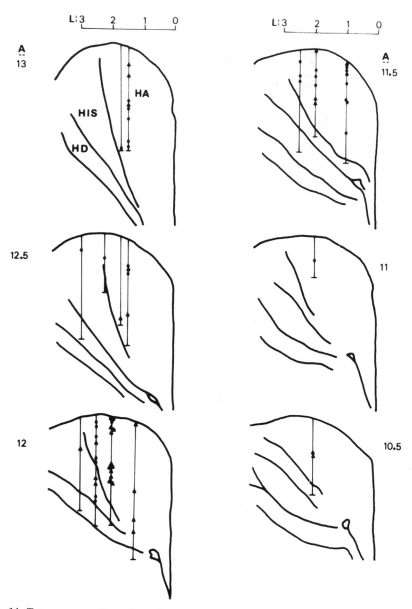

Fig. 14. Transverse sections through the pigeon's Wulst (from Karten and Hodos, 1967) showing the location of non-orientation-selective (●) and orientation-selective (▲) units examined for all microelectrode penetrations. *A,* Anterior planes; *L,* lateral coordinates (mm).

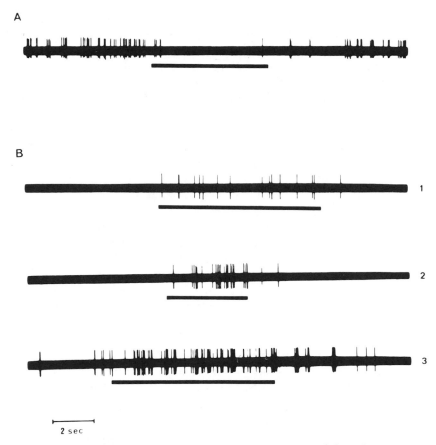

Fig. 15. Cells responding to tactile stimulation. A: Inhibition of the cell's spontaneous activity produced by brushing of the feathers on the animal's back. B: Visual and somesthethic unit: (1) response to visual stimuli randomly moved in the visual field; (2) response to light tactile stimulation applied to the leg extremities; (3) response produced by a combination of the visual and tactile stimuli.

worked on the anesthetized preparation (urethane), found visual units organized in columns oriented perpendicular to the HA-HIS boundary and in a more restricted region of the Wulst. It should also be noted that in O'Flaherty and Invernizzi's investigation 85.4% of Wulst units were driven by visual stimulation, compared with 53% in our experiments, while Revzin reported that only a fraction of the Wulst neuron population responded to visual stimulation.

The RFs of units in the pigeon Wulst have been described as circular or oval in shape, and the units exhibited either excitatory or inhibitory responses to visual stimulation. A larger number of the RFs mapped in the present study were rectangular in shape. Some RFs were composed of distinct antagonistic regions. Rectangular and circular RFs possessing antagonistic regions have also been reported in the Wulst of the owl (Pettigrew and Konishi, 1976).

In the pigeon Wulst, Revzin gave dimensions of RFs of between 3 and 80 deg^2 (2–10 deg diameter). Thirty-seven percent of the units mapped in the present investigation were comparable in size ($<$ 80 deg^2); the remainder showed sizes varying from 80 to 2530 deg^2, values which are in closer agreement with those provided by O'Flaherty and Invernizzi (oval-shaped RFs; 10–45 $\times$ 12–80 deg corresponding to a mean area of 1800 deg^2). For a given electrode penetration, Pettigrew and Konishi illustrated RF sizes varying from about 1 deg^2 to 180 deg^2.

O'Flaherty and Invernizzi noted that stimulus dimensions of 15–25 deg were the most effective in driving units; decreasing the stimulus size resulted in a reduction of the response, and, for sizes $<$5 deg, no response was obtained. Similar results were observed in the present study in the case of spot stimuli. By far, bar and edge stimuli were always more effective, suggesting that Wulst units are edge detectors rather than convexity detectors. Similarly, a very large proportion of the neurons in the owl Wulst were reported to respond optimally to moving edge stimuli (Pettigrew and Konishi). Revzin noted no marked preference for stimulus shape for most units, and O'Flaherty and Invernizzi made no mention of the shapes of stimuli employed in their investigation.

On the basis of their reponse to moving bar stimuli, the visual units here examined were divided into non-orientation selective and orientation selective. Among the latter group, approximately one-third (15%) showed direction selectivity. A similar proportion of units (12.5%) showing direction preference were reported by O'Flaherty and Invernizzi. Revzin described two units as horizontal line detectors (orientation-selective cells). Elsewhere, orientation and direction selectivity appear to be an important feature of Wulst units in the owl (Pettigrew and Konishi).

Velocity preference for stimulus movement has been recognized in Wulst units in the owl (Pettigrew and Konishi) and the pigeon (O'Flaherty and Invernizzi). In the latter study, the optimal velocities ranged from 28 to 100 deg/sec. Our results show the range of optimal velocities to be relatively lower, falling between 1 and 50 deg/sec.

One explanation offered by O'Flaherty and Invernizzi which could account for such differences in the findings is linked to changes in the general properties of visual units related to the mode of anesthesia employed, Revzin using urethane and Pettigrew and Konishi using ketamine. The investigations of O'Flaherty and Invernizzi, as well as our own, were carried out without using general anesthesia. Another explanation is related to the level of light adaptation in which the animal was placed as well as the stimulus parameters used (luminance, size, shape, and dynamic properties of the stimulus). Similarly the distribution of the recording sites in the Wulst and the location of the stimulated areas of the retina may well be other contributory factors.

GENERAL DISCUSSION

There is evidence that the Wulst is composed of functionally distinct regions and receives inputs which are other than visual. Karten et al. (1973) have reported projections, arising from nonvisual dorso-medial nuclei of the thalamus (DLM, DMA), to a more medial portion of HD, a system which is anatomically and functionally distinct from the DLA-Wulst system. Elsewhere, Delius and Bennetto (1972) have recorded both auditory and somesthetic evoked potentials in the rostral Wulst in front of hyperstriatal regions receiving visual information. Our finding of units in the pigeon's Wulst responding to visual and/or tactile stimulation indicates some degree of sensory overlap. Furthermore, the visual stimuli employed in the present study were ineffective in driving units in regions of the Wulst caudal to the coordinate A 10.5 mm. This coincided with areas of the Wulst where field potentials evoked by diffuse light stimulation were of rather low amplitude and long latency (Miceli and Gioanni, unpublished data). It is conceivable that this posterior region of the Wulst has functionally different properties from those of the more anterior region.

The anatomical data provided by the present study indicate that the highest density of Wulst fiber terminals attaining the DLL are located in the ventral portion of DLLd, an area which is both a major target of retinal fibers innervating the dorsal thalamus and at the origin of bilateral projections to the Wulst. Such an arrangement suggests that the thalamus–Wulst–thalamus system may be implicated in the processing of binocular information. Furthermore, it is interesting to note that the projection from the Wulst to the tectum appears to be denser in rostral and ventral regions of the tectum, an area coinciding with the representation of the red field of the pigeon's retina (Hamdi and Whitteridge, 1954; McGill et al., 1966) and probably encompassing a large segment of the binocular visual field.

Our electrophysiological investigation of the pigeon's Wulst demonstrated the presence of units with specific requirements for stimulus shape, preferring rectilinear over convex stimuli. In addition, Wulst units displayed selectivity for stimulus orientation and for direction and velocity of movement. These findings are comparable with previously reported data obtained in the owl Wulst where, in addition, units driven by binocular stimulation and selectivity for binocular disparity were reported (Pettigrew and Konishi, 1976). On the basis of similarities with the cell properties of the mammalian visual cortex, these authors have suggested an analogous function.

The present investigation also showed a high degree of complexity related to RF organization. Some of the units classed as orientation selective displayed RFs consisting of a rectangular excitatory region bounded on two opposite margins by inhibitory zones. The responses generated as a result of a change in the bar length used for the stimulation showed that the lateral inhibitory zones strongly reinforced the cell's specificity for stimulus orientation. Similar properties have been described to account for the behavior of some simple cells in the mammalian visual cortex (Henry and Bishop, 1972; Henry et al., 1974).

Other RFs examined in the present study appeared to be composed of several subregions generating polyphasic patterns of discharge to a moving, adequately oriented bar stimulus, a property which is compatible with the RF organization of "multimodal" units of the mammalian visual cortex (Pettigrew et al., 1968; Henry and Bishop, 1972; Sherman et al., 1976).

The presence of units displaying highly specific stimulus requirements at both the peripheral (Maturana, 1962; Maturana and Frenk, 1963; Pearlman and Hughes, 1976) and telencephalic visual system of the pigeon's thalamofugal pathway is in sharp contrast to the stepwise emergence of complex functions observed at the different levels of this pathway in the cat and the monkey. Nevertheless, the very specialized properties observed in the visual cortex are the result of the transformation of visual information, as such properties are not present at the LGN level, much in the same way as the properties of visual neurons in the avian Wulst do not only appear to reflect the activity of DLA neurons. The latter have been described as having concentric RFs, the majority of which responded to stationary spot stimulation (Jassik-Gerschenfeld et al., 1976; Pettigrew and Konishi, 1976), properties resembling those of LGN neurons.

ACKNOWLEDGMENTS. We wish to thank Dr. Jean-Pierre Raffin for his helpful cooperation; Dr. Yves Galifret for his support and useful comments and criticism of the manuscript; Mr. A. Gordon for his excellent technical assistance; and Mrs. F. Lanery and G. Sanchez for their secretarial assistance.

REFERENCES

Delius, J. D., and Bennetto, K.: Cutaneous sensory projections to the avian forebrain. *Brain Res.* **37:**205–221 (1972).

Edinger, L., Wallenberg, A., and Holmes, G.: Untersuchungen über die vergleichende Anatomie des Gehirns. 5. Untersuchungen über das Vorderhirn der Vögel. *Abh. Senckemb. Naturforsch. Ges.* **20:**343–426 (1903).

Galifret, Y.: Les diverses aires fonctionnelles de la rétine du Pigeon. *Z. Zellforsch. Mikrosk. Anat.* **86:**535–545 (1968).

Hamdi, F. A., and Whitteridge, D.: The representation of the retina on the optic tectum of the pigeon. *Q. J. Exp. Physiol.* **39:**111–119 (1954).

Henry, G. H., and Bishop, P. O.: Striate neurons: Receptive field organization. *Invest. Ophthalmol.* **11:**357–368 (1972).

Henry, G. H., Bishop, P. O., and Dreher, B.: Orientation axis and direction as stimulus parameters for striate cells. *Vision Res.* **14:**767–777 (1974).

Hunt, S. P., and Webster, K. E.: Thalamo-hyperstriate interrelations in the pigeon. *Brain Res.* **44:**647–651 (1972).

Jassik-Gerschenfeld, D., Teulon, J., and Ropert, N.: Visual receptive field types in the nucleus dorsolateralis anterior of the pigeon's thalamus. *Brain Res.* **108:**295–306 (1976).

Karten, H. J., and Hodos, W.: *A Stereotaxic Atlas of the Brain of the Pigeon (Columba livia).* Johns Hopkins Press, Baltimore (1967).

Karten, H. J., Hodos, W., Nauta, W. J. H., and Revzin, A. M.: Neural connections of the visual Wulst of the avian telencephalon: Experimental studies in the pigeon (*Columba livia*) and owl (*Speotyto canicularia*). *J. Comp. Neurol.* **150:**253–276 (1973).

Kuhlenbeck, H.: The ontogenetic development of the diencephalic centers in a bird's brain (chick) and comparison with the reptilian and mammalian diencephalon. *J. Comp. Neurol.* **66:**23–75 (1937).

Maturana, H. R.: Functional organization of the pigeon retina. In *22nd Int. Congr. Physiol. Sci., Leyden* (1962). Pp. 170–178.

Maturana, H. R., and Frenk, S.: Directional movement and horizontal edge detectors in the pigeon retina. *Science* **150:**977–979 (1963).

McGill, J. I., Powell, T. P. S., and Cowan, W. M.: The retinal representation upon the optic tectum and isthmo-optic nucleus in the pigeon. *J. Anat.* **100:**5–33 (1966).

Meier, R. E.: Autoradiographic evidence for a direct retino-hypothalamic projection in the avian brain. *Brain Res.* **53:**417–421 (1973).

Meier, R. E., Mihailović, J., and Cuénod M.: Thalamic organization of the retino-thalamo-hyperstriatal pathway in the pigeon (*Columba livia*). *Exp. Brain Res.* **19:** 351–364 (1974).

Miceli, D., Peyrichoux, J., and Repérant, J.: The retino-thalamo-hyperstriatal pathway in the pigeon (*Columba livia*). *Brain Res.* **100:**125–131 (1975).

Minelli, G.: Effeti delle degenerazioni sperimentali sulle corteccie e sui nuclei basali del telencefalo di Gallus e Coturnix. *Boll. Zool.* **31:**1273–1292 (1964).

O'Flaherty, J. J., and Invernizzi, G.: Organizzazione funzionale dei campi recettivi di singola unità visive del "Wulst" nel piccione. *Boll. Soc. Ital. Biol. Sper.* **158:**137–138 (1971).

Pearlman, A. L., and Hughes, C. P.: Functional role of efferents to the avian retina. Analysis of retinal ganglion cell receptive fields. *J. Comp. Neurol.* **166:**111–131 (1976).

Pettigrew, J. D., and Konishi, M.: Neurons selective for orientation and binocular disparity in the visual Wulst of the barn owl (*Typo alba*). *Science* **193:**675–678 (1976).

Pettigrew, J. D., Nikara, T., and Bishop, P. O.: Responses to moving slits by single neurons in the cat striate cortex. *Exp. Brain Res.* **6:**373–390 (1968).

Powell, T. P. S., and Cowan, W. M.: The thalamic projection on the telencephalon in the pigeon (*Columba livia*). *J. Anat.* **95:**78–109 (1961).

Rendahl, H.: Embryologische und morphologische Studien über das Zwischenhirn beim Huhn. *Acta Zool.* **5:**241–344 (1924).

Revzin, A. M.: A specific visual projection area in the hyperstriatum of the pigeon. *Brain Res.* **15:**246–249 (1969).

Sherman, S. M., Watkins, D. W., and Wilson, J. R.: Further differences in receptive field properties of simple and complex cells in cat striate cortex. *Vision Res.* **16:**919–927 (1976).

Webster, K. E.: Changing concepts of the organization of central visual pathway in birds. In Bellairs, R., and Grays, E. G. (eds.): *Essays on the Nervous System.* Oxford University Press, Oxford (1974). Pp. 258–298.

14

Neuroanatomical Aspects of the Vestibular System of the Pigeon

R. L. BOORD and H. J. KARTEN

INTRODUCTION

Recent studies on the anatomy of the avian vestibular nuclei and their afferent connections with the root fibers of the eighth cranial nerve have partially clarified discrepancies concerning the delineation of those cell groups that constitute the vestibular nuclear complex (VNC). For example, Boord and Karten (1974) have delimited those subdivisions of the VNC that receive an input from the lagenar component of the statoacoustic nerve of the pigeon. Wold (1975, 1976) has delineated the vestibular area of the chicken based on the simultaneous examination of cell and fiber stained normal material and experimental material processed by silver impregnation methods to reveal degenerating axons and terminals following lesions of the entire vestibular ganglion. Peusner and Morest (1977) have contributed to our knowledge of the topography and cellular structure of the tangential nucleus and its relations to vestibular root fibers of the chick embryo.

Despite these studies, the central projections of those components of the vestibular nerve that supply individual labyrinthine end organs remain uncertain. While the protocols used in the present series of

R. L. BOORD • School of Life and Health Sciences and Institute for Neuroscience and Behavior, University of Delaware, Newark, Delaware 19711.   H. J. KARTEN • Departments of Psychiatry and Behavioral Science and Anatomical Sciences, Health Sciences Center–School of Medicine, State University of New York, Stony Brook, New York 11794.
This work was supported by PHS Special Research Fellowship NS02088 and Grant NS 11272 to R. L. Boord.

experiments preclude a description of specific afferent cell connections of the various rami of the vestibular nerve, they did determine, to some degree, the differential projections of parts of the vestibular nerve within the VNC. Furthermore, as emphasized by Gacek (1969), it is essential to know the specific areas of the vestibular ganglion associated with particular nerves from labyrinthine receptors and the positional relationships of these nerves proximal to the ganglion in order to reliably interpret differential medullary projections of primary vestibular neurons. The anatomical organization of the vestibular nerve and its ganglion, as well as the topography of the superficial vestibular nerve roots, is therefore included.

THE STATOACOUSTIC NERVE AND GANGLION

The most favorable method to study the topographic organization of the statoacoustic nerve is by direct dissection following staining with Sudan black B of the otic capsule, containing the inner ear, and that segment of the medulla containing the superficial nerve root (Rasmussen, 1961). By this method, the various rami of the statoacoustic nerve can be traced from their end organs through the ganglion to their entrance into the medulla. The specific areas of the ganglion associated with the nerves from the labyrinthine receptors and the positional relationships of these nerves proximal to the ganglion can then be determined.

The statoacoustic nerve of the pigeon (Fig. 1) is divided into anterior, posterior, and cochleolagenar rami. The anterior ramus, equivalent to the superior vestibular nerve, consists of branches that innervate the cristae of the anterior and lateral semicircular canals and the utricular macula. The posterior ramus, equivalent to the inferior vestibular nerve, receives branches from the crista of the posterior semicircular canal, macula of the saccule, and crista neglecta. The cochleolagenar nerve consists of cochlear and lagenar components that innervate the papilla basilaris (organ of Corti) and macula of the lagena, respectively.

The neurons that constitute the statoacoustic nerve have their origin in four ganglionic masses that correspond to the four main branches, i.e., an anterior (superior) vestibular ganglion, a posterior (inferior) vestibular ganglion, and cochlear and lagenar ganglia. The cochlear and lagenar ganglia lie within the otic capsule, whereas both parts of the vestibular ganglion are situated within the internal auditory meatus medial to the entrance of the various vestibular branches through their foramina.

Fig. 1. Statoacoustic nerve of the pigeon mostly immediately proximal but partially through the ganglion, showing the positional relationships of the various vestibular nerve branches. The proximal cut ends of these branches correspond to those parts of the vestibular ganglion related to each branch. The cochleolagenar nerve lies in a groove in the posterior ampullary nerve as the latter swings over the for-

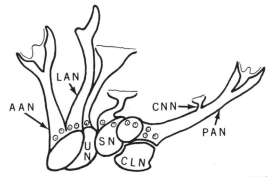

mer to reach the main vestibular nerve. Abbreviations: AAN, anterior canal nerve; CLN, cochleolagenar nerve; CNN, nerve of the crista neglecta; LAN, lateral canal nerve; PAN, posterior canal nerve; SN, saccular nerve; UN, utricular nerve.

Each branch of the vestibular nerve is a separate nerve that is traceable from its end organ through the ganglion to its entrance into the medulla. The cell bodies of origin of the posterior canal nerve occupy the caudal and dorsal part of the posterior vestibular ganglion, while those associated with the saccule lie within the rostral and ventral part. Some posterior canal ganglion cells are distributed along the proximal portion of the posterior canal nerve as the latter courses peripherally over the cochleolagenar nerve trunk. The cells of origin of those axons that innervate the crista neglecta are unknown.

The ganglion cells associated with the anterior and horizontal canal nerves comprise the rostrodorsal part of the anterior vestibular ganglion, and utricular ganglion cells occupy the caudoventral portion. The organization of the vestibular nerve at a level immediately proximal to the ganglion is shown in Fig. 1.

The proximal axons of the eighth nerve enter the brain stem in a slightly different sequence than the sequence of ganglion cells associated with each nerve component. The cochlear nerve enters most caudal and dorsal, followed by the lagenar nerve more ventral and rostral in position. The saccular nerve takes a straight course from its cells of origin in the rostroventral part of the posterior vestibular ganglion to enter the medulla immediately rostral and ventral to lagenar fibers. The posterior canal nerve swings over the cochleolagenar nerve trunk and beneath the saccular nerve to penetrate the medulla just ventral and rostral to the latter. The anterior and horizontal canal trunk enters the medulla just rostral and ventral to the posterior canal nerve. The utricular nerve enters caudal to the anterior and horizontal canal nerves.

The canal nerves are intimately associated with each other at their entrance into the medulla, but the macular nerves appear separated. The positional relationships of the superficial roots of the various branches of the statoacoustic nerve are shown in Fig. 2.

THE VESTIBULAR NUCLEAR COMPLEX (VNC)

The vestibular nuclear complex (VNC) of the pigeon can be subdivided into the following major territories, i.e., superior, medial, lateral (Deiters), descending, and tangential nuclei. However, several subdivisions of these main nuclei, as well as interspersed cell groups, are recognized by previous authors but are difficult to reliably identify due most likely to different planes of sections. The following brief survey is therefore correlated, insofar as is possible, with the terminology of previous authors, with the study of Nissl sections according to the standard stereotaxic planes of Karten and Hodos (1967), and with vestibular root fiber pathways within the VNC.

The tangential nucleus lies among vestibular root fibers and con-

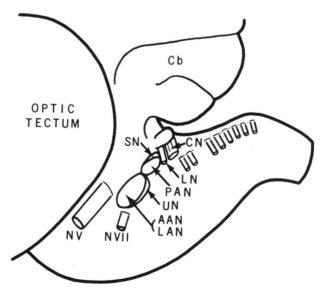

Fig. 2. Lateral view of the medulla showing the positional relationships of the various branches of the statoacoustic nerve at their entrance into the brain stem. Abbreviations: Cb, cerebellum; CN, cochlear nerve; LN, lagenar nerve; NV, trigeminal nerve; NVII, facial nerve; other abbreviations as in Fig. 1.

sists of two clusters, posterior (dorsal) and anterior (ventral), that are related to the anterior and posterior roots of the vestibular nerve, respectively. Each cluster appears to be divided into medial and lateral parts. The cellular composition of each is similar, but the cells of the former are smaller than those of the latter.

The lateral vestibular (Deiters) nucleus consists of dorsal and ventral divisions. The former division (the bigeminal or nucleus jumeaux of Ramón y Cajal) consists of large multipolar cells, and the latter consists of cells of diverse sizes and shapes. Cells are sparse in the ventral division at levels where vestibular fibers course medially through this nucleus and are oriented parallel to the incoming fibers.

The medial vestibular nucleus lies adjacent to the floor of the fourth ventricle for the greater part of its length, and its middle portion is divided into dorsomedial and ventrolateral parts by the dorsal cochlear decussation. However, both parts are similar cytoarchitectonically, and both receive medially directed branches of ascending and/or descending vestibular root fibers.

The descending vestibular nucleus consists of small to medium-sized, pale-staining cells of diverse shapes and is not obviously dissimilar to the medial vestibular nucleus; however, clusters of large, densely staining cells occur. Its rostral pole is capped by large, multipolar cells that receive incoming lagenar fibers. The cells in the remainder of this nucleus, as revealed in horizontal sections, appear to occur in rows conforming to the fascicles of descending vestibular root fibers.

The superior vestibular nucleus includes the nucleus quadrangularis that is elongated dorsoventrally and extends further caudally than other parts of the superior nucleus. At caudal levels, light-staining, small- to medium-sized cells predominate within the quadrangularis, but, at a level where it is continuous with the lateral cerebellovestibular process, larger cells not dissimilar to those in certain areas of the remainder of the superior nucleus are present.

The superior vestibular nucleus, exclusive of the quadrangular division, is the most difficult vestibular nucleus to identify and delineate because it varies, depending on the level, in shape and cellular composition. Homogeneous clusters of large, round cells are present, but these cells are not so large or so densely staining as the large cells of both parts of the lateral vestibular nucleus. Smaller, lighter-staining ovoid and fusiform cells predominate at the medial portions, but even here groups of large cells occur. The superior vestibular nucleus is therefore considered to include the lateral and medial divisions of the nucleus vestibularis dorsolateralis of Sanders (1929), the nucleus piriformis and the nucleus vestibulocerebellaris of Ramón y Cajal (1908), and the nucleus oralis of Bartels (1925). The superior vestibular nucleus as described by Sanders is not identifiable in pigeon material.

VESTIBULAR NERVE CENTRAL PATHWAYS

Destruction of the nerve cell bodies that compose the vestibular ganglion causes degeneration of both proximal and distal axons of these bipolar neurons. Following postoperative survival times of 2–6 days, the medullary projections can be revealed by silver axonal degeneration techniques (Fink and Heimer, 1967). Degenerating axons in the peripheral nerve can be seen by treating the otic capsules containing the inner ears with the Swank–Davenport modification of the Marchi method (Rasmussen, 1950). It is therefore possible to associate Marchi degeneration in the peripheral statoacoustic nerve with patterns of Fink–Heimer silver degeneration within the VNC.

Lesions placed in either the lagenar ganglion, posterior vestibular ganglion, or anterior vestibular ganglion show that each category of lesion results in different pathways and terminal fields within the various subdivisions of VNC. The central distribution of degenerating axons resulting from lesions that involve the lagenar and posterior vestibular ganglia is shown in Fig. 3.

The central projections of fibers from the macula of the lagena have previously been reported by Boord and Rasmussen (1963) and Boord and Karten (1974). Primary lagenar fibers distribute to specialized areas within the cochlear nuclei (the ventrolateral and ventral parts of the nuclei magnocellularis and angularis, respectively), the dorsolateral portion of the descending vestibular nucleus, including the magnocellular part of this nucleus, the dorsal portion of the caudal pole of the ventral part of the lateral vestibular nucleus, seemingly limited areas of the medial vestibular nucleus, and the quadrangular division of the superior vestibular nucleus from which fibers continue their ascending course to terminate within the lateral cerebellovestibular process. No lagenar fibers terminate within the dorsal (gigantocellular) part of the lateral vestibular nucleus nor in any part of the tangential nucleus. It is important to mention that the terminal field for lagenar fibers within caudal levels of the descending vestibular nucleus is ill-defined; there is evidence of terminals about the cells of the external cuneate nucleus, and no degenerating axons are confidently traceable to the deep cerebellar nuclei.

Lesions that involve the part of the posterior vestibular ganglion containing the nerve cell bodies whose axons comprise the posterior vestibular nerve result in different pathways and loci of termination within the VNC than those that involve the lagenar ganglion. Figure 3 shows the distribution of degenerating central axons resulting from a lesion that destroyed the posterior canal ganglion but very few cells of the saccular ganglion. Analysis of the peripheral nerve revealed so few degenerating saccular fibers that this projection can be reasonably interpreted as representing the crista of the posterior canal ganglion. These axons enter the medulla, immediately caudal and dorsal to anterior vestibular nerve root fibers, and rostral and ventral to lagenar fibers, at the level of the posterior division of the tangential nucleus. They traverse both medial and lateral parts of this nucleus and the entire width of the dorsal part of the ventral lateral vestibular nucleus to reach the medial vestibular nucleus. These root fibers give off collaterals that terminate about the cells of both medial and lateral parts of the tangential nucleus and the ventral division of the lateral vestibular nucleus. In the mediodorsal part of the ventral part of the lateral vestibular nucleus, posterior canal root fibers form a descending root and terminal field that occupies the dorsomedial part of the descending vestibular nucleus (medial to the descending lagenar root) throughout the greater part of its rostrocaudal length. Throughout its descending course, collaterals emanate from the parent root to terminate in the medial vestibular nucleus, substantially more in the dorsomedial than the ventrolateral portions at levels where it is divided by the dorsal cochlear decussation. Both posterior canal and lagenar fibers terminate diffusely, with some overlap in the caudal pole of the descending vestibular nucleus, but, in contrast to lagenar fibers, there is no evidence that posterior canal fibers terminate about the cells of the external cuneate nucleus.

The ascending root appears to leave the incoming posterior canal root fibers more lateral in position than the descending root, and courses rostrally and dorsally to enter the medial division of the superior vestibular nucleus. Abundant terminals occur in a large-celled subgroup at caudal levels of the superior vestibular nucleus that is situated ventrolateral to the dorsal gigantocellular part of the lateral vestibular nucleus and that is interpreted as the vestibulocerebellar nucleus of Ramón y Cajal. Collaterals emanate from the ascending root as it courses through the superior vestibular nucleus, and course medially to terminate in the medial vestibular nucleus. No fibers terminate about the cells within the lateral (quadrangular) division of the superior vestibular nucleus. Furthermore, the ascending posterior canal projection is confined to caudomedial parts of the superior vestibular nucleus (few extend farther rostrad than shown in Fig. 3a), and, at these levels, modest numbers of fibers are traceable to intermediate and lateral cerebellar nuclei.

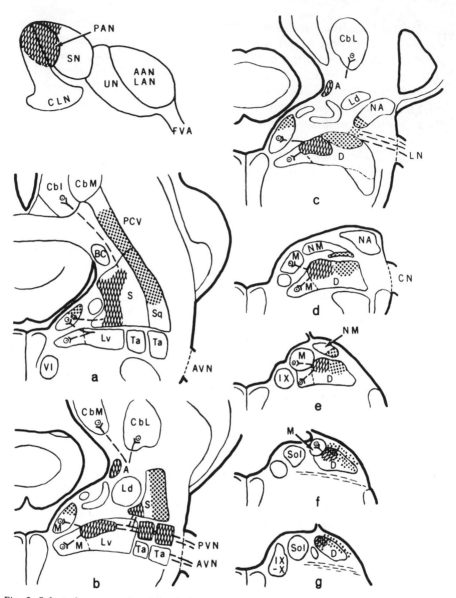

Fig. 3. Selected cross-sectional levels (a-g) through the vestibular nuclear complex of the pigeon showing the terminal fields of the posterior vestibular nerve (cross-hatched) and lagenar nerve (dotted). The diagram of the proximal stump of the statoacoustic nerve (upper left) shows the position of peripheral degenerating axons (cross-hatched) following a lesion in the caudal part of the posterior vestibular ganglion. These are represented within the cross-section diagrams by the same symbol. Note some overlap of lagenar and posterior vestibular (posterior canal) fibers at caudal levels of the descending vestibular nucleus. Anterior vestibular nerve root fibers distribute within those areas of Ta,

Destruction of the anterior vestibular ganglion results in the degeneration of utricular, anterior canal, and lateral canal axons that compose the anterior vestibular nerve. Degenerating anterior vestibular nerve axons enter the medulla rostral and ventral to the posterior vestibular nerve, and traverse both medial and lateral parts of the anterior division of the nucleus tangentialis and the rostroventral portion of the ventral lateral vestibular nucleus. These medially directed root fibers give off terminals within the above nuclei and continue at this level to terminate in the medial vestibular nucleus. Descending branches and terminal field are confined to the ventral half of the descending vestibular nucleus. Medially directed collaterals emanate from descending root fibers to terminate within the medial vestibular nucleus. The ascending pathway is limited to the more central portions of the superior vestibular nucleus between lagenar and posterior canal pathways, but it occupies more rostral portions of the superior nucleus than the latter. Collaterals from the ascending anterior vestibular root course medially to terminate within the medial vestibular nucleus. Some root fibers continue through the superior nucleus to the intermediate deep cerebellar nuclei.

CONCLUDING REMARKS

The VNC of the pigeon can be divided into six major territories similar to those delineated by Wold (1975, 1976) in the domestic hen and seemingly comparable to those of mammals. It is technically extremely difficult, by the methods used in this study, to determine the precise afferent connections of primary vestibular neurons that supply individual labyrinthine receptors; however, it did prove possible to show a topographic representation of axons arising from anterior and posterior vestibular ganglia and from the lagenar ganglion within the ipsilateral VNC, i.e., within the superior, ventral part of the lateral,

---

Lv, D, and S that contain no symbols. Abbreviations: AAN, anterior canal nerve; A, cell group A of Wold; AVN, anterior vestibular nerve; BC, brachium conjunctivum; CbI, internal cerebellar nucleus; CbL, lateral cerebellar nucleus; CbM, medial cerebellar nucleus; CLN, cochlear nerve; D, descending vestibular nucleus; FVA, facial vestibular anastomosis; IX, glossopharyngeal nucleus; IX-X, glossopharyngeal nucleus and dorsal motor nucleus of the vagus; LAN, lateral canal nerve; Ld, dorsal part of the lateral vestibular nucleus; LN, lagenar nerve; Lv, ventral part of the lateral vestibular nucleus; M, medial vestibular nucleus; NA, nucleus angularis; NM, nucleus magnocellularis; PA, posterior canal nerve; PCV, lateral cerebellovestibular process; PVN, posterior vestibular nerve; S, Superior vestibular nucleus; SN, saccular nerve; Sol, solitary nucleus; Sq, quadrangular part of superior vestibular nucleus; Ta, tangential nucleus; UN, utricular nerve.

tangential, and descending vestibular nuclei. Terminal fields are not as well defined within the medial vestibular nucleus, and the dorsal gigantocellular part of the lateral vestibular nucleus is consistently free of degenerating terminals. This is not to suggest that each terminal field emanating from each lesion category is restricted exclusively to particular areas within the VNC, because there is much evidence to indicate that some overlap occurs (Wilson and Felpel, 1972; Gacek, 1969). Moreover, fragmented axons and terminals are not restricted exclusively from each category of lesion to the terminal fields specified.

Furthermore, the VNC receives afferents from other than first-order vestibular neurons and consists of more than simple sensory relay nuclei (Brodal, 1972). Remaining to be determined, in the pigeon, are the relationships of the various cellular subgroups that occur within or are associated with the major vestibular nuclei to particular parts of the vestibular ganglion or to nonvestibular afferents and efferents.

REFERENCES

Bartels, M.: Über die Gegend des Deiters- und Bechterewskernes bei Vögeln. Z. Anat. Entwicklungsgesch. **77**:726–784 (1925).
Boord, R. L., and Karten, H. J.: The distribution of primary lagenar fibers within the vestibular nuclear complex of the pigeon. Brain. Behav. Evol. **10**:228–235 (1974).
Boord, R. L., and Rasmussen, G. L.: Projection of the cochlear and lagenar nerves on the cochlear nuclei of the pigeon. J. Comp. Neurol. **120**:463–475 (1963).
Brodal, A.: Some features in the anatomical organization of the vestibular nuclear complex in the cat. Prog. Brain Res. **37**:31–53 (1972).
Fink, R. P., and Heimer, L.: Two methods for selective silver impregnation of degenerating axons and their synaptic endings in the central nervous system. Brain Res. **4**:369–374 (1967).
Gacek, R. R.: The course and central termination of first order neurons supplying vestibular endorgans in the cat. Acta Oto-laryngol. Suppl. **254**:1–66 (1969).
Karten, H. J., and Hodos, W.: A Stereotaxic Atlas of the Brain of the Pigeon (Columba livia). Johns Hopkins Press, Baltimore (1967).
Peusner, K. D., and Morest, D. K.: The neuronal architecture and topography of the nucleus vestibularis tangentialis in the late chick embryo. Neuroscience **2**:189–207 (1977).
Ramón y Cajal, S.: Les ganglions terminaux du nerf acoustique des oiseaux. Trab. Inst. Cajal Invest. Biol. **6**:195–225 (1908).
Rasmussen, G. L.: Method for studying Wallerian degeneration of the cochlear nerve. Anat. Rec. **106**:120 (1950).
Rasmussen, G. L.: A method of staining the statoacoustic nerve in bulk with Sudan black B. Anat. Rec. **139**:465–470 (1961).
Sanders, E. B.: A consideration of certain bulbar, midbrain and cerebellar centers and fiber tracts in birds. J. Comp. Neurol. **49**:155–222 (1929).

Wilson, V. J., and Felpel, L. P.: Specificity of semicircular canal input to neurons in the pigeon vestibular nuclei. *J. Neurophysiol.* **35:**253–264 (1972).

Wold, J. E.: The vestibular nuclei in the domestic hen *(Gallus domesticus).* I. Normal anatomy. *Anat. Embryol.* **149:**29–46 (1976).

Wold, J. E.: The vestibular nuclei in the domestic hen *(Gallus domesticus).* II. Primary afferents. *Brain Res.* **95:**531–543 (1975).

15

Identification of Tectal Synaptic Terminals in the Avian Isthmooptic Nucleus

W. J. CROSSLAND

INTRODUCTION

The system of efferents to the avian retina is interesting to investigators in a number of disciplines, including the behavioral, physiological, anatomical, and neurobiological sciences. Many species of vertebrates are thought to possess centrifugal fibers in their optic nerves (Ogden, 1968); however, the source of the centrifugal fibers has been demonstrated anatomically only in birds (see Cowan, 1970, for review) and reptiles (Halpern et al., 1976). The avian centrifugal system has been investigated more thoroughly in terms of anatomy (Cowan and Powell, 1963; Cowan, 1970; LaVail and LaVail, 1974; Crossland and Hughes, 1978), physiology (Miles, 1971; Holden and Powell, 1972; Miles, 1972a,b,c,d; Pearlman and Hughes, 1976), and development (see Cowan and Clarke, 1976, for review). In spite of the research interest in the avian centrifugal system in recent years, there are still several anatomical issues regarding the morphology of cells in the centrifugal pathway and the synaptic arrangements on these cells which require further study.

W. J. CROSSLAND • Department of Anatomy, Wayne State University School of Medicine, Detroit, Michigan 48201. This research was begun in the Department of Anatomy at Washington University in St. Louis, where it was supported under Grant EY-01225 from the National Eye Institute. The work was supported at Wayne State University by Grant EY-01796 from the National Eye Institute.

It has been known for some time (McGill et al., 1966a,b) that the optic tectum in the bird projects topographically on the isthmooptic nucleus (ION) of the caudal midbrain. The ION, in turn, makes a topographic projection on the retina, ending on the principal processes of amacrine cells at the junction of the inner nuclear layer and inner plexiform layer (Dowling and Cowan, 1966). Furthermore, recent experiments (Crossland and Hughes, 1978) demonstrated the origin of the tectoisthmal projection to be from a single lamina of cells in the stratum griseum et fibrosum superficiale of the optic tectum at the junction of sublaminae h and i, according to the nomenclature of Cowan et al. (1961). Other than the precise topography of the projection (McGill et al., 1966a; Crossland et al., 1974; Crossland and Hughes, 1978), very little is known about the way in which tectal afferents end within the neuropil of the ION.

The present investigation of the mode of termination of tectal input to the ION had three primary goals: (1) to make some observations on the form of ION neurons based on Golgi preparations as an aid to interpreting subsequent electron microscopic (EM) data, (2) to report on the normal synaptic arrangements within the ION neuropil, and (3) to identify the synaptic terminals of tectal origin following partial ablation of the optic tectum.

MATERIALS AND METHODS

The termination pattern of the tectoisthmal fibers was studied by EM observation of degenerating synapses in the chick ION. Ten 2-month-old chicks were used in these experiments. Each was anesthetized with chloral hydrate and placed in a stereotaxic head holder, and the tectum was exposed. After removal of the dura and stripping away of the pia–arachnoid, large portions of the lateral aspect of the left tectum were removed by aspiration. Care was taken to avoid damaging the dorsomedial aspect of the tectum close to the ION and the rostromedial aspect along the course of the isthmooptic tract. Approximately 30–60% of the tectal surface was removed in the operated animals. Following the operation, the lesioned area was packed with cotton and Gelfoam and sprinkled with antibiotic powder, and the skin was sutured. Two animals were sacrificed 3 days after the operation, one on day 5, six on day 7, and one on day 11. Two normal animals of the same age were also sacrificed.

At the time of perfusion, each animal received an overdose of chloral hydrate, the heart was exposed, and 1 ml of 1% sodium nitrite was injected intracardially. After clamping of the descending aorta, transcardiac perfusion was initiated with 75–100 ml of a solution at room temperature containing 1% paraformaldehyde and 0.02 mM CaCl$_2$ in 0.12 M cacodylate buffer at pH 7.4. This solution was followed by 300 ml of a solution containing 3% glutaraldehyde, 3% paraformaldehyde, and 0.02 mM CaCl$_2$ in 0.12 M cacodylate buffer, pH 7.4. The brain was immediately removed and placed in a solution of the concentrated fixative for a period of 4 hr. After this period of fixation, 2-mm slices were hand-cut in the frontal plane with a razor blade. The sections containing the ION were then identified under a dissecting microscope. A small piece of tissue containing the nucleus was cut out of the slice and placed in a solution of 0.12 M cacodylate buffer, 0.02 mM CaCl$_2$, and 7% dextrose.

The pieces of tissue were then washed in several changes of buffer and sucrose, postfixed 2 hr in 2% OsO$_4$, made up in 0.12 M cacodylate buffer and 7% dextrose, dehydrated in ethanol, and embedded in an epon–araldite mixture. Sections from the embedded material were cut at 2 μm, stained with toluidine blue, and examined until the nucleus could be identified in the block. Following final trimming, thin sections showing silver interference colors were cut on a diamond knife, picked up on uncoated 200-mesh copper grids, stained with lead citrate and uranyl acetate, and examined on a Siemens Ia or Phillips 201 electron microscope.

A number of posthatch chicks were prepared either following the Golgi–Cox procedure of van der Loos (1956) and counterstained with thionine or by the rapid Golgi method of Valverde (1970). The observations described in this chapter are from newly hatched (rapid Golgi) or 1-month posthatch chicks (Golgi–Cox) cut in the frontal or parasagittal planes. The Golgi material was used to characterize the normal neuronal morphology of the ION and to facilitate the interpretation of EM profiles in the nucleus.

RESULTS

Observations on Golgi Material

Each ION neuron has an oval or round cell body 12–16 μm in its longest dimension. The contours of the cell body are not smooth. Many of the neurons have a lumpy appearance, and several types of appendages can be seen protruding from the soma (Figs. 1, 2, and 3). The appendages may be filiform, with or without swellings along their length, or they may have the form of pedunculated spines of variable dimensions (compare appendages in Fig. 3A and Fig. 3C). Such appen-

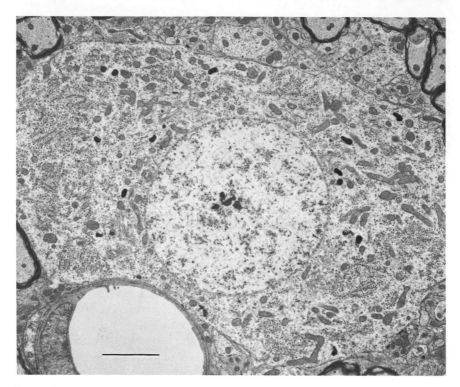

Fig. 1. Low-power electron micrograph to illustrate the appearance of a typical ION principal cell. These cells contain a large eccentric nucleus and moderate volumes of cytoplasm. Many organelles, among them a large number of dense lysosomelike inclusions, many mitochondria, and abundant Nissl substance, are evident within the cytoplasm. The background matrix of the ION contains many myelinated fibers with scattered islands of neuropil. Calibration bar, 3 μm.

dages are seen infrequently along the shafts of dendrites between branch points.

The axon typically leaves the soma from a small axon hillock, but may leave from one of the dendrites at a point near the cell body (see arrows in Figs. 2 and 3). Some axons have been impregnated for up to 75 μm in the Golgi–Cox material. These axons quickly assume a diameter of 2–3 μm after leaving the hillock, then follow a fairly straight course for 10–50 μm, at which point impregnation ceases. No collateral axonal branches have been noted in any of our material.

The most striking feature of the Golgi preparations is their involuted dendritic arborization. Each major dendrite (one to four have been observed, but there are typically two) arises from a broad conical expansion of the cell body, which tapers rapidly proximal to the cell body, then more gradually distal to the cell body, where it assumes a diameter of 2–4 μm. Typically, the dendrite does not branch within 10–20 μm of the perikaryon.

The branch points of the ION cells (Fig. 3) are characterized by a local broadening and partial flattening of the dendritic trunk. One or two large branches, which are somewhat smaller in diameter than the dendritic segment leading into the branch point, may extend for an-

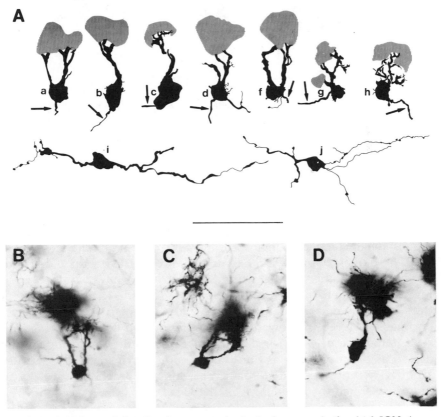

Fig. 2. A: (a–h) Seven Golgi–Cox-impregnated principal neurons in the chick ION. Axons are indicated by arrows. Major dendrites leave the cell body to branch in a zone approximately 50–75 μm from the soma. A densely impregnated mass resembling a protoplasmic astrocyte always was impregnated among the branching dendrites, indicated here by stippling. (i, j) Two neurons lying along the perimeter of the ION. Thick processes appear to be dendritic; fine processes possessing swellings along their length are suspected to be axonal. The processes were seen running parallel to the perimeter of the nucleus. B, C, D: Photographs of three Golgi-impregnated ION principal neurons illustrating the densely impregnated mass atop the dendrites. Calibration bar for A–D, 100 μm.

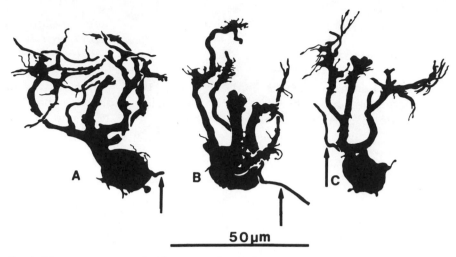

Fig. 3. Three neurons traced with a camera lucida from rapid Golgi preparations of newly hatched chicks. These preparations show the dendritic patterns of the neurons more clearly than the Golgi–Cox material. Several of the dendrites in each case were not drawn to facilitate detailed presentation of other branches. Axons are marked by arrows. Note in (A) that the dendrites tend to branch within a central area. Also observe that branch points frequently are somewhat widened and flattened as well as fringed by numerous appendages.

other 10–20 μm before branching again. The enlarged branch points are also characterized by many sessile and filiform appendages which give the branch point a macelike appearance. If the dendrite does not continue to another branch point, it often will end abruptly with a number of spinelike and filiform appendages at the terminus. Some of these abruptly ending branches appear to be similar to the "clawlike" endings described by Cowan (1970) in the pigeon ION.

As may be observed in Figs. 2 and 3, the initial trajectory of the dendrites often changes at the branch points such that the dendrites arborize within a delimited spherical volume approximately 50 μm in diameter. Since the branching of the dendrites is frequent within a small volume of tissue, the network of branches and appendages is very difficult to observe clearly (see photographs in Fig. 2B,C,D), especially in the Golgi–Cox material. It is possible that in the Golgi–Cox material there may be simultaneous impregnation of protoplasmic astrocyte processes among the dendrites as well, especially in view of the intimate relation between astrocytic processes and the synaptic endings in the neuropil to be discussed below. It is important to stress that no other neurons in these chick brains were observed to have such an association between protoplasmic astrocytes and their dendrites. However, in our rapid Golgi specimens it was possible to isolate some of the dendrites clearly. Figure 3 shows that the dendrites intertwine to give rise to much of the dense tangle appearing in the cells drawn in Fig. 2A,a-h.

On occasion in the Golgi-stained material, a second type of cell was found along the perimeter of the nucleus (Fig. 2A, i and j). This cell has a similar cell-body diameter and shape as the other principal cells of the nucleus. The appearance of the cell processes is entirely different, however. Two sets of processes leave opposite poles of the soma and run roughly parallel to the perimeter of the ION for 100–200 μm. Some of these processes project away from the nucleus, while some project within the boundaries of the ION. The stout, gradually tapering processes leaving the soma appear to be dendritic. Unlike the other ION neurons, they branch relatively infrequently, appear to have regular surface contours, and lack spines completely. Fine processes of uniform diameter bearing swellings along their length and at their ends were observed to leave the cell body or the dendrites. Such processes could be locally ramifying axons. No axonal process was seen leaving the soma similar to the 2- to 3-μm-diameter process of the principal ION cells. Since this category of cells could not be found within the central portion of the nucleus, there is a possibility that these cells are from a non-ION population. Their occurrence around the entire perimeter of the nucleus, however, argues against this interpretation. Unfortunately, we have no EM data on these cells.

Observations on EM Material

Normal Appearance of ION Neurons. At the EM level, the ION is filled with many myelinated axons and a fairly uniform population of large neurons (Fig. 1). The neuronal cell body profiles contain an eccentric nucleus with a prominent nucleolus. Within the cytoplasm of the ION cells are stacks of rough endoplasmic reticulum, many scattered polyribosomes, mitochondria with somewhat dilated cisternae, occasional microtubules, a prominent Golgi apparatus, and many dense, membrane-bound inclusions which resemble secondary lysosomes. Areas of neuropil are scattered among the cell bodies and networks of myelinated axons. The dilations of the ION cell mitochondria cristae were useful features for differentiating ION cell processes from those of extrinsic cell processes found within the nucleus (Fig. 4A). Glial cell mitochondria had similarly dilated cristae, although their background matrix tended to stain more densely than that found in ION cell mitochondria.

The outline of the principal ION cell bodies is irregular along much

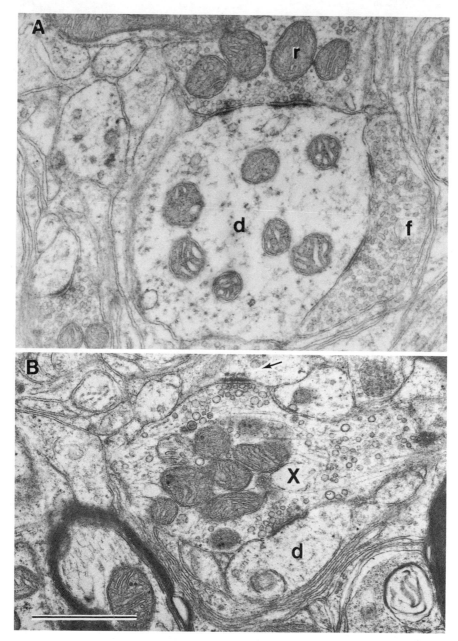

Fig. 4. A: Axodendritic synapse configuration in unoperated animals. Axodendritic synapses are made by two R-type terminals (r) containing round synaptic vesicles as well as by an F-type terminal (f) containing pleomorphic vesicles. Note the greater asymmetry of the R terminal synaptic membrane with respect to the F terminal. Also note the difference in mitochondrial morphology between the ION cell dendrite (d) and the R

of their extent (Fig. 2A, a-h, Fig. 3) when studied with either Golgi or EM techniques. Folds and protrusions of various sizes could sometimes be seen in electron micrographs extending out several microns into the surrounding neuropil. Presumably these profiles correspond to the filiform spinous processes which leave the somata of Golgi-impregnated neurons and occasionally end in terminal enlargements (Fig. 2A, a-h). The few processes we have seen in electron micrographs which were in continuity with the soma all received synapses and hence may function as miniature dendrites.

In two cases we have observed longitudinally cut profiles which followed a straight course away from the cell body for 30 μm and maintained a uniform diameter of 2 μm. Since these profiles contained more neurotubules than are ordinarily found in dendrites, and since there was a sharp decrease in the number of ribosomes in the vicinity of the presumed axon hillock, the profiles were tentatively identified as axon initial segments. However, the profiles also contained occasional ribosomal rosettes and short segments of rough endoplasmic reticulum. It is possible that these processes are some type of somatic filiform protrusion, although the somatic protrusions of this type seen in Golgi preparations are on the order of 0.5 μm in diameter. The processes received numerous synaptic contacts of all types (R, F, and S).

Distribution of Synapses in the ION. In EM preparation of the ION, the distribution of synapses on profiles of individual somata of ION cells is patchy. Large portions of the cell perimeter remain synapse free. These areas usually have smooth contours and are wrapped in one or more glial lamellae (astrocytic) (Fig. 5B) similar to the wrapping of Purkinje cell bodies by Fañanas cells (Peters et al., 1970). At times, cell-body profiles rest against one another; under these conditions, the glial wrapping is not present. Other portions of the cell membrane, especially those areas near the proximal dendrites, are of irregular contour and may be densely covered by synapses.

The neuropil, largely composed of axodendritic synapses and a relatively small number of axosomatic synapses, is characterized by the

terminal mitochondria. F terminal mitochondria closely resemble those of the R terminal. Layers of astrocytic cytoplasm may be seen along one side of the synaptic terminals. B: Degenerating terminal (X) in the ION 5 days after tectal lesion. The terminal contains many swollen synaptic vesicles (compare with vesicles in R terminal in A) and a relatively large number of neurofilaments surrounding a central core of mitochondria. The terminal makes two synaptic contacts. One contact in the lower portion of the picture is made on a small profile surrounded by several layers of glial cytoplasm. In the upper half of the picture, the terminal synapses on another small profile which contains a postjunctional complex (arrow). Calibration bar, 1 μm for both electron micrographs.

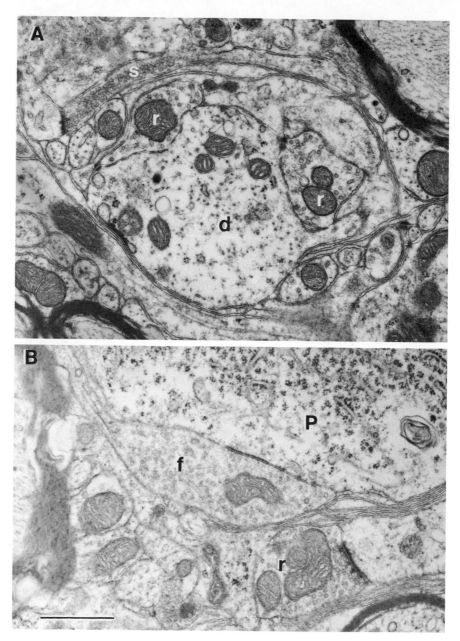

Fig. 5. A: Configuration of the glomerulus in the ION of an unoperated animal. A central dendrite (d) is contacted by two terminals (r). Surrounding the synaptic complex are several layers of glial cytoplasm. Also shown in the upper left portion of the field is an S-type terminal (s) synapsing on a spinelike profile. Note the narrowness of the S terminal and the high packing density of the synaptic vesicles. B: An F-type terminal (f) making synaptic contact with the perikaryon (P) of an ION neuron in an unoperated animal. Nearby an R terminal can be seen contacting a small profile to the right. Note the glial lamellae separating the R and F terminals. The glial lamellae continue along the cell body to the right. Calibration bar, 1 μm for both electron micrographs.

presence of glial wrappings around relatively small assemblages of synaptic contacts (Fig. 5A, also Fig. 4A,B), similar to the glomerular-type contacts reported by many authors in the lateral geniculate body (Rafols and Valverde, 1973; Szentágothai, 1963; Wong-Riley, 1972), superior colliculus (Lund, 1969), ventrobasal complex (Ralston and Herman, 1969), and elsewhere. In the ION, these glomeruli are formed by a central large dendrite contacted by several axon terminals (Figs. 4A and 5A) or, less commonly, by a central axon terminal synapsing on one or more small dendrites (Fig. 4B). Glial wrappings are also found separating an axodendritic synapse from a cell body lying only a few tenths of a micrometer away (Fig. 5B). Many other synapses occur which are not apparently involved in glomerular assemblages.

Two additional points should be emphasized. First, there were no postsynaptic profiles which contained synaptic vesicles such as are seen in the processes of intrinsic neurons of the lateral geniculate nucleus (Rafols and Valverde, 1973). Second, there were no presynaptic elements which contained mitochondria of the same distinct form as those found in ION cells.

Three types of synapses can be recognized in the ION neuropil. Their distribution on cell bodies and dendrites is summarized in Table 1. The R-type synapse (Figs. 4A and 5B) is more or less bulbous, 1–3 μm in diameter, with round synaptic vesicles in a clear background matrix. The R type makes asymmetrical synapses with large (greater than 1 μm) and small (less than or equal to 1 μm) dendrites or dendritic appendages. The terminal sometimes contains a postjunctional complex similar in appearance to those described by other investigators (Akert et al., 1976; Milhaud and Pappas, 1966; Waxman and Pappas, 1970) in the postsynaptic element. It is interesting to note that a degenerating synapse pictured in Fig. 4B which is presynaptic to two other profiles has a postjunctional body in only one of the postsynaptic profiles. However, postjunctional bodies were never seen postsynaptic to any other type of presynaptic terminal. This type of terminal accounts for

Table 1. Frequency of Different Types of Synaptic Terminals in the Isthmooptic Nuclei of Two Control Chicks

Postsynaptic structure	R type	F type	S type	Total
Dendrite >1 μm	223	115	32	370
Dendrite ≤1 μm	209	46	28	283
Soma	13	22	5	40
Total	445	183	65	693

Table 2. Frequency of Different Types of Synaptic
Terminals in the Isthmooptic Nucleus of a Chick 5
Days after an Ipsilateral Tectal Lesion

Postsynaptic structure	R type	F type	S type	Degen.	Total
Dendrite >1 μm	18	34	6	56	114
Dendrite ≤1 μm	42	24	10	46	122
Soma	3	5	3	0	11
Total	63	63	19	102	247

64% of all the synapses found in the ION and 74% of all the synapses found on small dendrites. The second, less common, F-type terminal (Figs. 4A and 5B) is more flattened in appearance and frequently forms a thin concave profile in cross section 1–3 μm in diameter as it enwraps the postsynaptic element. The terminal contains pleomorphic vesicles, somewhat smaller in size than those found in the R terminal, with an electron-lucent background matrix. The synapses formed by this terminal are more symmetrical than the R type, although they are still slightly asymmetrical. The F terminals were more frequently found on large dendrites (66% of the F terminals) than on smaller ones (19%). Although these terminals account for only 22% of all the terminals in the ION, they composed 46% of the axosomatic terminals. The third and least frequent type of terminal, the S type (Fig. 5A), which makes asymmetrical synaptic contacts, is small, with a dense background matrix tightly packed with small, moderately electron-dense, pleomorphic synaptic vesicles. Because of the variability in the shape of synaptic vesicles found in different S-type terminals, it is possible that this group actually represents two or more subpopulations of terminal. The low frequency of occurrence of S terminals has prevented their study in detail and hence they will be treated here as a single group. The terminals were found contacting the ION cell perikarya and small protrusions from the cell bodies as well as other small processes. These terminals accounted for only 10% of the synapses in the ION but constituted 38% of the axosomatic synapses.

Terminal Degeneration in the ION. Much has been written about the pattern of degeneration of axon terminals in the vertebrate CNS (Cuénod et al., 1970; Gray and Hamlyn, 1962; Guillery, 1970; Jones and Powell, 1970; Jones and Rockel, 1973). While the exact details of the degeneration process and its time course differ among species and neural systems, we will only briefly describe the general appearance of the degeneration process for the tectoisthmal fibers as we outline the location of degenerating terminals.

The 2-month posthatch chicks were sacrificed at either 3, 5, 7, or 11 days following lesions of the lateral tectal surface. Since only partial tectal removals were possible in these animals, and since the tectum projects topographically on the ION, it was necessary to scan through different portions of the nucleus to find the areas which contained degenerating terminals. Areas which did not contain degenerating terminals were excluded from the sample. Once an area of neuropil containing degenerating terminals was located, it was photographed in a closely spaced series of negatives without regard to the occurrence of degeneration in any given photographic field. This method of choosing photographic fields was not random; hence the statistical data to be presented below should be considered as only an indication of the actual proportions of events in the sampling distribution.

Although some signs of degeneration were found in the 3-day animals, especially swollen synaptic vesicles (Cuénod et al., 1970), the signs of degeneration were not well developed until day 5. At this time, several forms of degenerating terminals could be recognized. It must be emphasized that all terminals described here possessed synaptic vesicles and made unequivocal synaptic contacts with some structure. The majority of degenerating terminals contained aggregations of swollen vesicles (Figs. 4B and 6A) along the presynaptic thickening. The morphology of the mitochondria was not appreciably altered until the stage of electron densification described below. In some terminals, a large number of neurofilaments surrounded a central core of mitochondria and synaptic vesicles (Figs. 4B and 6A). The terminals which were undergoing these phases of degeneration had the general form of the R-type terminals and frequently were found within the boundaries of a glomerulus (Fig. 4B). In cross-section, the synapses made by these terminals are asymmetrical and sometimes the postsynaptic structure contains a postjunctional complex (Figs. 4B and 6B). Table 2, showing the distribution of synapses in the 5-day-postoperative animal, has been included for comparison with the control animals seen in Table 1. Two points emerge on comparison of these two tables. First, the number of R synapses decreased in frequency so that by the fifth day they were equal in number to the F-type synapses. Second, if one takes the sum of all the synaptic types, including degenerating synapses, and computes the percentage of the total made up of the F synapses (63/247), one finds that F synapses compose 25% of the total vs. 22% for a similar comparison in the control case. If one combines the total of R-type synapses in the 5-day-postoperative animal with the total number of degenerating synapses, one finds that this proportion of the total

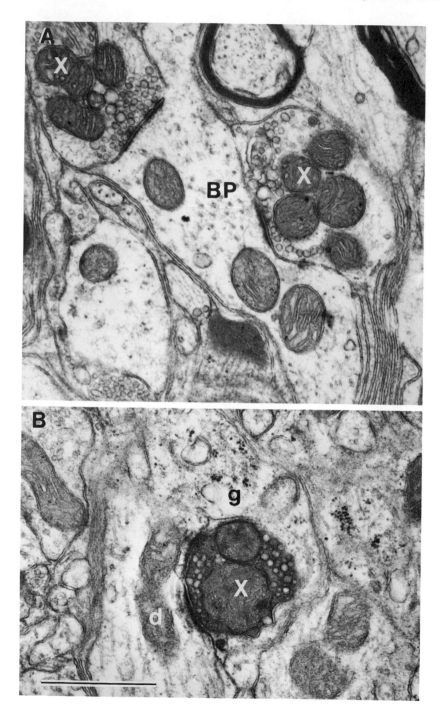

number of synapses in the tally (165/247), 67%, is very similar to the proportion of R-type synapses in the control animals (64%). The S-type synapses remain relatively unchanged.

By the seventh day following tectal lesion, many of the terminals were electron dense and had irregular borders (Fig. 6B). Electron-lucent profiles, presumably the remains of swollen synaptic vesicles, were visible in some of these terminals. At the seventh-day and especially at the 11th-day survival periods, many of the electron-dense profiles were partially surrounded by electron-lucent, glycogen-containing processes, presumably originating from reactive astrocytes. At no time during the 11th-day-postoperative survival period was there any sign of "vacated" postsynaptic thickenings on the ION cell processes.

On the seventh postoperative day, the R-type terminals represented only 20% of all the terminals, including those which were degenerating, while the F type had risen to 31%. In the control case, there were three R-type terminals for every F type, whereas there were only 0.7 R-type terminals for each F type on the seventh day of postoperative survival. S-type terminals continued to remain 10-15% of the population, including the degenerating terminals.

Results for the 11-day case, although not presented in detail here, were consistent with those of the 7-day animals, including a further decrease in the ratio of S:F terminals (0.4:1). There was also a further increase in the proportion of electron-dense degenerating synaptic terminals.

On the seventh postoperative day and later survival periods, some changes were noted in the F terminals. Many of the F terminals demonstrated a proliferation of synaptic vesicles and an increased background density within the terminal. Longer survival times would be required to determine whether or not these changes in the appearance of the F terminals were transient or whether further changes might be forthcoming.

Fig. 6. A: Two degenerating profiles (X) contacting an elongated dendritic profile (BP) seen on the fifth postoperative day. Both degenerating profiles contain many neurofilaments and swollen synaptic vesicles. The presence of a pedunculated spinous process at the top of the elongated dendritic process suggests that this is a section through one of the branch points of the dendrite. B: An electron-dense degenerating terminal seen 11 days after operation. Note the irregular boundary of the terminal and the presence of round electron-lucent vesicles, suggestive of synaptic vesicles surronding electron-dense mitochondria. A glial cell process (g) containing glycogen can be seen surrounding the terminal on three sides. The synaptic region in contact with a dendrite (d) is still intact. Calibration bar, 1 μm for both electron micrographs.

DISCUSSION

The Golgi investigations of the normal chick ION indicate the cells of the ION have a very limited volume of neuropil occupied by their dendritic arborizations but the complex branching patterns of the ION neurons give rise to a large dendritic surface area. In addition, the EM investigations indicate that the synaptic contacts on dendrites are frequently isolated from neighboring synapses by means of glial wrappings to form glomeruli and perisomatic lamellae. The dendritic pattern of ION cells is peculiar in that the dendritic trunks may initially radiate away from each other, then change course, and ultimately arborize in the same locality. This branching pattern appears to be unique to ION neurons, although it bears a superficial resemblance to some of the small ganglion cell dendritic branching patterns seen in the mammalian retina (Ramón y Cajal, 1972).

From our rapid Golgi material, the dendritic branching pattern seems more complex than that reported for the pigeon (Cowan, 1970). In the chick, the branch points are marked by a proliferation of appendages and by a broadening and flattening of the dendritic trunk. Such features were not described in the pigeon. However, both chick and pigeon appear to be similar in the general form of ION neurons and in their dendritic terminations.

The densely impregnated matrix in the regions of extensive dendritic branching in the Golgi–Cox preparations has some of the characteristics of impregnated astrocytes. Since the glomerular wrapping of the synapses is made by astrocyte processes, it is possible that portions of the astrocytic branches in intimate contact with the impregnated neuron may have also become impregnated. One observation which favors this hypothesis is that, on occasion, impregnated afferent terminals were observed contacting ION cell dendrites, and it was not unusual to find portions of impregnated axon arborizations meandering along the edges of the impregnated dendritic mass. It would seem unlikely that in *every* case astrocytic processes would be impregnated among the dendrites, especially since we have not observed this to occur with any other neurons in the chick brain.

The EM observations of the ION have brought out several points. First, there are several types of input to the ION based on terminal and synaptic vesicle morphology. The synaptic targets of the R- and F-type terminals appear to be the same: large and small dendrites and cell bodies. The F type is predominantly found on large dendrites and cell bodies, while the R type is most frequently found among glomerular-type synaptic complexes contacting small dendrites. S-type terminals are rarely found within the glomeruli but are often seen contacting small processes in the vicinity of the cell body or contacting the cell body itself.

Second, on the basis of light or electron microscopic material, there does not appear to be any evidence of local circuit neuron or cell processes which both make and receive synaptic contacts (Rafols and Valverde, 1973; Szentágothai, 1963; Wong-Riley, 1972) within the nucleus. Moreover, there is no direct evidence in our Golgi material that ION cells give off intrinsic axon collaterals. EM evidence bearing on this point, however, is negative; there is no type of terminal observed in the present material which contains mitochondria of the same morphology as those found in the soma and dendrites of ION cells. It would be expected that if the ION cells gave off intrinsic collaterals their terminals would contain mitochondria of the same appearance as those in the cell body. It is possible that the cells lying along the perimeter of the nucleus possessing tangentially oriented dendrites may function as interneurons since they do not appear to have axons which project for long distances. These neurons will require further study in both Golgi and EM preparations before their roles can be ascertained.

Third, the presumed extrinsic origin of the F- and S-type synapses provides the only modulation of tectal input. The flattened or pleomorphic vesicles and nearly symmetrical pre- and postsynaptic thickenings of the F synapse are suggestive of an inhibitory function (Uchizono, 1965). The distribution of this type of synapse along the soma and major dendritic processes would underline the possibility that it plays a major role in whatever integrative processes are carried on by the ION. It is important to the future understanding of the centrifugal system to discover the origin of these processes.

The relatively low density of S-type terminals and their possible location on somatic spinelike processes suggest that they function in an important fashion: they are very close to the presumed site of action-potential generation, yet they occupy only relatively few synaptic sites. If their distribution can be shown to be restricted to somatic spinelike process and the region of the soma, as seems likely from the present observations, then they also possess considerable potential influence over the firing of the ION neurons.

Last, the small diameter of receptive fields of ION neurons (Miles, 1971; Holden and Powell, 1972), which is on the same order of size as the receptive fields of the superficial layers of the optic tectum (Hughes and Pearlman, 1974), is consistent with the anatomical observations made here. First, the tectoisthmal fibers arborize in narrow domains within the ION (Cowan and Powell, 1963; McGill et al., 1966a; Crossland and Hughes, 1978). Second, the ION cell dendrites in turn arborize within a very small volume. Third, the ION cells do not have any obvious influence over their neighbors by means of interneurons or axon collaterals observed thus far. The structure of the ION seems well adapted to preserve the precision of the retinotopic map in addition to its other, as yet unexplained, functions.

ACKNOWLEDGMENTS. It is a pleasure to acknowledge the help of Mark Connelly at Washington University and Wes Heiple at Wayne State University for their assistance with the electron microscopy and to thank Linda Stephenson and Carol Uchwat for their technical assistance. I would also like to thank Dr. J. A. Rafols for his advice and helpful comments on the manuscript.

REFERENCES

Akert, K., Pfenninger, K., and Sandri, C.: The structure of synapses in the subfornical organ of the cat. Z. Zellforsch. Mikrosk. Anat. 81:537–556 (1976).
Cowan, W. M.: Centrifugal fibers to the avian retina. Br. Med. Bull. 26:1–28 (1970).
Cowan, W. M., and Clarke, P. G. H.: The development of the isthmo-optic nucleus. Brain Behav. Evol. 13:345–375 (1976).
Cowan, W. M., and Powell, T. P. S.: Centrifugal fibers in the avian visual system. Proc. R. Soc. London Ser. B 158:232–252 (1963).
Cowan, W. M., Adamson, L., and Powell, T. P. S.: An experimental study of the avian visual system. J. Anat. 95:545–563 (1961).
Crossland, W. J., and Hughes, C. P.: Observations on the afferent and efferent connections of the avian isthmo-optic nucleus. Brain Res. 145:239–256 (1978).
Crossland, W. J., Cowan, W. M., Rogers, L. A., and Kelly, J. P.: The specification of the retino-tectal projection in the chick. J. Comp. Neurol. 155:124–164 (1974).
Cuénod, M., Sandri, C., and Akert, K.: Enlarged synaptic vesicles as an early sign of secondary degeneration in the optic nerve terminal of the pigeon. J. Cell Sci. 6:605–613 (1970).
Dowling, J. E., and Cowan, W. M.: An electron microscope study of normal and degenerating centrifugal fiber terminals in the pigeon retina. Z. Zellforsch. Mikrosk. Anat. 71:14–28 (1966).
Gray, E. G., and Hamlyn, L. H.: Electron microscopy of experimental degeneration in the avian optic tectum. J. Anat. 96:309–316 (1962).
Guillery, R. W.: Light and electron microscopic studies of normal and degenerating axons. In Nauta, W. J. H., and Ebbesson, S. O. E. (eds.): Contemporary Research Methods in Neuroanatomy. Springer-Verlag, New York (1970). Pp. 77–105.
Halpern, M., Wang, R. T., and Colman, D. R.: Centrifugal fibers to the eye of a non-avian vertebrate: Source revealed by horseradish peroxidase studies. Science 194:1185–1188 (1976).
Holden, A. L., and Powell, T. P. S.: The functional organization of the isthmo-optic nucleus in the pigeon. J. Physiol. 233:419–447 (1972).
Hughes, C. P., and Pearlman, A. L.: Single unit receptive fields and cellular layers of the pigeon optic tectum. Brain Res. 80:365–377 (1974).
Jones, E.G., and Powell, T. P. S.: An electron microscopic study of the laminar pattern

and mode of termination of afferent fiber pathways in the somatic sensory cortex of the cat. *Philos. Trans. R. Soc. London Ser. B* **257**:45–62 (1970).

Jones, E. G., and Rockel, A. J.: Observations on complex vesicles, neurofilamentous hyperplasia and increased electron density during terminal degeneration in the inferior colliculus. *J. Comp. Neurol.* **147**:93–118 (1973).

LaVail, J. H., and LaVail, M.: The retrograde intra-axonal transport of horseradish peroxidase in the chick visual system: A light and electron microscopic study. *J. Comp. Neurol.* **157**:303–358 (1974).

Lund, R. D.: Synaptic patterns of the superficial layers of the superior colliculus of the rat. *J. Comp. Neurol.* **135**:179–208 (1969).

McGill, J. I., Powell, T. P. S., and Cowan, W. M.: The retinal representation upon the optic tectum and the isthmo-optic nucleus in the pigeon. *J. Anat.* **100**:5–33 (1966a).

McGill, J. I., Powell, T. P. S., and Cowan, W. M.: The organization of the projection of the centrifugal fibers to the retina in the pigeon. *J. Anat.* **100**:35–49 (1966b).

Miles, F. A.: Visual responses of centrifugal neurons to the avian retina. *Brain Res.* **25**:411–415 (1971).

Miles, F. A.: Centrifugal control of the avian retina. I. Receptive field properties of retinal ganglion cells. *Brain Res.* **48**:65–92 (1972a).

Miles, F. A.: Centrifugal control of the avian retina. II. Receptive field properties of cells in the isthmo-optic nucleus. *Brain Res.* **48**:93–113 (1972b).

Miles, F. A.: Centrifugal control of the avian retina. III. Effects of electrical stimulation of the isthmo-optic tract on the receptive field properties of retinal ganglion cells. *Brain Res.* **48**:115–129 (1972c).

Miles, F. A.: Centrifugal control of the avian retina. IV. Effects of reversible cold block of the isthmo-optic tract on the receptive field properties of cells in the retina and isthmo-optic nucleus. *Brain Res.* **48**:131–145 (1972d).

Milhaud, M., and Pappas, G. D.: The fine structure of neurons and synapses of the habenula of the cat with special reference to sub-junctional bodies. *Brain Res.* **3**:158–173 (1966).

Ogden, T. E.: On the function of efferent retinal fibers. In von Euler, Skolung, and Soderberg (eds.): *Structure and Function of Inhibitory Neuronal Mechanisms. Proc. 4th Int. Meet. Neurobiologists.* Pergamon Press, Oxford (1968). Pp. 89–109.

Pearlman, A. L., and Hughes, C. P.: Functional role of efferents to the avian retina. II. Effects of reversible cooling of the isthmo-optic nucleus. *J. Comp. Neurol.* **166**:123–132 (1976).

Peters, A., Palay, S. L., and Webster, H. D.: *The Fine Structure of the Nervous System.* Harper and Row, New York (1970).

Rafols, J. A., and Valverde, F.: The structure of the dorsal lateral geniculate nucleus in the mouse: A Golgi and electron microscope study. *J. Comp. Neurol.* **150**:303–332 (1973).

Ralston, H., and Herman, M.: The fine structure of neurons and synapses in the ventrobasal thalamus of the cat. *Brain Res.* **14**:77–97 (1969).

Ramón y Cajal, S.: *The Structure of the Retina.* S. A. Thorpe and M. Glickstein (transl.) Charles C Thomas, Springfield, Ill. (1972). Pp. 76–92.

Szentágothai, J.: The structure of the synapse in the lateral geniculate body. *Acta Anat.* **55**:166–185 (1963).

Uchizono, K.: Characteristics of excitatory and inhibitory synapses in the central nervous system of the cat. *Nature (London)* **207**:642–643 (1965).

Valverde, F.: The Golgi method. A tool for comparative structural analyses. In Nauta, W. J. H., and Ebbesson, S. O. E. (eds.): *Contemporary Research Methods in Neuroanatomy.* Springer-Verlag, New York (1970). Pp. 12–31.

van der Loos, H.: Une combinaison de deux vieilles méthodes histologiques pour le système nerveux central. *Monatsschr. Psychiatr. Neurol.* **132:**330–334 (1956).

Waxman, S. G., and Pappas, G. P.: Synaptic organization of the oculomotor nucleus: A comparative electron microscopic study. *Biol. Bull.* **139:**142 (1970).

Wong-Riley, M. T.: Neuronal and synaptic organization of the normal dorsal lateral geniculate nucleus of the squirrel monkey. *J. Comp. Neurol.* **144:**25–60 (1972).

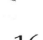

16

Visual Pigments and Oil Droplets in the Pigeon Retina, as Measured by Microspectrophotometry, and Their Relationship to Spectral Sensitivity

J. K. BOWMAKER

INTRODUCTION

The retinas of diurnal birds are characterized by a relatively high ratio of cones to rods, the cones containing prominent oil droplets in the ellipsoid. The oil droplets are brightly colored and highly variable in color, size, and location within the retina of a single species and between species. Since the oil droplets interpose between the incoming light and the visual pigment of the cone outer segment, they must play a significant role in avian color vision. With three differently colored droplets, red, orange, and yellow, acting as cutoff filters, it is possible to construct a color system based on a single visual pigment such as the P562 measured by Liebman (1972) in the retinas of the chicken, pigeon, and gull. However, in the turtle *Chelonia mydas*, which also possesses colored oil droplets in its cones, Liebman and Granda (1971)

J. K. BOWMAKER • MRC Vision Unit, Centre for Research on Perception and Cognition, University of Sussex, Falmer, Brighton, BN1 9QG, East Sussex, England. Present address: Department of Zoology and Comparative Physiology, Queen Mary College, London E 1 4NS, England.

identified three cone visual pigments (P562, P502, and P440) whose spectral sensitivity will be modified by the transmission of their respective oil droplets.

In recent studies using microspectrophotometry (MSP) on the retinas of the chicken (Bowmaker and Knowles, 1977), the pigeon (Bowmaker, 1977), and the rook (Bowmaker, unpublished data), as well as the highly nocturnal tawny owl, *Strix aluco* (Bowmaker and Martin, 1978), we have identified three groups of cone visual pigments absorbing maximally in the yellow, green, and blue. We have also distinguished at least five types of oil droplets characterized primarily by their λ_{T50} (absorbance at which 50% transmission occurs). By determining the combination of visual pigment and oil droplet in each cone and from the absorbance characteristics of both the visual pigment and the droplet, it is possible to derive the relative spectral sensitivity of each cone type.

In the pigeon, the retina can be divided into two regions, a dorsal-posterior sector dominated by cones containing either multiple red or single orange droplets (Pedler and Boyle, 1969) and the remainder of the retina dominated by yellow oil droplets. Since considerable data are available on the spectral sensitivity of the pigeon, an attempt has been made to relate the sensitivities of the pigeon's individual cone types from both the red and yellow fields with the modulator-type spectral sensitivities isolated from ganglion cells (Donner, 1953) and electroretinographically (Ikeda, 1965), with the spectral sensitivities of rotundal units of the thalamus (Granda and Yazulla, 1971; Yazulla and Granda, 1973) and tectal units (King-Smith, quoted by Muntz, 1972), as well as with the overall photopic sensitivities determined both from electroretinography and behavorial studies (Granit, 1942; Blough, 1957; Graf, 1969; Blough et al., 1972; Norren, 1975; Romeskie and Yager, 1976).

MATERIALS AND METHODS

Adult pigeons (*Columba livia*) were dark-adapted overnight. A bird was then decapitated and the eyes were removed. Under dim red light, the front of the eye and the lens were removed and the eye cup was oriented, using the pecten as a guide. The eye was then cut into four sections: the posterior-dorsal section comprising primarily the so-called red sector, and the other three sections comprising primarily the yellow sector.

The method of preparation of the specimens for MSP, the design of the instrument, and the method of analysis of the spectra have been described previously (Bowmaker et al., 1975). Because of the extreme smallness of the diameter of the cone outer segments, in general less than 2 μm, a beam of only 1.5 × 2.5 μm was used; even so, some light leakage around the receptors could not always be avoided. This causes an apparent decrease in the absolute absorbance of the pigment, thereby decreasing the signal-to-noise ratio. The λ_{max}'s of the pigments are difficult to determine from such records; therefore, they were determined from selected records with good signal-to-noise ratios, i.e., with a maximum absorbance greater than about 0.02.

The MSP is designed to measure absorbances of less than 1.0, so the absorbance spectra of the oil droplets that apparently have extremely high absorbances cannot be measured in full but only in the region where the absorbance rises rapidly to 1.0. Liebman and Granda (1975) experienced similar difficulties in measuring the absorbances of colored oil droplets in two species of turtle. When light leakage around small droplets (less than 3 μm) did occur, broad, flat absorbance curves were recorded, with a maximum absorbance considerably less than 1.0.

RESULTS

Rods

A typical absorbance spectrum of a pigeon rod outer segment is shown in Fig. 1. The λ_{max}, determined from five records, was 503 ± 1

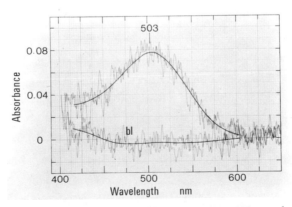

Fig. 1. Absorbance spectrum of a pigeon rod outer segment measured with the microspectrophotometer. Bl, Baseline. The smooth line is the absorbance of a rhodopsin of λ_{max} 503 nm calculated from the Dartnall nomogram and corrected for the irregularities in the baseline. The diameter of the outer segment was about 4 μm.

nm, and the spectrum can be closely fitted by the Dartnall nomogram, λ_{max} 503 nm (Wyszecki and Stiles, 1967), the curve shown superimposed on the record in Fig. 1. In general, the rod outer segments were 3–4 μm in diameter and about 30 μm long, with a specific absorbance of 0.018 ± 0.003 μm^{-1}.

Oil Droplets—Red Sector

By recording spectra with the MSP, five types of oil droplets could be distinguished in the red sector (Fig. 2). Since they were similar to those found previously in the chicken retina (Bowmaker and Knowles, 1977), the same notation has been used, i.e., the oil droplet of the double cone was termed B type and those of the single cones were termed Clear, A, C, and Red, depending on their absorbance spectra. The oil droplets appear to act as cutoff filters, with the A-, C-, and Red-type droplets having λ_{T50} at about 473, 570, and 610 nm. The Clear oil droplets showed no appreciable absorbance above about 450 nm, but showed some evidence of rising absorbance below this wavelength. Their small size (often less than 2 μm in diameter) made it difficult to measure the absorbance spectrum below about 450 nm. Only the chief

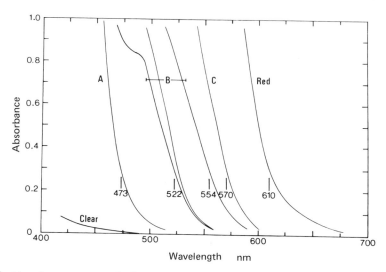

Fig. 2. Absorbance spectra of oil droplets from the red sector of the pigeon retina. Clear, A, C, and Red occur in single cones and B is the chief member of the double cone. The absorbance of the B droplet varies within the range shown and is apparently dependent on the area of the red sector in which the cone is situated. The wavelengths shown are the 50% transmission points of the droplets. No droplet is present in the accessory member of the double cone.

member of the double cone contained an oil droplet, and the absorbance of this B-type droplet varied considerably between different areas of the red sector. In some cases, the droplets appeared orange under the light microscope, and could be distinguished from the orange C-type droplets only by their different position in the retina, the inner segments lying below those of the Red and C types. However, the absorbance spectra were clearly distinguishable since the λ_{T50} of the orange B type was about 554 nm compared with 570 nm in the C type (Fig. 2). In other areas of the red sector, the B-type droplets appeared yellow under the light microscope, with a λ_{T50} at about 525 nm. In some areas, the absorbance spectrum had a shoulder at about 485–490 nm, with an absorbance of 0.8–0.9 and a λ_{T50} at about 522 nm (Fig. 2).

Oil Droplets—Yellow Sector

Five types of oil droplets could also be distinguished in the yellow sector (Fig. 3). The λ_{T50}'s of the oil droplets in the single cones were up to 10 nm shorter than those in the red sector, being about 470, 562, and 600 nm for the A, C, and Red types, respectively. Clear-type single cones were also present, their oil droplets showing a rise in absorbance below about 400–425 nm. The double cones contained a droplet only

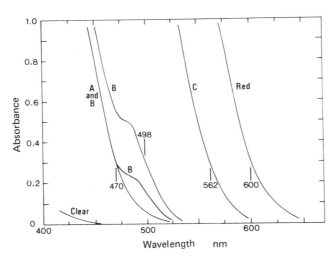

Fig. 3. Absorbance spectra of oil droplets from the yellow sector of the pigeon retina. Clear, A, C, and Red occur in single cones and B is the chief member of the double cone. The absorbance of the B droplet varies within the range shown and is apparently dependent on the area of the yellow sector in which the cone is situated. The wavelengths shown are the 50% transmission points of the droplets. No droplet is present in the accessory member of the double cone.

in the chief member, the absorbance of which varied considerably over the area of the yellow sector. The B-type spectrum was characterized by a shoulder at about 485 nm that had an absorbance ranging up to about 0.5 with a λ_{T50} at about 498 nm. At the periphery of the zone, the absorbance of the B-type droplet showed almost no shoulder, with a λ_{T50} at about 470 nm, and was almost identical to the absorbance of the A-type droplet.

Cone Visual Pigments

Absorbance spectra were obtained from 103 intact cones, that is, cones in which both the oil droplet and the visual pigment absorbance spectra could be obtained. Of these, 91 contained a yellow-absorbing pigment with λ_{max} between 560 and 575 nm, nine contained a green-absorbing pigment with λ_{max} between 510 and 520 nm, and three contained a blue-absorbing pigment with λ_{max} between 450 and 475 nm. By analyzing the records with a high signal-to-noise ratio, the λ_{max} of the long-wave-absorbing pigment was determined to be 567 ± 3 nm. The bandwidth of the spectrum at 50% absorbance was 3900 ± 200 cm^{-1}, that is, narrower than the 4150 cm^{-1} given by the Dartnall nomogram (Fig. 4). The green- and blue-absorbing pigments were best fitted by nomograms with λ_{max} at 514 and 461, nm respectively.

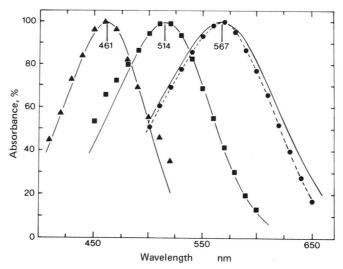

Fig. 4. Absorbance spectra of the three cone visual pigments. ●--●, Yellow absorbing; ■, green abosrbing; ▲, blue absorbing. The full lines are the Dartnall nomogram curves with λ_{max} 567, 514, and 461 nm.

The P567 was the dominant pigment located in retinal cones containing the red oil droplet and in both members of the double cone (Fig. 5-I), as well as in some of the cones containing the A-type droplet. The P514 was located in cones containing the C-type droplet and in some of the cones containing the A-type droplets in the yellow sector of the retina (Fig. 5-II) but apparently only in cones containing the C-type droplet in the red sector. The P461 was found only in the red sector and associated with the A-type oil droplet (Fig. 5-III). No pigment other than the P567 was ever found in the Red-type single cones or either member of the double cones, and no pigment other than the P514 was found in the C-type single cones.

The single cones containing the clear oil droplets were very small with outer segments often less than 1 μm in diameter, making measurement of the visual pigment almost impossible. Only on one occasion was a photosensitive pigment successfully detected in these receptors, and it proved to be the P567. However, the possibility of a further pigment being present in this class of receptor cannot be excluded. The combinations of pigments and oil droplets in the two sectors of the retina are summarized in Table 1.

Table 1. *Oil Droplets and Visual Pigments in the Pigeon Retina*

Oil droplet		Outer segment	Oil droplet–visual pigment combination[a]		
Type	λ_{T50} (nm)	Pigment λ_{max} (nm)	Effective λ_{max} (nm)	Bandwidth at half peak height (cm^{-1})	Approximate % of total cones[b]
			Red Sector		
Red	610	567	619	1417	23
C	570	514	575	1712	27
B	554	567	589	2376	30
	(522)	(567)	(570)	(3124)	
A$_r$	476	567	567	4157	
A$_b$	476	460	485	2561	20
Clear	?	567?	567?	4526?	
			Yellow sector		
Red	600	567	613	1592	12
C	562	514	567	1785	12
B	499[c]	567	567	3608	51
A$_r$	470	567	567	4299	
A$_g$	470	514	525	3537	25
Clear	?	?	?	?	

[a] Calculations based on an end-on absorbance of 0.30 for the cone outer segment.
[b] From Waelchli (1883).
[c] Can be as low as 470 nm at periphery of yellow sector.

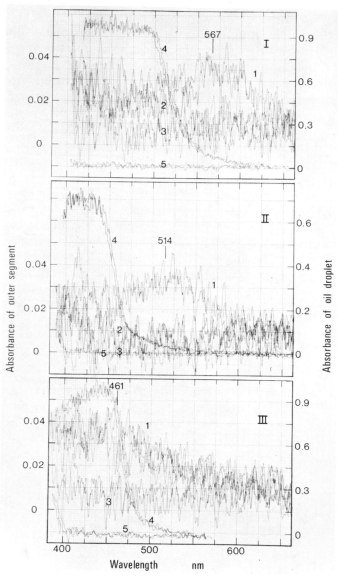

Fig. 5. Absorbance spectra of the visual pigments in the outer segments and the associated oil droplets in three pigeon cones measured with the MSP. I: Chief member of a double cone from red sector with P567 plus the B-type droplet. II: Single cone from yellow sector with P514- plus A-type droplet. III: Single cone from red sector with P461- plus A-type droplet. Curve 1 is the absorbance of the outer segment (left-hand scale); curve 2 is the same after a white bleach; curve 3 is the baseline with the same scale expansion as curves 1 and 2; curve 4 is the absorbance of the oil droplet (right-hand scale); curve 5 is the baseline with the same scale expansion as curve 4.

DISCUSSION

The pigeon retina has been shown to be composed of rods and five types of cones—a double and four singles characterized by the absorbance of their oil droplets—and four visual pigments, a P503 in the rods and P567, P514, and P461 in the cones. The P503 and P567 have been reported previously from MSP studies by Liebman (1972), although he found the λ_{max} to lie at slightly shorter wavelengths. The P514 and P461 have not been previously reported. A comparison of the cone visual pigments of the pigeon with those so far detected by MSP in other birds is shown in Table 2.

The absorbance spectra of the oil droplets in the pigeon retina have been determined previously by Strother (1963) and King-Smith (1969). The present data are in good agreement with those of King-Smith, who similarly found that the λ_{T50}'s of the droplets in the yellow sector were about 10 nm shorter than in the red sector. King-Smith also found great variability in the absorbance of the yellow droplets, with λ_{T50} ranging from about 470 nm to 530 nm. The variability of the B-type droplet reported in this chapter covers a similar range, and it would seem probable that there is a gradation of absorbances of the double-cone oil droplet from a λ_{T50} of 554 nm in the center of the red sector to a λ_{T50} of 500 nm in the yellow sector and to a λ_{T50} of about 460 nm in the periphery of the yellow sector.

Scotopic Sensitivity

The scotopic sensitivity of the pigeon, mediated by the rods, can be predicted from the λ_{max} and specific absorbance of the rod visual pigment. The rod outer segments in the pigeon are about 30 μm long

Table 2. λ_{max} of Visual Pigments of Birds Measured by MSP[a]

	Pigeon	Chicken	Rook	Owl	Laughing gull
Rod	503	506	504	503	
	500*	500*			508*
"Red" cone	567	569	565	555	
	562*	562*			562*
"Green" cone	514	497	497	503	—
"Blue" cone	461	—	—	463	—

[a] Source of data: *, Liebman (1972). Other data: pigeon, Bowmaker (1977); chicken, Bowmaker and Knowles (1977); rook, Bowmaker (unpublished data); owl, Bowmaker and Martin (1978).

and contain the P503 with a specific density of 0.018 μm^{-1}, giving an approximate end-on absorbance of 0.5. The absorptance spectrum (percentage of light absorbed) of the rods, plotted on a log basis, is shown in Fig. 6 and compared with the scotopic sensitivity of the pigeon (expressed on an equal quantum basis) as determined from electroretinography (Donner, 1953; Ikeda, 1965; Graf and Norren, 1974), pupillary measurements (Alexandridis, 1967), and measurements in isolated thalamic units (Granda and Yazulla, 1971). The excellent fit of the data illustrates the direct relationship between the rod visual pigment absorptance and scotopic sensitivity.

Cone Spectral Sensitivities

Since the cone oil droplets interpose between the incident light and the cone visual pigments, the cutoff of the droplets will determine the effective spectral sensitivities of the pigments. From the MSP results, it is therefore possible to derive the effective spectral sensitivities of the various cone types. For these calculations, the cones were taken

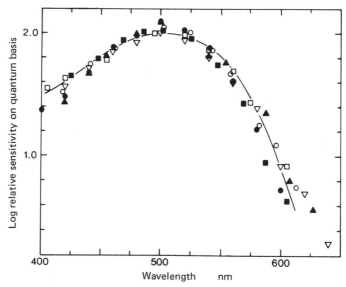

Fig. 6. Scotopic sensitivity of the pigeon. Full line is the scotopic sensitivity derived from the percentage of light absorbed by a P503 in a 30-μm-long rod outer segment. Symbols are experimentally determined scotopic sensitivities: ○, from Donner (1953); ●, ■, from Ikeda (1965); □, from Alexandridis (1967); ▽, from Granda and Yazulla (1971); ▲, from Graf and Norren (1974). The experimental data have been displaced in the vertical axis to obtain the greatest coincidence on the two limbs of the curve.

as being 20 μm long, with an end-on absorbance of 0.30, the specific density being about 0.015 μm^{-1}.

As a general rule, the effect of an oil droplet in a given cone is to displace the effective maximum sensitivity of the cone to a wavelength longer than the λ_{max} of the visual pigment, to reduce the bandwidth of the spectral sensitivity of the visual pigment by cutting off the shorter wavelengths, and to reduce the absolute sensitivity of the cone at its λ_{max} from that of the visual pigment λ_{max}. Thus in the red sector of the pigeon retina the red oil droplet cuts off light below about 560 nm and displaces the effective maximum sensitivity of the P567 to about 619 nm, reduces the absolute sensitivity at 619 nm to about 38% of the sensitivity of the visual pigment at 567 nm, and reduces the bandwidth of the spectral sensitivity to about 30% of that of the P567 (Fig. 7, Red curve). Similarly, the C- and A-type droplets also will affect the sensitivity of their respective pigments (Fig. 7). The effective spectral sensitivity of the double cones will vary depending on the transmission characteristics of the different B-type droplets: the orange-colored drop-

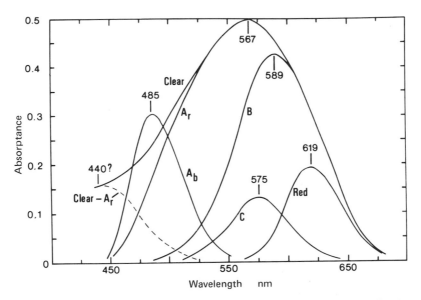

Fig. 7. Calculated absorptance for the pigment–oil droplet combinations in the six recognized cone types in the red sector of the pigeon retina, assuming an end-on absorbance of 0.30 for the cone outer segments. Clear, absorptance of a cone having the clear oil droplet with P567 in the outer segment; A_r, A-type droplet with P567; A_b, A-type droplet with P461; B, B-type droplet (λ_{T50} 554 nm) with P567; C, C-type droplet with P514; Red, red droplet with P567. The dashed line indicates the possible response, maximal at about 430–440 nm, derived by interaction between the Clear and A_r-type cones.

lets ($\lambda_{T50}=544$) displacing the effective maximum sensitivity to considerably longer wavelengths than the yellow droplets ($\lambda_{T50}=522$).

In the yellow sector of the retina a similar pattern is found, but with the effective maximum sensitivities of the cones being at slightly shorter wavelengths than those in the red sector (Fig. 8). The Red- and C-type cones have maxima at about 613 and 567 nm, respectively, compared with 619 and 575 nm in the red sector. The A-type plus P461 combination has not been found in the yellow sector and is replaced by an A-type plus P514 combination that has an effective maximum sensitivity at about 525 nm (Fig. 8, curve A_g). The characteristics of all the cone types are shown in Table 1.

Photopic Sensitivity

Although the relationship between the rod visual pigment and scotopic sensitivity is straightforward, the relationship between cone visual pigments and photopic sensitivity must be more complex because of the variety of the cone types present. In a previous paper

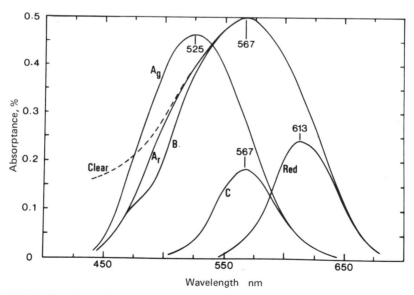

Fig. 8. Calculated absorptance for the pigment–oil droplet combinations in the six recognized cone types in the yellow sector of the pigeon retina, assuming an end-on absorbance of 0.30 for the cone outer segments. Clear (dashed line), possible absorptance of a cone having the clear oil droplet with P567 in the outer segment; A_r, A-type droplet with P567; A_g, A-type droplet with P514; B, B-type droplet with P567; C, C-type droplet with P514; Red, red droplet with P567.

(Bowmaker and Knowles, 1977) it was suggested that, in the chicken, a direct summation of the spectral sensitivities of the individual cone types, in the ratio of the number of each cone type present in the retina, gave an overall spectral sensitivity that was well matched to the photopic sensitivity as determined experimentally.

No attempt was made in the present study to obtain counts of each type of receptor in the pigeon retina. However, the relative numbers of the cone types in the chicken retina determined in the previous study were found to be in good agreement with the data of Waelchli (1883), so his data on the relative numbers of cone types in the red and yellow fields of the pigeon were used in the present study. The data are presented in Table 1. The yellow sector of the retina is similar in composition to the chicken retina, being dominated by the double cones ("large green" of Waelchli) accounting for about half of the total cone population, with approximately equal numbers of Red- and C-type cones (red and orange of Waelchli). In the red sector, according to Waelchli, there are approximately equal numbers of red and two orange types of oil droplets separated by their level in the retina (C-type and B doubles; see Results) that make up about 80% of the total cone population. Using the direct-summation method and the relative numbers of the cone types from Waelchli (1883), photopic sensitivities have been determined for both the red and yellow sectors of the retina.

For the yellow sector, a photopic sensitivity was derived by summing the Red-, C-, B-, and A- plus P514–type cones of the yellow sector in the ratio $1.2:1.2:5.1:1.0$, respectively (Table 1). The resulting sensitivity curve has a maximum at 560–570 nm and is shown as the full curve in Fig. 9. Although the A- plus P514-type receptor was not identified by Waelchli, it must represent a proportion of his 25% "small green" type cones. Varying the relative numbers of these cones does not greatly affect the overall sensitivity spectrum since it is dominated by the B-type double cones. The sensitivity spectrum below about 530 nm is determined primarily by the transmission spectrum of the B-type droplets; the dashed lines in Fig. 9 show a possible range of sensitivities depending on the variety of B-type droplet used (see Fig. 3).

The photopic sensitivity of the pigeon has been determined by a number of workers either from electroretinography (Granit, 1942; Donner, 1953; Ikeda, 1965; Blough et al., 1972; Graf and Norren, 1974; Norren, 1975), from thalamic (Granda and Yazulla, 1971; Yazulla and Granda, 1973) and tectal units (King-Smith quoted by Muntz, 1972), or behaviorally (Blough, 1957; Graf, 1969; Romeskie and Yager, 1976). Unfortunately, it is not always clear from which area of the retina the results were obtained, because the photopic sensitivity of the red and

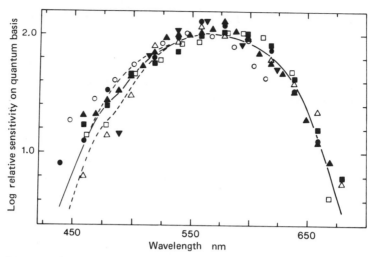

Fig. 9. Photopic sensitivity of the pigeon. Full line is the spectral sensitivity for the yellow sector of the retina derived from the absorptance of the Red-, C-, B-, and A- plus P514-type cones (Fig. 8) summed in the ratio 1.2 : 1.2 : 5.1 : 1.0, respectively (Table 1). Dashed lines represent the effect of using the different transmission characteristics of the B-type droplets in the yellow sector. Symbols are experimentally determined photopic sensitivities: ■, from Granit (1942); □, from Donner (1953); ●, from Blough (1957); ○, from Ikeda (1965); ▲, from Graf (1969); △, from Blough et al. (1972);▼, from King-Smith quoted by Muntz (1972). The experimental data have been displaced in the vertical axis to obtain the greatest coincidence on the two limbs of the curve.

yellow sectors clearly will differ because of the different types and relative numbers of the cones present in each area. Only the data of King-Smith (Muntz, 1972) are specifically from tectal units stimulated from either the red or yellow fields. However, the data from the majority of determinations of photopic sensitivity are in broad agreement, showing a maximum sensitivity between 560 and 580 nm, and are similar to the photopic sensitivity recorded by King-Smith for the yellow-field tectal units. These data are shown in Fig. 9, expressed on an equal quantum basis and adjusted in the vertical axis to obtain the greatest coincidence of the limbs of the sensitivity spectrum but not necessarily of the peak. The photopic sensitivity derived from the data presented in this chapter is in broad agreement with the experimental photopic sensitivities, although there is considerable variation in the data from the different laboratories.

In the red sector, 80% of the cones are made up of Red, C, and B types, with λ_{max} of 619, 575, and 589 nm, respectively. These were summed in the ratio 2.3 : 2.7 : 3.0 (Table 1) to give the spectral sensitivity shown as the full curve in Fig. 10, with a maximum sensitivity between

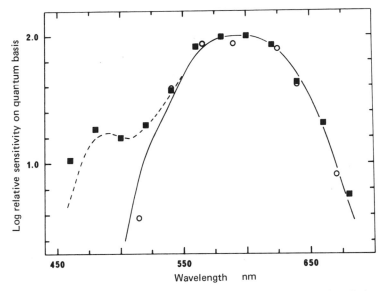

Fig. 10. Photopic sensitivity of the red sector of the pigeon retina. Full line is the spectral sensitivity for the red sector derived from the absorptance of the Red-, C-, and B-type cones (Fig. 7) summed in the ratio 2.3 : 2.7 : 3.0, respectively (Table 1). Dashed line represents the effect of the addition of the A- plus P461-type cones in the ratio of 1.0. ■, photopic sensitivity from Romeskie and Yager (1976); ○, sensitivity of tectal units stimulated from the red sector from King-Smith quoted by Muntz (1972).

580 and 600 nm. This curve does not include the blue cones since the percentage of these is not known, although they will be a fraction of the 20% clear cones of Waelchli (Table 1). Assuming a figure of about 10% and therefore adding the blue cones (λ_{max} = 485 nm) in a ratio of 1.0, the dashed line in Fig. 10 is obtained with a secondary peak between 480 and 490 nm. The data of King-Smith (Muntz, 1972) for the red-sector tectal units and the psychophysical data obtained from the red field by Romeskie and Yager (1976) are shown for comparison. The fits are excellent and suggest that the tectal units recorded by King-Smith do not receive information from the blue cones.

Cone Sensitivities and Color Channels

In studies on the photopic sensitivity of the pigeon, a number of wavelength-dependent mechanisms have been isolated. Donner (1953) identified blue, green, and red modulator units from ganglion cell recordings with maxima at about 480, 540, and between 596 and 613 nm. Ikeda (1965) isolated similar mechanisms from electroretinographic

studies with maxima at about 550 nm and 605 nm, and Granda and
Yazulla (1971) also identified single units in the nucleus rotundus of
the pigeon with maximum sensitivities at about 540 nm and 600–620
nm. In Fig. 11 an attempt has been made to relate these modulator
curves to the spectral sensitivities of individual cone types. Fig. 11-I

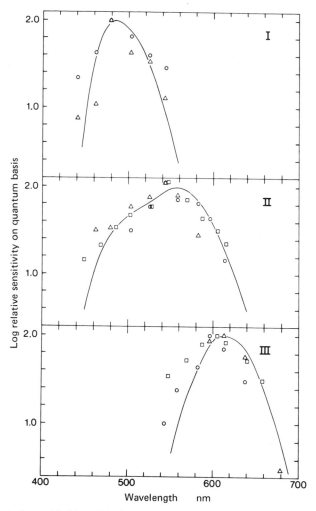

Fig. 11. Spectral sensitivities of individual cone types. I: Full curve, sensitivity of A-
plus P461-type cone of the red sector: ○, △, blue modulator sensitivity recorded from
ganglion cells (Donner, 1953). II: Full curve, sensitivity of A- plus P514-type and C-type
cones from the yellow sector summed in the ratio 1.0 : 1.2: ○, △, green modulator
sensitivity recorded from ganglion cells (Donner, 1953); □, sensitivity determined from
electroretinogram (Ikeda, 1965). III: Full curve, sensitivity of red cone from yellow sector:
○, △, red modulator sensitivity recorded from ganglion cells (Donner, 1953); □, sensitivity determined from electroretinogram (Ikeda, 1965).

shows the spectral sensitivity of the P461- plus A-type cone found in the red sector compared with the blue modulator of Donner (1953). As pointed out previously, addition of this unit to the overall sensitivity of the majority receptors in the red field will fit the secondary peak found by Romeskie and Yager (1976) and will similarly fit the 480-nm-sensitive system isolated by Norren (1975).

The green modulators identified by Donner (1953) and Ikeda (1965) are shown in Fig. 11-II. The data peak between 540 and 550 nm, but are too broad to fit either of the spectral sensitivities of the A- plus P514-type cone and the C-type cone in the yellow sector (λ_{max} = 525 and 567 nm). However, summing these two in the ratio of 1.0:1.2 (as used in the estimation of the overall sensitivity of the yellow sector) results in the spectral sensitivity shown in Fig. 11-II, full line, that is a reasonable fit to the green modulator sensitivity. In Fig. 11-III the red modulator data of Donner (1953) and Ikeda (1965) are compared to the spectral sensitivity of the red cone in the yellow sector with λ_{max} of 613 nm.

Blue Sensitivity

Considerable evidence has accumulated for a further blue-sensitive mechanism maximal between 400 and 440 nm in diurnal birds (Yazulla and Granda, 1973; Graf and Norren, 1974; Norren, 1975; Romeskie and Yager, 1976; Govardovskii and Zueva, 1977); a visual pigment with λ_{max} about 420 nm has been postulated to account for this sensitivity. No such visual pigment has been directly measured in birds. However, with MSP it is not possible to say that a certain visual pigment is not present, only that it is probably not present when it has not been found after records have been taken from large numbers of cones in the retina. However, in the pigeon there is a population of cones that are too small for MSP measurement which may contain a still unidentified visual pigment, although the recordings that have been obtained from these cones suggest that at least some contain the P567.

Nevertheless, blue sensitivity can be achieved by interaction between cones containing the P567 with the clear oil droplets and the P567 with the A-type droplets. Interaction of this type will produce a sensitivity maximal at wavelengths below about 440 nm (Fig. 7, Clear -A_r), and, indeed, Yazulla and Granda (1973) have recorded from opponent units in the pigeon thalamus that reponded either positively to blue and negatively to yellow, or the reverse, with maxima at 420–440 nm and about 560 nm. These were the only opponent units that they found, all the other units being either excitatory or inhibitory (Granda and Yazulla, 1971).

From the data presented above, it would appear that the effective absorbance spectra of the cone types found in the retina of the pigeon can be directly related to the photopic sensitivity of the pigeon as measured both behaviorally and electrophysiologically. The narrowband modulator-type sensitivities can be obtained by the cutoff filtering of the oil droplets associated with the different visual pigments, while the overall photopic sensitivities of the red and yellow sectors of the retina can be derived by a simple summation of the individual cone sensitivities in the same ratio as the relative numbers of each cone type in each area of the retina. Short-wave length blue sensitivity may be achieved through an opponent mechanism between two cone types containing the same visual pigment but different oil droplets.

REFERENCES

Alexandridis, E.: Pupillographische Untersuchung der Netzhautempfindlichkeit des Taubenauges. *Arch. Ophthalmol.* **172**:139-151 (1967).

Blough, D. S.: Spectral sensitivity in the pigeon. *J. Opt. Soc. Am.* **47**:827-833 (1957).

Blough, P. M., Riggs, L. A., and Schafer, K. L.: Photopic spectral sensitivity determined electroretinographically for the pigeon eye. *Vision Res.* **12**:477-485 (1972).

Bowmaker, J. K.: The visual pigments, oil droplets and spectral sensitivity in the pigeon. *Vision Res.* **17**:1129-1138 (1977).

Bowmaker, J. K., and Knowles, A.: The visual pigments and oil droplets of the chicken retina. *Vision Res.* **17**:755-764 (1977).

Bowmaker, J. K. and Martin, G. R.: Visual pigments and color vision in a nocturnal bird, *Strix aluco* (tawny owl). *Vision Res.* **18**:1125-1130 (1978).

Bowmaker, J. K., Loew, E. R., and Liebman, P. A.: Variation in the λ_{max} of rhodopsin from individual frogs. *Vision Res.* **15**:977-1003 (1975).

Donner, K. O.: The spectral sensitivity of the pigeon's retinal elements. *J. Physiol. (London)* **122**:524-537 (1953).

Govardovskii, V. I., and Zueva, L. V.: Visual pigments of chicken and pigeon. *Vision Res.* **17**:537-543 (1977).

Graf, V. A.: A spectral luminosity function in the pigeon determined by flicker photometry. *Psychon. Sci.* **17**:282-283 (1969).

Graf, V. A., and Norren, D. V.: A blue sensitive mechanism in the pigeon retina: λ_{max} 400 nm. *Vision Res.* **14**:1203-1209 (1974).

Granda, A. M., and Yazulla, S.: The spectral sensitivity of single units in the nucleus rotundus of the pigeon. *J. Gen. Physiol.* **57**:363-384 (1971).

Granit, R.: The photopic spectrum of the pigeon. *Acta Physiol. Scand.* **4**:118-124 (1942).

Ikeda, H.: The spectral sensitivity of the pigeon (*Columba livia*). *Vision Res.* **5**:19-36 (1965).

King-Smith, P. E.: Absorption spectra and function of the coloured oil drops in the pigeon retina. *Vision Res.* **9**:1391-1401 (1969).

Liebman, P. A.: Microspectrophotometry of photoreceptors. In Dartnall, H. J. A. (ed.): *Handbook of Sensory Physiology, VII/1.* Springer-Verlag, Berlin (1972).

Liebman, P. A., and Granda, A. M.: Microspectrophotometric measurements of visual pigments in two species of turtle, *Pseudemys scripta* and *Chelonia mydas*. *Vision Res.* **11**:105-114 (1971).

Liebman, P. A., and Granda, A. M.: Super dense carotenoid spectra resolved in single cone oil droplets. *Nature (London)* **253**:370-372 (1975).

Muntz, W. R. A.: Inert absorbing and reflecting pigments. In Dartnall, H. J. A. (ed.): *Handbook of Sensory Physiology, VII/1*. Springer-Verlag, Berlin (1972).

Norren, D. V.: Two short wavelength sensitive cone systems in pigeon, chicken and daw. *Vision Res.* **15**:1164-1166 (1975).

Pedler, C., and Boyle, M.: Multiple oil droplets in the photoreceptors of the pigeon. *Vision Res.* **9**:525-528 (1969).

Romeskie, M., and Yager, D.: Psychophysical studies of pigeon color vision. I. Photopic spectral sensitivity. *Vision Res.* **16**:501-505 (1976).

Strother, G. K.: Absorption spectra of retinal oil globules in turkey, turtle and pigeon. *Exp. Cell Res.* **29**:349-355 (1963).

Waelchli, G.: Zur Topographie der gefärbten Kugeln der Vogelnetzhaut. *Arch. Ophthalmol.* **29**:205-223 (1883).

Wyszecki, G., and Stiles, W. S.: *Colour Science.* Wiley, New York. Pp. 584. (1967).

Yazulla, S., and Granda, A. M.: Opponent-color units in the thalamus of the pigeon (*Columba livia*). *Vision Res.* **13**:1555-1563 (1973).

17

Retinal Oil Droplets and Vision in the Pigeon (*Columba livia*)

G. R. MARTIN and W. R. A. MUNTZ

INTRODUCTION

There is increasing evidence that the retinal oil droplets of the avian retina act as light filters selective at the individual receptor level, affecting the absorbance spectra of only the individual cone in whose inner segment the droplet is situated. Oil droplets do not appear to act as general filters in the same sense as other intraocular filters (cornea, lens, macular pigment) which affect the spectral composition of the whole (or part) of the retinal image. See Muntz (1972) and Wolbarsht (1976) for recent reviews of the various theories of the function of retinal oil droplets.

In the pigeon (*Columba livia*), the retina can be divided into separate areas according to the proportions of the different oil droplet types contained in them. The red field occupies the whole of the dorsotemporal quadrant and about half of the adjoining dorsonasal quadrant. The remainder of the retina constitutes the yellow field (Galifret, 1968). The oil droplet types of these fields have been described by King-Smith (1969) and Bowmaker (1977), and estimates of their relative abundance have been made by Waelchli (1883) and Bloch and Maturana (1971).

Since it would seem that avian photopic spectral sensitivity (at least at wavelengths greater than 450 nm) can be reasonably well modeled by assuming direct summation of the spectral sensitivities of the

G. R. MARTIN and W. R. A. MUNTZ • Laboratory of Experimental Psychology, University of Sussex, Falmer, Brighton, Sussex, England.

individual cone types (cone pigment–oil droplet combinations at their known absorbances) in the ratio of their approximate numbers in the retina (Bowmaker, 1977, this volume; Bowmaker and Knowles, 1977; Bowmaker and Martin, 1978), it would be predicted that the spectral sensitivities of these two retinal areas differ.

In addition, consideration of optics and eye position indicates that the red field is used by the pigeon for frontal viewing and hence is the field used to guide pecking behavior, while the yellow field is that part of the retina used for lateral viewing. It seems reasonable to suggest that these fields serve different visual functions and that these are related to photic factors in the ecological niche occupied by the species.

Romeskie and Yager (1976) presented results which they interpreted as showing a difference in the spectral sensitivity of the red and yellow fields of the pigeon. Photopic spectral sensitivity was determined behaviorally, and the maximum sensitivity was found to be shifted to longer wavelengths, compared to Blough's (1957) function. They suggested that sensitivity in their experiment was determined by the red field, while sensitivity in Blough's experiment was determined by the yellow field. The difference in field stimulated was considered to have arisen as a result of differences in the loci of response and stimulus in the two experiments. However, the experimental procedures used in the two experiments also differed in another important variable—the light adaptation which the subjects received. In Romeskie and Yager's experiment the birds were constantly light adapted, while in Blough's experiment data were obtained during the early stages of dark adaptation. The spectral distribution and high luminance level of the adapting light used by Romeskie and Yager could well have resulted in a shift in spectral sensitivity toward the red end of the spectrum. King-Smith is reported (Muntz, 1972) to have detected a difference in the locus of maximum spectral sensitivity between tectal neurons having receptive fields in the yellow and red fields of the pigeon. No details of the experimental procedures are available, however, and hence it is not possible to evaluate these results fully.

It would therefore seem of value to investigate whether differences in visual capacity can be detected between the two droplet fields of the pigeon retina. This has been done by determining spectral sensitivity functions for the two fields in the same eye under identical conditions.

METHODS

Subjects

Two pigeons (*Columba livia*) from the laboratory's colony of homing pigeons were used. They were maintained at 80% of their free-feeding weight on a standard laboratory diet of grain and vitamin additives.

Apparatus and Procedure

General. The pigeons were trained to make a pecking response, reinforced by the presentation of grain, in response to light stimuli presented at fixed loci inside a dome-shaped headgear bolted to the bird's skull. The stimuli were delivered to this "dome" through light guides which were positioned so that they fell in either the red or the yellow field. A two-choice discrete-trials simultaneous discrimination procedure was used in which the subjects were trained to respond to one of the keys when a stimulus light was presented and to the other key in the absence of the stimulus light. Sensitivities to monochromatic stimuli of different wavelengths were determined by constructing psychophysical functions (curves showing percent correct response vs. intensity). A pigeon wearing the dome device is shown in Figs. 1 and 2. Figures 3 and 4 show general views of the apparatus, and diagrammatic representations are shown in Figs. 5 and 6.

Behavioral Apparatus. The birds were restricted within the small response chamber (indicated by the grid floor in the diagrams and photographs) by a shaped partition which allowed them to stretch forward to reach the response keys and feed from the hopper, but not to enter the area where these were situated. The response keys were constructed of translucent perspex and transilluminated by achromatic light. They were placed symmetrically above the food hopper. The chamber wall below the response key was concave so that the birds could feed freely from the hopper while wearing the dome. The hopper was a modified standard pigeon grain hopper in which grain was presented in an open-ended, square-section tube (10 by 10 mm) which was raised vertically through the floor of the pigeon chamber below the response keys. Grain in the hopper was replenished by a modified rat pellet dispenser which delivered a measured amount of grain into the hopper while in its lowered position. Two speakers were mounted on either side of the response chamber and delivered white noise. All surfaces were painted matt gray. The whole of the response area of the chamber was covered by a large, transparent perspex hemisphere. The hemisphere was covered by a translucent plastic sheeting material and the whole apparatus was covered by a large light box. The inner surfaces of the light box were painted matt white, and four tungsten strip lamps (60 W) were mounted symmetrically on each of the four walls. This box and hemisphere arrangement ensured homogeneous lighting conditions within the apparatus.

Pigeon Headgear. The pigeon headgear is shown diagrammatically in Fig. 7. It consisted of an aluminum frame supporting two transparent perspex hemispheres on each of which were mounted two small perspex blocks. Each of these blocks was mounted above a hole in the perspex hemispheres to hold in place a 3-mm-diameter ball bearing in

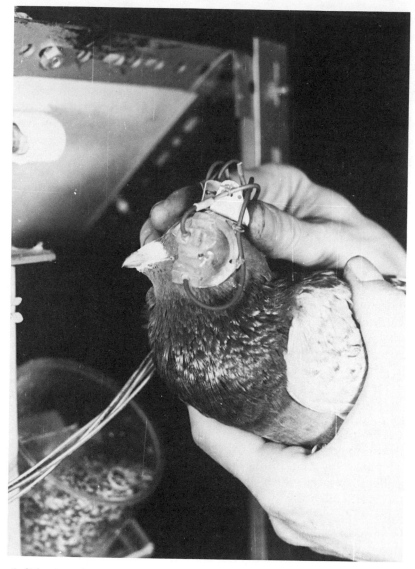

Fig. 1. Side view of a pigeon wearing the aluminum and perspex dome bearing the fiber optic light guides.

which the fiber optic light guides were embedded. A small section cut out of the aluminum frame and perspex hemisphere on each side allowed the bird to see clearly along the line of its bill. The whole assembly weighed 4.6 g and was attached to the bird's head by two stainless steel bolts which were fixed into a stainless steel plate held

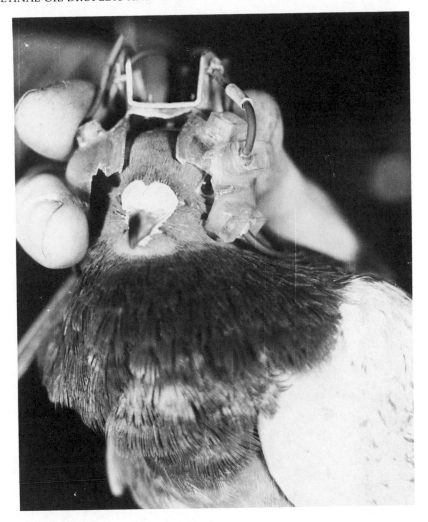

Fig. 2. Front view of a pigeon wearing the aluminum and perspex dome, showing the section cut away to allow the bird to see clearly along the line of its bill.

by dental acrylic to the bird's skull. This arrangement enabled the head-gear to be easily detached and transferred from pigeon to pigeon. Each light guide consisted of a 1-m length of a resheathed bundle of six individual fibers (Crofon, Rank). The resheathing material was silicone rubber electrical sleeving, which permitted a higher degree of flexibility than the original manufacturer's sheathing. The fibers were held at their ends by embedding them in epoxy resin. The embedded ends were filed smooth and polished. At the dome end, they were inserted in a hole drilled through the ball bearing. The ball bearing arrangement

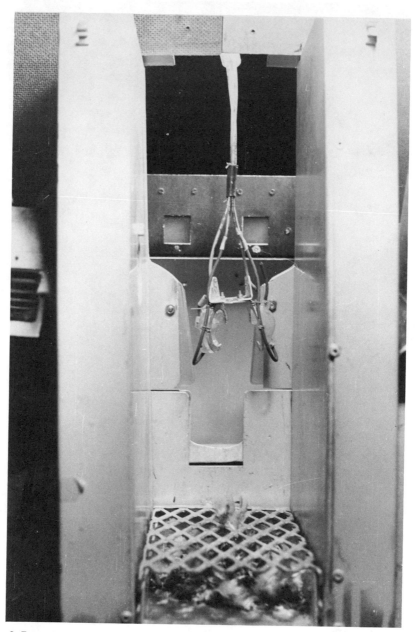

Fig. 3. Rear view into the response chamber. The grid floor indicates the area into which the pigeon was restrained by the shaped partition. The pigeon headgear is hanging centrally, supported by the fiber optic light guides, and the response keys can be seen beyond the restraining partition.

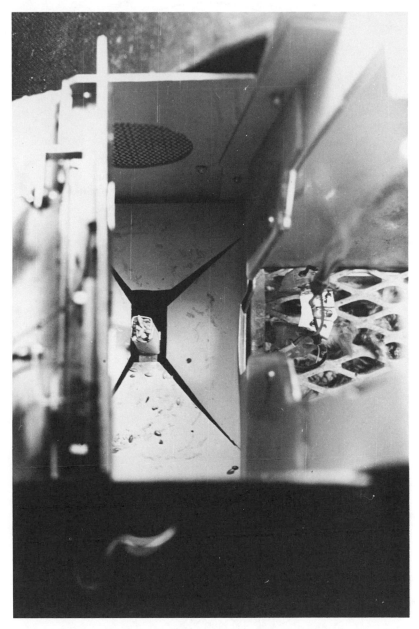

Fig. 4. Plan view of the response chamber. The restraining partition and headgear are to the right. The grain hopper is raised up through the floor of the chamber and the response keys are to the left.

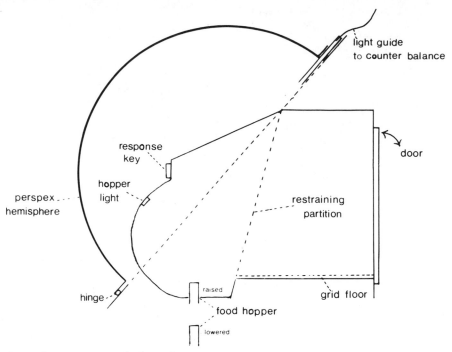

Fig. 5. Diagrammatic side view of the apparatus. Note the concave shape of the chamber wall below the response key and the perspex hemisphere used to produce homogeneous illumination within the chamber.

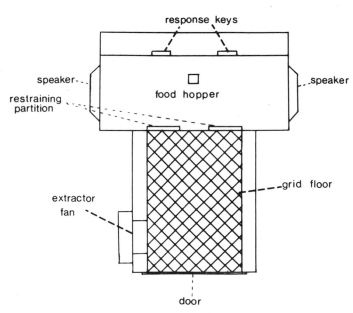

Fig. 6. Diagrammatic plan view of the response chamber.

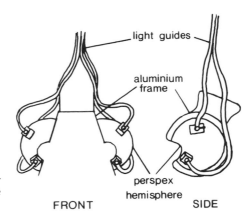

Fig. 7. Diagrammatic views of the aluminum and perspex dome worn by the pigeons.

enabled the light guides to be swiveled to a desired position and then locked by a set screw. Each light guide was fastened to the aluminum frame of the dome, and the four guides passed out of the top of the apparatus below the rim of the light-adapting hemisphere to a counterbalance device. This allowed the pigeon to move freely in the apparatus while the slack in the light guide was kept to a minimum. The light guide was positioned in the bird's dome by projecting light through it at high illuminance onto the bird's eye and swiveling the ball bearing until the illumination lit the eye symmetrically (i.e., the light guide was pointing directly at the eye). The ball bearing was then locked in position and a small piece of tracing paper was fixed across the end of the light guide. The effect was to produce a small light patch approximately 2 mm diameter on the inside surface of the dome. In each eye, one light guide was positioned so that it stimulated the red-droplet field and was close to the bird's line of sight along its bill, and the other so that it delivered light to the yellow-droplet field from a position above the horizontal in the lateral visual field. It was not possible to measure the exact distance between the stimulus spot and the pigeon's eye. However, the approximate angle subtended by the stimuli at the cornea was 12 deg of arc.

Optical Apparatus and Calibration. The optical apparatus is shown diagrammatically in Fig. 8. The stimulus light was provided by a quartz-halogen lamp (Atlas, AI/180,24 V) run from a constant-current supply. Wavelength was controlled by interference filters (Balzars, B40) (IF) and intensity was controlled by Kodak Wratten neutral density filters (ND). A bank of four ND filters of nominal value 0.2, 0.4, 0.8, and 1.6 was mounted on solenoids so that the light intensity could be changed between trials by steps of 0.2 over a range of 3.0 log units. A fixed ND filter was also used to bring the intensity within the desired

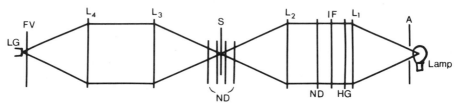

Fig. 8. Diagram of optical apparatus. Abbreviations: A, aperture; L_1–L_4, lenses; IF, interference filter; HG, heat glass; ND, neutral density filter; S, shutter; FV, flicker vane; LG, light guide.

range. A silently operating shutter (S) was positioned at the first focus of the optical system. This consisted of a small piece of aluminum foil, painted matt black, mounted on the arm of a galvanometer. Just before the second focus of the system, a flicker vane (FV) was positioned which caused the stimulus to flicker at 5 Hz with equal light/dark ratio. The light guide (LG) was mounted at the second focus.

The relative energy available through the different interference filters was measured with a Hilger-Schwartz FT17 thermopile placed at the second focus of the system. The ND filters were calibrated with a combination of instruments: the thermopile, an EMI photomultiplier, and an SP500 spectrophotometer. The transmission of the IF filters was calibrated with a Shimadzu scanning spectrophotometer. The luminance of the light-adapting hemisphere was measured with an SEI photometer and equaled 1.8 log mL.

Procedure. The headgear was first introduced to the birds following hopper training. The birds were trained to key-peck, reinforced by the presentation of food, under a schedule of continuous reinforcement. Reinforcer presentation was indicated by the extinction of the adapting and key lights, the switching on of the hopper light, and the sound of a buzzer. The hopper remained in position for 7 sec. The amount of grain eaten in this time was limited by the depth that the bill could reach into the hopper tube rather than the length of presentation. The intertrial interval equaled 10 sec. The birds were trained to peck the left-hand key if a stimulus light was present within the dome and to peck the right-hand key if no light was present. The position of the stimulus light in the visual field was irrelevant. Ninety-six trials per daily session were given, half of which were stimulus trials, the order being determined by a Gellerman sequence. Extensive training was necessary before discriminative performance reached asymptote at over 85% correct. However, once it had reached this level, stimulus control remained high. This was checked by recording the number of false-positive responses per session (i.e., subject responding that a stimulus was present in its absence). False-positive responses were usually only about 4% of all trials, and data from those sessions in which false-positive trials exceeded 15% were not used.

Psychophysical functions were constructed by plotting the number of correct trials at each stimulus intensity, and thresholds were determined by interpolating at the 50%-correct level. The stimuli were presented at the same wavelength but at different retinal loci on alternate days, in the same eye. Stimuli were presented at eight different intensities according to a modified method of constant stimuli (i.e., six trials at each intensity per session) and psychophysical functions were constructed from between 24 and 36 trials at each intensity.

RESULTS

Psychophysical functions were derived for both birds at nine test wavelengths for the two stimuli positions in the same eye. These functions indicated a high degree of stimulus control, with discriminative performance varying almost linearly with log stimulus intensity over the range from about 70% to 20% correct. Sample psychophysical functions for the two birds at 568 nm (yellow field) are shown in Fig. 9. Spectral sensitivity functions (equal quantum intensity base) for each

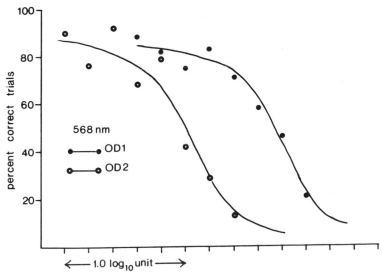

Fig. 9. Sample psychophysical functions for the two subjects at 568 nm in the yellow field. Abscissa, relative density; ordinate, percent correct trials. Thresholds were determined by interpolating the functions (best fit by inspection) at the 50%-correct point. The curves have been displaced along the abscissa for clarity.

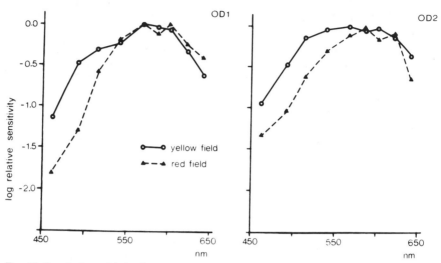

Fig. 10. Spectral sensitivity functions for the red and yellow droplet fields in two pigeons. The curves have been equated at their maxima.

bird at both retinal loci are shown in Fig. 10. Figure 11 shows the mean function for the two birds. Numerical values are given in Table 1.

DISCUSSION

Clear differences are evident between the two spectral sensitivity functions of each subject (Fig. 10). It is very likely that these differences can be attributed to a difference in the sensitivity of the red and yellow

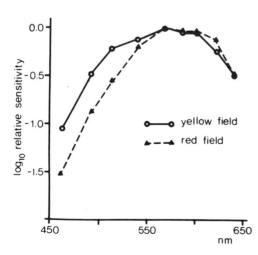

Fig. 11. Mean spectral sensitivity functions for the red and yellow droplet fields in two pigeons. The curves have been equated at their maxima.

Table 1. Log Relative Sensitivity of the Two Pigeons in the Red and Yellow Oil Droplet Fields

λ	Subject OD1 droplet field		Subject OD2 droplet field		Mean droplet field	
	Red	Yellow	Red	Yellow	Red	Yellow
462	−1.81	−1.15	−1.32	−0.95	−1.52	−1.05
493	−0.80	−0.48	−1.03	−0.48	−0.87	−0.48
514	−0.58	−0.31	−0.62	−0.13	−0.55	−0.22
540	−0.20	−0.23	−0.30	−0.02	−0.20	−0.13
568	0.00	0.00	−0.10	0.00	0.00	0.00
586	−0.12	−0.02	0.00	−0.05	−0.01	−0.04
601	0.00	−0.06	−0.15	−0.04	−0.03	−0.05
623	−0.25	−0.33	−0.07	−0.13	−0.11	−0.23
643	−0.41	−0.62	−0.64	−0.36	−0.48	−0.49

fields. While it was not possible to specify exactly the retinal locus stimulated by each stimulus patch, the position of the patches within the dome worn by the birds made it highly likely that they were stimulating the dorsotemporal quadrant (red field) and the ventral-temporal/nasal area (yellow field) of the retinas in both birds. Adaptation conditions were identical throughout the experiment and hence are unlikely to have been responsible for the differences detected here. The light guides were identical, and selective transmission by them cannot therefore account for the differences found.

The spectral sensitivity functions for the two subjects (Fig. 10), while differing in a number of ways, show the following similarities: (1) the red-field functions are narrower than those of the yellow field; (2) the yellow field is more sensitive than the red field at wavelengths below about 550 nm; and (3) the two fields show similar relative sensitivity at wavelengths beyond 600 nm.

Since it is unlikely that the stimulus patch stimulated exactly equivalent retinal loci in the two subjects, it is not possible to determine with certainty to what extent the differences found between the subjects can be ascribed to individual differences in the sensitivity of the red and yellow fields.

Comparison With Other Spectral Sensitivity Functions for the Pigeon

Among the behaviorally determined spectral sensitivity functions that have previously been reported for the pigeon, those of Graf (1969) and Blough (1957) show good overall agreement in both shape and locus of maximum sensitivity. The behaviorally determined function of Romeskie and Yager (1976) differs from these two functions in both of these features. Figure 12 shows the spectral sensitivity functions of

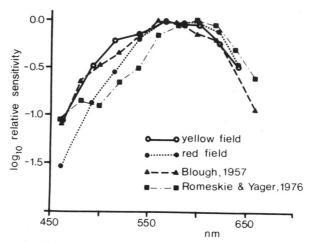

Fig. 12. Mean red and yellow spectral sensitivity functions for the two pigeons and the pigeon spectral sensitivity functions of Blough (1957) and Romeskie and Yager (1976). The functions have been equated at their maxima.

Blough (1957) and Romeskie and Yager (1976) and the two mean spectral sensitivity functions recorded here. The yellow-field spectral sensitivity shows reasonable similarity to the function of Blough. Both functions exhibit the same overall shape, and the maximum sensitivity is similarly located in both cases. The main discrepancy between the two functions is at about 520 nm, where the sensitivity in this experiment was found to be slightly higher than in Blough's function.

The function of Romeskie and Yager shows some similarity to that of the red field at wavelengths greater than 600 nm, but differs considerably below this wavelength. The two functions intersect at about 500 nm, with the red field being relatively less sensitive below this wavelength and more sensitive above it. The reasons for these differences are not clear. It is not possible to establish with certainty from these results whether Romeskie and Yager were in fact recording spectral sensitivity from the red field, as they suggest, or whether the relative sensitivity below about 580 nm was depressed in their experiment as a result of the adaptation conditions they employed. In support of this latter interpretation is the large difference in relative sensitivity between the red field and Romeskie and Yager's function at about 460 nm, coupled with the fact that, at this wavelength, Romeskie and Yager's function coincided with the present yellow-field sensitivity function.

Theoretical Interpretations of the Spectral Sensitivity Curves

A number of models have been proposed for the mechanisms underlying photopic spectral sensitivity in birds (see Graf, this volume). However, these models are often unsatisfactory because of the number of degrees of freedom involved in setting the models' parameters. Bowmaker (1977, this volume) has examined the pigeon retina by microspectrophotometry (MSP) and determined the characteristics of the pigment-droplet combinations to be found in the red and yellow fields. He estimated the effective spectral sensitivity of each cone type by assuming that the droplets selectively filter the light reaching the outer segment of the cone in which they are situated. It was then possible to model the majority of the published pigeon spectral sensitivity functions (Granit, 1942; Donner, 1953; Blough, 1957; Ikeda, 1965; Graf, 1969; Blough et al., 1972) by a direct summation of the spectral sensitivities of the individual cone types in the ratio of their numbers in the yellow-droplet field (cf. Bowmaker, Fig. 9, this volume). Bowmaker's modeled yellow-field curve is well matched by the yellow-field spectral sensitivity function found here (Fig. 13). This reinforces the hypothesis that oil droplets do indeed act in such a way as to alter the effective spectral sensitivity of each cone type individually.

Figure 13 also shows a comparison of Bowmaker's modeled red-field spectral sensitivity function with the red-field function deter-

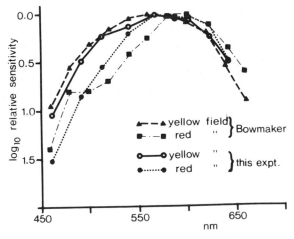

Fig. 13. Mean red and yellow field spectral sensitivity functions for the two pigeons and the modeled red- and yellow-field spectral sensitivity functions of Bowmaker (1977). The functions have been equated at their maxima.

mined in this experiment. Here, the match between modeled and experimental data is not so good. Two possible explanations may be advanced for this discrepancy: (1) Bowmaker modeled his function to take account of Romeskie and Yager's sensitivity function (in which a shoulder appears at about 480 nm) by assuming a somewhat arbitrary value for the abundance of the blue cones ($\lambda_{max} = 485$ nm) in this sector (there being no data on the proportion of such receptors, although they are probably less than 20% of the total receptor population). (2) There is a large variation in the transmission of the B-type oil droplets. The shoulder in the absorbance spectrum and the λ_{T50} (wavelength at which 50% transmission occurs) of this droplet type has been found to vary in all three avian species examined in detail with MSP (Bowmaker and Knowles, 1977; Bowmaker, 1977; Bowmaker and Martin, 1978). In the pigeon, the λ_{T50} of the B-type droplet was also found to vary considerably across the retina, with a gradation of absorbance from λ_{T50} of 554 nm in the center of the red sector to a λ_{T50} of 500 nm in the yellow sector, and a λ_{T50} of about 470 nm in the yellow-sector periphery. The B-type droplet is associated with the P567 pigment, and the maximum of the resultant cone spectral sensitivity can vary between 570 and 589 nm in the red field. In his modeled function, Bowmaker chose to use a cone spectral sensitivity of 589 nm. Clearly, the relative sensitivity will be increased at wavelengths below the modeled maximum if a cone sensitivity maximum of 570 nm is assumed. The variation in B-type oil droplet transmission may also explain the slight discrepancy between the yellow-field sensitivity function and Blough's (1957) function referred to above (Fig. 12).

It is instructive to note, however, that both the red-field and yellow-field spectral sensitivity functions of subject OD2 (Fig. 10) show good agreement with Bowmaker's modeled functions. This suggests that, even within a given droplet field, spectral sensitivity varies, and that this variation is probably attributable to the variation in the transmission spectrum of the B-type droplets. Hence it would seem that, even with a knowledge of the actual visual pigments and droplet types and of their relative abundances in the retina, the successful modeling of the spectral sensitivity functions still depends on a judicious choice of parameter values.

In spite of these minor variations, these findings provide good support for the hypothesis that avian spectral sensitivity can be explained by a direct summation model of the type put forward by Bowmaker, in which account is taken of the actual cone sensitivities and their number present at a given retinal locus, at least for wavelengths greater than about 450 nm. Such a summation model, however, cannot account for the high blue sensitivity reported by Delius and Emmerton (this volume), Graf (this volume), and Kreithen (this volume). Bowmaker failed to detect any cones with a pigment λ_{max} below 460 nm, but because of sampling considerations their presence in the pigeon retina cannot be entirely ruled out. If they do exist, as has been suggested by Graf and Norren (1974), Govardovskii and Zueva (1977), and Graf (this volume), their contribution to overall sensitivity must be inordinately disproportionate to their relative abundance within the retina. The high blue sensitivity reported could perhaps be accounted for by an interaction between two longer-wavelength cones (Bowmaker, 1977). However, if this is the case, it is difficult to understand how the mechanism can be isolated under intense red or yellow adaptation (Graf and Norren, 1974; Norren, 1975).

Function of the Droplet Fields

It is difficult to determine whether the differences in spectral sensitivity between the two droplet fields found here are indeed functional (that is, of adaptive significance) or merely epiphenomena. There is little doubt that in a general sense the photopic spectral sensitivity of terrestrial species is matched to the spectral distribution of daylight. However, it would seem particularly problematic to attempt to define slight differences in the spectral distribution of light associated with the two visual fields normally scanned by the red and yellow droplet fields of the pigeon. This is especially problematic with the homing pigeon since its ecological niche and hence behavior in the natural environment are somewhat poorly understood (see Chapter 1). The rather subtle differences in sensitivity found here would seem to suggest that the primary function of the droplet fields is not concerned with spectral sensitivity.

Bowmaker (this volume) found six and five cone types in the red and yellow fields of the pigeon, respectively. The bandwidths of the spectral sensitivity of some of these cone types are much narrower than that of the pigment alone, and can be identified with the various modulator-type functions detected by electrophysiology (Donner, 1953; Ikeda, 1965). Both the red and yellow fields of the pigeon are in fact dominated by near-identical cone types with a broad bandwidth and a λ_{max} at about 570 nm. The cones containing the B- and A-type droplets in both fields have approximately the same resultant cone spectral sensitivity (Bowmaker, this volume, Figs. 7 and 8). In addition to the broad-bandwidth cones, four narrow-bandwidth cones have been postulated to exist in the red field, while only three have been postulated for the yellow field. There is some uncertainty as to the actual number of narrow-bandwidth cone functions due to the variability of the λ_{T50} of the B-type droplet. Depending on the λ_{T50} of the droplet, the resultant cone functions become broader or narrower with a parallel shift in the locus of maximum sensitivity. It would thus seem that, as a first approximation, the red and yellow fields can be viewed as retinal areas with a similar underlying spectral sensitivity function (the broadband cones) which is subtly modified by the presence of cone mechanisms with narrow bandwidths. The primary function of these latter cones is probably in the coding of color information. Since these narrowband cone types probably differ in number, and certainly differ in locus of maximum sensitivity, it would be hypothesized that the fields differ in their capacity for color discimination, the red field probably being capable of more subtle discrimination than the yellow field.

Thus the primary function of the differences between the receptor populations of the two droplet fields would seem to lie in the mediation of differences in color discrimination and not in spectral sensitivity. Just what these differences are and how they relate to ecological and behavioral variables is clearly worthy of investigation. It is perhaps worth noting in this connection that the function of color vision in a behavioral-ecological sense is in the discrimination of objects which cannot be distinguished on a brightness basis alone. Therefore, a difference in color vision ability between the red and yellow droplet fields suggests a difference in the ability to discriminate objects. Hence, to determine fully the sensory-ecological function of the droplet fields, cognizance must also be taken of possible differences in the visual acuity of the two retinal areas.

It can perhaps be concluded that the primary function of the colored oil droplets rests on the production of narrowband sensitivity channels for the mediation of color discrimination, the droplets performing at the level of individual receptors a function similar to the spectral "sharpening" of color vision mechanisms performed at the retinal neural level in other vertebrate classes such as fish. This is not to suggest that the selective filtering of the oil droplets is essential for color vision in birds, but rather that the droplets provide a mechanism for sharpening the discrimination between colored stimuli. Such an analysis is in accord with Wallman's (this volume) finding that color vision in quail is still maintained, although slightly changed, when the oil droplets of the animal are rendered colorless, and that this slight change is reversed when color returns to the droplets.

A number of other functions have also been proposed for retinal oil droplets in avian and other species, and when account is taken of the phylogenetic distribution of retinal oil droplets (Muntz, 1972) it would seem likely that they subserve different and possibly multiple functions in different classes and species. Among such functions are the reduction of chromatic aberration, the removal of the cis peak in the cone visual pigment absorption function (Wolbarsht, 1976), and the storage of chemical nutrients (Hailman, 1976). The optical properties and possible function in funneling light into the receptor outer segments do not appear to have been investigated. Thus the oil droplets of the avian retina would seem to pose a number of questions which are clearly worthy of further investigation.

REFERENCES

Bloch, S., and Maturana, H. R.: Oil droplet distribution and color discrimination in the pigeon. *Nature (London) New Biol.* **234**:284–285 (1971).

Blough, D. S.: Spectral sensitivity in the pigeon. *J. Opt. Soc. Am.* **47**:827–833 (1957).

Blough, P. M., Riggs, L. A., and Schafer, K. L.: Photopic spectral sensitivity determined electroretinographically for the pigeon eye. *Vision Res.* **12**:447–485 (1972).

Bowmaker, J. K.: The visual pigments, oil droplets and spectral sensitivity in the pigeon. *Vision Res.* **17**:1129–1138 (1977).

Bowmaker, J. K., and Knowles, A.: The visual pigments and oil droplets of the chicken retina. *Vision Res.* **17**:755–764 (1977).

Bowmaker, J. K., and Martin, G. R.: Visual pigments and color vision in a nocturnal bird, *Strix aluco* (tawny owl). *Vision Res.* **18**:1125–1130 (1978).

Donner, K. O.: The spectral sensitivity of the pigeon's retinal elements. *J. Physiol. (London)* **122**:524–537 (1953).

Galifret, Y.: Les diverses aires fonctionnelles de la rétine du pigeon. *Z. Zellforsch. Mikrosk. Anat.* **86**:535–545 (1968).

Govardovskii, V. I., and Zueva, L. V.: Visual pigments of chicken and pigeon. *Vision Res.* **17**:537–543 (1977).

Graf, V. A.: A spectral luminosity function in the pigeon determined by flicker photometry. *Psychon. Sci.* **17**:282–283 (1969).

Graf, V. A., and Norren, D. V.: A blue sensitive mechanism in the pigeon retina: λ_{max} 400 nm. *Vision Res.* **14**:1203–1209 (1974).

Granit, G.: The photopic spectrum of the pigeon. *Acta Physiol. Scand.* **4**:118–124 (1942).

Hailman, J. P.: Oil droplets in the eyes of adult anuran amphibians: A comparative survey. *J. Morphol.* **148(4)**:453–468 (1976).

Ikeda, H.: The spectral sensitivity of the pigeon (*Columba livia*). *Vision Res.* **5**:19–36 (1965).

King-Smith, P.E.: Absorption spectra and function of the colored oil droplets of the pigeon retina. *Vision Res.* **9**:1391–1399 (1969).

Muntz, W. R. A.: Inert absorbing and reflecting pigments. In Dartnall, H. (ed.): *Handbook of Sensory Physiology VII/I*. Springer-Verlag, Berlin (1972).

Norren, D. V.: Two short wavelength sensitive cone systems in pigeon, chicken and daw. *Vision Res.* **15**:1164–1166 (1975).

Romeskie, M., and Yager, D.: Psychophysical studies of pigeon color vision 1. Photopic spectral sensitivity. *Vision Res.* **16**:501–505 (1976).

Waelchli, G.: Zur Topographie der gefärbten Kugeln der Vogelnetzhaut. *Arch. Ophthalmol.* **29**:205–223 (1883).

Wolbarsht, M. L.: The function of intraocular color filters. *Fed. Proc.* **35**:44–50 (1976).

18

Role of the Retinal Oil Droplets in the Color Vision of Japanese Quail

JOSH WALLMAN

INTRODUCTION

For an animal to obtain information about the wavelength of light independent of information about the light's intensity (that is, to have color vision), it is necessary that the animal possess more than one class of visual receptor, each with different spectral sensitivity. In birds, the inner segment of each cone contains an intensely colored inclusion, the oil droplet, which filters the light before it reaches the visual pigment. Since oil droplets of several different colors are found in the retina, they could act as color separation filters, dividing the cones into different populations with different wavelengths of maximum sensitivity, even if all the cones contain the same visual pigment.

Although the involvement of the oil droplets in color vision was proposed over a century ago, it remains controversial despite a large amount of evidence both pro and con. This chapter will review the published evidence and then describe experiments showing that, by dietary manipulation, birds can be produced whose retinas contain

JOSH WALLMAN • Biology Department, City College, City University of New York, New York, New York 10031. The experimental part of this chapter was part of a Ph.D. dissertation (Wallman, 1972) from the Biology Department of Tufts University, Medford, Massachusetts. Preliminary results were published in abstract form (Wallman, 1970) and were presented at a meeting of the American Society of Zoologists in December 1970. The work was supported by predoctoral fellowships from NASA and NIH.

only one type of oil droplet. These birds still have color vision, although it is different from the color vision of normal birds.

AVIAN COLOR VISION

In light of the apparent significance of colors in the courtship displays of some birds (e.g., peacock, English robin, pheasant), it may seem almost superfluous to demonstrate that birds have color vision. Nonetheless, much early research tried to show that birds have color vision, until Lashley (1916) established it beyond question for the chicken. Later, Hamilton and Coleman (1933) determined the wavelength discrimination function for the pigeon. Despite the unreasonably high thresholds these investigators obtained and the peculiar training methods they used, their work has been the standard for nearly 40 years. Recently, Wright (1972a) measured the pigeon wavelength discrimination function with much greater precision and without the methodological peculiarities of Hamilton and Coleman, and obtained rather different results. His results (maximum wavelength discriminability at 500, 540–550, and 600 nm) have been supported in part by a number of studies: Schneider (1972) used multidimensional scaling techniques on data obtained from pigeons required to discriminate among 15 spectral lights to obtain a color space for the pigeon, which agrees quite well with Wright's wavelength discrimination data; Bloch and Martinoya (1971), in a less extensive study, obtained similar curves around 500 and 600 nm; Blough (1972) showed data on wavelength generalization that support the existence of a peak in discrimination at 540 and 600 nm, as do Wright and Cumming's (1971) data on color naming in the pigeon. Using a rather different technique, Riggs et al. (1972) measured the electroretinogram in response to phase reversals of a grating in which adjacent stripes differed in wavelength but not in luminance. These data yielded functions generally similar to those just discussed but with some differences.

All of these results are compatible with the idea that pigeons have trichromatic color vision. There is some evidence that pigeons have tetrachromatic color vision (that is, have four color mechanisms). Jitsumori (1976) used an anomaloscope procedure in which pigeons matched a yellow light to various mixtures of red and green lights. The resulting functions were similar in shape to those of trichromatic human observers, but no combination of red and green matched the yellow light very well. Although the author offers several possible explanations for this, that of tetrachromatic color vision remains attractive. Romeskie and Yager (1976b) measured a function related to the spectral saturation of lights of different wavelengths (the photochromatic interval function) and found that their results could be fitted reasonably well by a theoretical curve based on four color mechanisms.

ROLE OF THE OIL DROPLETS

The principal efforts to show the role of the oil droplets in color vision have attempted either to relate measurements of color vision to the transmission spectra of individual oil droplets or to relate differences in color vision to differences in the relative abundance of the different types of oil droplets.

Studies of the Transmission Characteristics of Oil Droplets

The transmission spectra of the oil droplets have long been known to have the form of cutoff filters transmitting the longer wavelengths (Roaf, 1929; Fujimoto et al., 1957; Strother, 1963). (Roaf, 1933, one of the early discoverers of this fact, was so taken with it that he proposed a theory of human color vision based on hypothetical receptors with absorption spectra similar to the oil droplet transmission spectra.) More recently, Liebman and Granda (1975) have shown that turtle (and probably bird) oil droplets can have maximum optical densities of 50–90, implying extremely concentrated pigments. The red and orange droplets apparently contain the same pigment in different concentrations. Since the optical densities of the oil droplets are extremely high, the spectral composition of light passing through the oil droplets must be dramatically changed. Although the cutoff wavelengths of the different oil droplets differ somewhat from species to species (Strother, 1963; Mayr, 1972), as well as from study to study (Konishi, 1965), the similarities among species are more striking.

Because until recently there was no good evidence that birds had more than one visual cone pigment, several authors (LeGrand, 1962; King-Smith, 1969; Muntz, 1972; Donner, 1960) attempted to make models of various features of avian color vision on the basis of one visual pigment and three oil droplets. Recent work (see below) requires making a new start on models of this sort.

Newly hatched precocial birds show very distinctive color preferences (Kear, 1964; Nyström, 1969a; Oppenheimer, 1968; Hailman, 1967; Delius et al., 1972), and several authors attempted to explain these preferences by reference to the transmission characteristics of the oil droplets. An example of why one might expect a simple explanation of these preferences can be found in the results of Hailman (1966). He found that the curve of pecks directed at stimuli of different colors against an achromatic background is exactly the mirror image of that for achromatic stimuli against colored backgrounds, a result reminiscent of opponent-color neurons.

Hailman (1964, 1967) hypothesized some simple neural interactions which, together with the transmission characteristics of the oil droplets, accounted quite precisely for the wavelength preference curve of newly hatched laughing gulls. Delius et al. (1972) performed similar experiments on different species of gulls and obtained slightly different results. Using a more elaborate optical system, they were also able to do several color-matching experiments and use the results to test several hypothetical mechanisms. Although none of the models worked very well, the model based on the oil droplets worked least well.

There are several factors that complicate the analysis of retinal mechanisms that account for these color preferences. First, the experiments of Impekoven (1969) suggest that black-headed gull chicks have different color preferences when in different motivational states. Also, there is evidence that the preferences are affected by the type of stimulus presentation—simultaneous or successive (Nyström, 1969a)—and that preferences change very rapidly after hatching and are quite sensitive to experiential effects (Taylor et al., 1969; Nyström, 1969b).

Since there is considerable diversity in the color preferences of newly hatched birds of different species (Kear, 1964; Nyström, 1969a; Taylor et al., 1969) but relatively little diversity in the oil droplet transmission spectra of different species, if the oil droplet transmission spectra are to explain the preferences, one would have to invent for each species different hypotheses of the neural interactions necessary to produce the observed preferences. For the present, it seems wiser to regard color preferences of newly hatched birds as brought about by those mysterious central nervous system processes responsible for other preferences, rather than by a simple peripheral mechanism.

Studies of the Relative Abundance of the Different Oil Droplets

Another feature of oil droplets which has attracted much attention is that the frequencies of the different types of oil droplets vary dramatically both from species to species and from one part of the retina to another. Several authors have related these variations in oil droplet distribution to variations in color vision. Peiponen (1963) determined the color preferences of three species of birds and showed that the birds preferred Munsell color chips matching their own feathers. He provided some evidence that the difference in color preferences can be related to the oil droplet distribution in certain parts of the retina. Later, Peiponen (1964) showed a general relation between the oil droplet distribution across the retina of 44 species of diurnal birds and the ecology of the birds.

A more specific relation of the oil droplets to the ecology of the animal comes from the work of Cullen (Muntz, 1972), who studied the oil droplets in a number of aquatic species. He found that those species with high frequencies of red oil droplets shared the behavioral characteristic of looking into the water from air.

None of these studies necessarily answers the question of whether the oil droplets are important factors in color vision, since even if the oil droplets only slightly modified the birds' color vision it might be reasonable to have more oil droplets of colors behaviorally significant to the bird.

Bloch and Maturana (1971) approached the problem of whether the color vision of pigeons is influenced by the part of the retina that is used, since the oil droplet distribution varies dramatically in this species. They trained birds to make color discriminations, then tested them with the same stimuli on a different part of the retina and found that the discriminations always transferred. This might indicate that the different oil droplet distribution did not noticeably alter the birds' color vision were it not for the fact that the discriminations tested were very crude (only four colors were used). Since the discriminations tested were not close to the birds' threshold for wavelength discrimination, one cannot conclude from these negative results that different parts of the retina have no effect on color discrimination.

An entirely new perspective of the role of the oil droplets in the behavior of birds was offered by the experiments of Pézard (cited by Mayr, 1970) which showed that hormonal states affect not only color preferences in chickens but also the frequency of the different types of oil droplets. He suggested, for example, that capons have fewer red oil droplets, thereby being less sensitive to the red combs of other chickens, and thus are less aggressive. Dücker (1970) and Mayr (1970) tested these surprising results in another species, *Euplectes orix*. Dücker determined the color preferences under a variety of hormonal conditions, while Mayr measured the frequencies of the different oil droplets. They were unable to show any correlation between color preference and oil droplet frequency distribution. Mayr suggests that Pézard's results could be accounted for by small errors in the retinal location of the samples examined and refers to other data which throw Pézard's results into question.

Avian Visual Pigments

If the oil droplets are not responsible for avian color vision, one should expect to find several different visual pigments in the cones of birds. A number of studies have found no evidence for more than a single visual pigment either by microspectrophotometry of cone outer segments (in pigeon, chicken, and gull, Liebman, 1972) or by chemical extraction of the visual pigments (in turkey, Crescitelli et al., 1964; in chicken, Wald et al., 1955; in pigeon, Bridges, 1962, and Sillman, 1969).

Very recently, however, two sets of studies have shown more than one visual pigment in the cones of pigeons and chickens. By microspectrophotometry of cone outer segments, Bowmaker and Knowles (1977) found two pigments in the chicken (λ_{max} about 569 nm and 497 nm), and Bowmaker (this volume) found three pigments in the pigeon (λ_{max} about 567, 515, and 460 nm). By very different methods, Govardovskii (1976) and Govardovskii and Zueva (1977) found four visual pigments in both chicken and pigeon, at least three of them presumably cone pigments (λ_{max} about 561, 509, 465, and 415 nm). They illuminated isolated retinas from the receptor side so that the light was absorbed by the visual pigment without passing through the oil droplets. They demonstrated the visual pigments by two techniques, both of which rely on the fact that the amplitude of the early receptor potential is linearly related to the visual pigment concentration. The first method involves measuring the efficacy of different long-wavelength-pass filtered lights[1] at bleaching the visual pigment, compared to their efficacy at bleaching a known visual pigment. For example, if a red light bleached an unknown pigment more rapidly than it bleached frog rhodopsin, we can infer that the absorption curve of the unknown pigment lies at longer wavelengths than frog rhodopsin. If we assume that the unknown pigment has the same-shaped absorption curve as rhodopsin, we can compute its λ_{max}. The seond method simply involves measuring the spectral sensitivity curves of the early receptor potential after bleaching with different wavelengths.

The discovery of a cone pigment absorbing maximally at short wavelengths confirms studies using behavioral measurements of spectral sensitivity (Romeskie and Yager, 1976a; Graf, this volume), electroretinographic measurements of spectral sensitivity (Graf and Norren, 1974; Norren, 1975), single-unit electrophysiology (Yazulla and Granda, 1973), and behavioral measurements of spectral saturation (Romeskie and Yager, 1976b).

The fact that Bowmaker (this volume) found a 460 nm pigment in

---

[1] There appears to be an error in the original paper (Govardovskii and Zueva, (1977), which refers to "long-wave cutoff" filters.

the pigeon but not in the chicken suggests the possibility of a species difference. Govardovskii and Zueva (1977), however, found the same visual pigments in chicken and pigeon, and Norren (1975) found no difference between chicken, pigeon, and daw in the wavelength maximum of either the 415 nm or the 480 nm mechanism.

Other Functions for Oil Droplets

The fact that birds possess several cone visual pigments means that the oil droplets cannot be the sine qua non of avian color vision, but it says nothing about whether they are involved in color vision, either by permitting two types of cone mechanisms that use the same visual pigment or by changing the spectral characteristics of the cones.

Walls and Judd (1933) argued against droplets being involved in color vision because they did not find all types of oil droplets in the fovea. Mayr (1972), however, has found all types of oil droplets in the fovea of several species of weaver finches.

Pedler and Boyle (1969) make a different argument against the role of oil droplets in color vision. They argue that each oil droplet would act as a very short focal length lens, defocusing the light that passes through it and spreading it into several cone outer segments. It would seem that to make this argument convincing would require a more sophisticated analysis of the optics involved than is available.

Walls and Judd also proposed other functions for the oil droplets, including correction of chromatic aberrations (but see Peiponen, 1964, p. 283) and attenuation of the short wavelengths which impair acuity by light scattering. Such functions could be served by the oil droplets, whether or not they also are involved in color vision, and might also account for differences in the proportions of different oil droplets in different species and in different parts of the retina. One can imagine different species with different proportions of the three types of receptors, but with similar color vision.

Wolbarsht (1976) suggested that the function of the oil droplets (as well as of the macular pigment and lens pigment in other animals) is to prevent short-wavelength light from being absorbed by the secondary absorption peak (the β or cis peak) of the visual pigment molecules. Although this absorption peak is usually presumed not to have important visual functions because of its small size and extreme short-wavelength position, Wolbarsht argues that if such absorption of short-wavelength light did take place, it would enhance the effect of chromatic aberration in degrading acuity and, unless compensated for neurally, would cause confusions between short and long wavelengths.

Conclusion

Despite the relatively large literature on oil droplets and color vision in birds, almost all the evidence has been indirect. Although we now know from the work on avian visual pigments that the oil droplets cannot by themselves be responsible for color vision, there has been no experiment done with birds that matches the directness of Orlov and Maksimova's (1964) asserted demonstration that a turtle, *Emys orbicularis*, appeared to be a tetrachromat to light entering the eye through the lens but a dichromat to light entering through the back of the eye and thereby bypassing the oil droplets.[2]

PRODUCTION OF BIRDS WITH COLORLESS OIL DROPLETS

One aspect of the oil droplets which has not been exploited in attempts to clarify their function is that the precursors of the oil droplet pigments cannot be synthesized by the bird de novo. The pigments in the oil droplets are carotenoids of relatively long chain length compared to vitamin A (Wald and Zussman, 1938; Bridges, 1962) and apparently are biologically essential only as a source of vitamin A. As a result, they can be removed from the diet without bad effects as long as vitamin A is supplied, as shown by numerous experiments on carotenoid depletion in chickens (e.g., Ganguly et al., 1953). There do not seem to be metabolic pathways from vitamin A back to the long-chain carotenoids which color the oil droplets.

If a bird can be deprived of these carotenoids long enough to deplete the oil droplets of pigment, comparing such a bird's color vision with that of a bird on a normal diet would be a direct test of the role of the oil droplets in color vision. This would be particularly true if administration of exogenous carotenoids reversed the changes in color vision in the oil droplets.

Methods

For the experiments reported here, the Japanese quail (*Coturnix coturnix japonica*) was chosen because diets consisting of highly puri-

[2] These results are based on experiments involving heterochromatic substitutions of lights adjusted to give minimal electroretinogram responses. Such experiments, of course, assess a retinal correlate of color vision rather than color vision per se. Intriguing as these results are, one has cause for some skepticism, since no data are offered in support of these results, although they form the principal point of the authors' paper; data on other minor points are provided.

fied ingredients had been worked out for it (Fox and Harrison, 1964), and the birds are small enough not to require too much of these diets. There are several reasons why depleting the oil droplet carotenoids is substantially more difficult than depleting the general body stores of carotenoids: (1) The oil droplet carotenoids are particularly stable. My observations show that birds maintained without carotenoids for many months still have pigmented oil droplets. (2) Eggs contain large amounts of carotenoids. Birds whose mothers were fed normal diets are hatched with colored oil droplets and retain them even after long periods of carotenoid deprivation. (3) Quail appear to have a prodigious ability to concentrate trace amounts of dietary carotenoids. For these reasons, the experimental birds were raised for at least two generations on highly purified diets which used vitamin-free casein as a protein source. (Even the most purified soybean protein contains easily detectable amounts of carotenoids.)

The diets were basically those of Fox and Briggs (1960), with modifications suggested by Dr. Fox (personal communication), and were formulated by General Biochemicals, Inc., Chagrin Falls, Ohio. The basic diet for the chicks was diet C50 of Fox and Briggs except that the casein was 27%, calcium pantothenate was 40 mg/kg, and 8 g/kg L-arginine HCl, 20 mg/kg Santoquin, and 50 g/kg torula yeast displaced equivalent amounts of glucose. The vitamin A concentration was twice that of diet C50. The adults were fed the same diet except that 33 g/kg of glucose was replaced by 7 g/kg dibasic calcium phosphate and 25 g/kg calcium carbonate; also, all "vitamin" concentrations except that of choline chloride were doubled.

The birds raised on the purified diets showed reasonable growth and reproduction but appeared less fit than those on natural food diets, an effect previously reported for other purified diets by Gough et al. (1968). Examination of a bird's retina involved dark-adapting the bird for 2 hr and then giving it an overdose of sodium pentobarbital. The retina was excised, placed on a microscope slide with the receptor surface up, and covered with a coverslip.

Results and Discussion

A comparison of the appearance of the retinas of normal birds and birds raised on the carotenoid-deficient diet for at least two generations is shown in Fig. 1a,d. Although the black-and-white reproductions do not show the color of the oil droplets, it is clear that the carotenoid-deprived birds have only one type of oil droplet, whereas the normal birds have three principal types. (In the photographs there seem to be

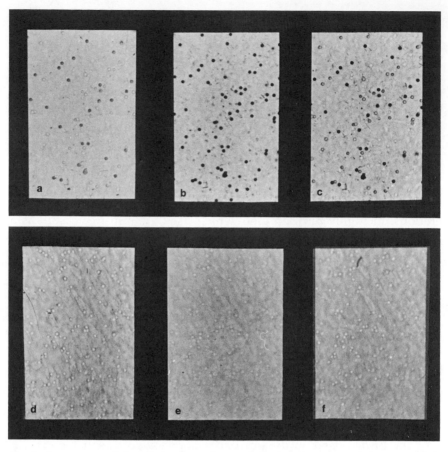

Fig. 1. Appearance of the oil droplets of normal (a-c) and carotenoid-deprived (d-f) birds. From left to right, the illumination is white, blue-green, green. Original photographs were taken under the same conditions and on the same roll of film.

many types, but this is due to different oil droplets being focused on at different levels.)

A more demanding test takes advantage of the fact that the oil droplets behave as long-wavelength-transmitting cutoff filters, the different types of oil droplets cutting off sharply at different wavelengths (Fujimoto et al., 1957; Strother, 1963). Viewing a normal retina through a microscope illuminated through a monochrometer, one finds that all oil droplets transmit long-wavelength light and that as the wavelength of the light is decreased the different types of oil droplets become opaque in three well-defined regions. This phenomenon is simulated (with broadband filters) for green light in Fig. 1c and for blue-green light in Fig. 1b. By comparing individual oil droplets, one can see that, for example, the yellow oil droplets transmit green light but are opaque to blue-green light, while the red oil droplets are opaque to both. All the oil droplets of the carotenoid-deprived bird, on the other hand, transmit throughout the spectrum (Fig. 1f,e). More precisely, at no wavelength from 700 to 425 nm did the density of any oil droplets become different from that of others.

An incidental observation made in the course of these carotenoid-deprivation experiments was that red oil droplets are the first to disappear. Konishi (1965) found that, embryologically, the red oil droplets are the last to appear. It is not clear to what extent the cutoff characteristic of the red oil droplet reflects a difference in pigment concentration rather than a difference in composition, as is probably the case in turtles (Liebman and Granda, 1975). [In the rump feathers of certain tanagers a color range from lemon-yellow to scarlet is produced by a single carotenoid present in different concentrations (Brush, 1970).]

BEHAVIORAL TESTS FOR COLOR BLINDNESS

To test the carotenoid-deficient birds for color blindness, a technique was developed which is based on the optomotor response of the animals. The notion underlying the technique is this: If a bird is placed in a rotating, vertically striped cylinder, it will follow the movement of the stripes with its eyes or head (optomotor response). This response will occur whether the stripes contrast with each other in brightness or color. Thus, in a cylinder made up of alternating red and green stripes of precisely equal luminance (to the animal), an animal with color vision would respond well, whereas a completely color-blind animal (a monochromat) would not respond, since the stripes would have zero contrast. This difference would constitute a positive test for a lack of color vision. This test, however, would be unable to distinguish an animal with minimal color vision from a normal animal, since both might respond to the stripe movement at all ratios of red/green luminance.

To make the test more sensitive, it would be desirable to measure the apparent contrast to the animal of the colored stripes as one varied the relative red/green luminance. In a nearly color-blind animal, the apparent contrast of the stripes would be almost completely dependent on the luminance ratio of the two kinds of stripes. In an animal with good color vision, the apparent contrast of the stripes would be less affected by changes in the red/green luminance, since the animal would always see a strong chromatic contrast between the stripes. In this way, one can estimate the extent to which color cues are used by the animal.

To measure the apparent contrast of the stripes, the colored stripes were superimposed on another grating (called the reference grating) moving in the opposite direction. In this situation, the animal followed whichever grating had greater apparent contrast. The contrast of the reference grating was then adjusted so that the animal followed neither grating. At this point, the apparent contrast of the two gratings was considered to be equal. Since the reference grating was achromatic and could be easily calibrated, this procedure permitted assessment of the apparent contrast of the red/green grating by matching it to a grating of known contrast.

Methods

Apparatus. This apparatus and its calibration are described in detail in a separate paper (Wallman, 1975). The apparatus is shown in Fig. 2. The inner plexiglas cylinder has mounted on it a grating consisting of alternate strips of Wratten filters 58 (green: dominant wavelength about 535 nm) and 25 (red: dominant wavelength about 616 nm). These are relatively broadband filters with very little overlap in their transmission bands.[3] The outer cylinder has flexible rear-projection-screen material mounted on it, and on top of that a grating consisting of alternate strips of polarizer and Wratten 0.2 neutral density filters. All strips are ½ inch wide and 5 inches long. The bird views the grating from a small plexiglas cylinder in the center of the other two cylinders. Each stripe subtends about 5 deg horizontally and moves at about 12 deg/sec. The two annular mirrors above and below the gratings make the stripes appear longer than they in fact are.

The cylinders are illuminated from without by five 500-W slide projectors, the optical axes of which lie on radii of the cylinders 60 deg apart. (The experimenter occupies the place where the sixth projector would go.) In front of each projector is a round polarizer which determines the contrast of the outer, achromatic grating. These polarizers are mounted on synchros which are connected in parallel to a larger, control synchro which the experimenter adjusts.

The relative luminance of the red and green stripes of the colored grating was altered by changing the relative amount of red and green

---

[3] The transmission characteristics of the filters were checked with a Beckman Acta II spectrophotometer. The green filter has a transmission peak of 54% at 530 nm with a half-peak-transmission bandwidth of 50 nm. The red filter is a low-wavelength cutoff filter with half-peak transmission at 610 nm. Except for these peaks, each filter had a density of at least 3.6 A from 200 to 700 nm. This assures that the results reported are not due to ultraviolet radiation affecting the birds' color matches, as Wright (1972b) has shown in pigeons.

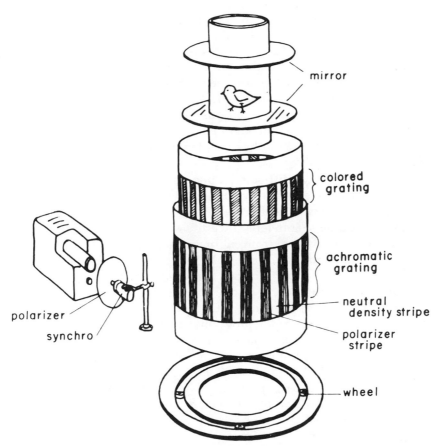

Fig. 2. Exploded diagram of apparatus for studying optomotor responses. The cylinders move in opposite directions. Not shown: four other projectors, motor driving one of the wheels, platform on which bird stands.

light in the projectors' output. This was done by placing calibrated cyan or red Wratten color correction filters in front of the projector lenses.

Contrast Calibration. The method of contrast calibration has been described in detail elsewhere (Wallman, 1975); it involves measuring the objective contrast at a variety of angles to the optical axis of the projectors and then measuring the animals' responses to a series of calibrated achromatic gratings. This procedure produces a contrast calibration corrected for contrast variation due to varying angles between stripes and projectors and for inaccuracies due to artifacts such as imperfections in the grating.

Illumination Calibration. The equation of the color temperature of the different projectors and the calibration of the filters used to change and luminance ratio of the two colors of stripes both present the same difficulty: quantification of the "luminances" of the colored stripes as they appear to the bird. Since the stripes are made from relatively broadband filters, the use of a light detector with an arbitrary spectral response function can cause serious errors, particularly in the long wavelengths. This objection also applies to the use of the human eye as the detector, since it too has a different spectral response function from that of the quail.

To circumvent this difficulty, a photometer with approximately the spectral characteristics of the eye of the Japanese quail was constructed. The basic detector was a calibrated RCA 935 vacuum photodiode connected to a digital voltmeter. Since the spectral response function of the phototube was known from calibrations made with monochromator and thermopile, and that of the quail was known from measurements using the flicker electroretinogram (unpublished data), it was easy to compute the transmission characteristics of the filter necessary to convert spectral response function of the phototube into that of the photopic quail eye. A computer program considered the possible combinations of 45 Wratten filters taken up to four at a time, computing the standard deviation of the logarithm of the ratio of the transmittance of the combination filter to that of the desired filter. The best filter combination (of the 187,000 possible) of greater than 5% peak transmittance was attached to the phototube. Before each experimental run, this photometer was used to determine the ratio of "luminances" of the red and green stripes when illuminated by each of the five projectors. After each run, the ratios were remeasured. If this criterion for equality was no longer met, the run was discarded.

The luminance of the stimuli was determined by a Macbeth illuminometer to be approximately 75 mL.

Procedures. Before each experimental run, the subject was light adapted for at least 2 hr to 9000 lux light from cool-white fluorescent bulbs to assure that all animals were in the same state of adaptation and to minimize the possible effect of receptor contraction or elongation (Detweiler, 1943).

Before the subject was placed in the apparatus, the contrast of the achromatic grating was set to its minimal value. The bird was then put into the apparatus and the cylinders were rotated. Invariably, the bird's optomotor responses showed that it was tracking the movement of the colored grating. The contrast of the achromatic grating was then increased until the bird completely ceased to track the colored grating, and the polarizer angle at which this occurred was recorded. Next the cylinders were stopped, the achromatic grating contrast was increased to maximum, and the procedure was repeated, except this time the achromatic grating contrast was decreased until the bird no longer followed the achromatic grating. After two such trials (taking less than 10 min), the bird was replaced in the light-adapting environment for 10 min.

This inverted method of limits was used because many birds become increasingly agitated when subjected to the stimulation of both gratings being of equal contrast and they pay little attention to either grating.

The polarizer angles recorded during the experiments were converted to the calibrated contrast values[4] and plotted by computer.

The data were statistically analyzed using a four-way factorial design analysis of variance. The factors were the diet (carotenoid deficient or normal), the red/green ratio, the subjects (replications), and whether the point represented the upper or lower limit of the region of contrast equality of the two gratings.

Results and Discussion

The results of performing this experiment with normal and carotenoid-deprived birds are shown in Fig. 3. The most prominent result is that in the carotenoid-deprived birds, as in the normals, the minimum apparent contrast that the red/green grating attained (when luminance cues are presumably balanced out) is not zero. That this was not due to artifacts in the grating was tested by making the colored grating only from strips of the green filter. In fact, the minimum contrast seems similar to that of normal birds. This implies that the carotenoid-deprived birds are not color-blind. The curves of a completely color-blind animal would have two characteristics: (1) their shape would be determined solely by the luminance contrasts of the grating, and (2) the null would be at zero contrast, i.e., when the red and green stripes are matched in luminance, the stripes should seem to virtually disappear.

Although the carotenoid-deprived birds do not meet these criteria, the curves of Fig. 3b are clearly not normal. The major difference between the curves is that those of the carotenoid-deprived birds show a very distinct, deep null, indicating that the contrast of the colored grating is strongly luminance dependent for these birds compared to normal birds.

In summary, the normal birds respond mainly to the color contrast

---

[4] Contrast is defined conventionally: $(L_a - L_b)/(L_a + L_b)$, where L_a and L_b are the luminances of adjacent stripes in the grating.

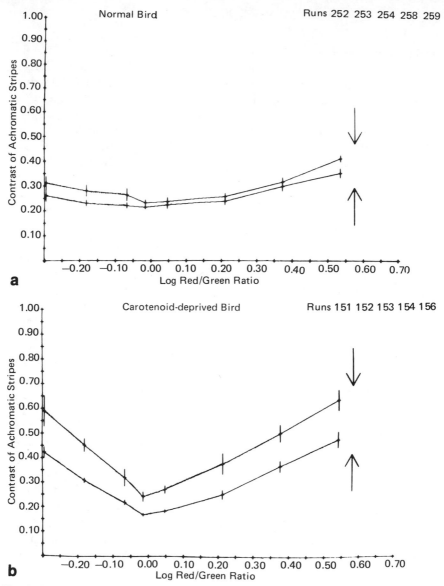

Fig. 3. Results of optomotor response experiment. Influence of different red/green luminance ratios on contrast of red/green grating as indicated by the optomotor response. (a) Normal birds, (b) carotenoid-deprived birds. Photopic conditions. The lower line represents the values obtained by increasing the contrast of the achromatic grating (see arrow) until the bird stopped tracking the motion of the red/green grating. The upper line represents the values obtained by decreasing the contrast until the bird stopped following the achromatic grating. Thus, for example, the area under the lower line represents the combinations of contrasts of the achromatic grating (vertical axis) and the red/green grating (horizontal axis) at which the bird follows the red/green grating. The area between the lines represents combinations where neither grating is followed. Vertical bars are ±1 standard error.

of the grating, while the carotenoid-deprived birds respond mainly to the brightness contrast. This difference is expressed statistically by the interaction of the factors diet and red/green ratio, and is highly significant ($F = 15.3$, $df = 7/124$, $p < 0.001$).

It seemed useful to compute a parameter that reflects the extent of luminance dependence of the response, since this is the most important difference between the groups. To do this, the curve expected if a bird were responding only to luminance contrast was calculated by assuming that the red and green stripes are of equal luminosity at that red/green ratio at which the null occurs in Fig. 3b, and, from this, calculating the luminance contrast of other red/green ratios. Once this luminance-contrast-only curve was obtained, each of the experimental curves could be compared to it by calculating the slope of the line between each data point and the null, expressing it as a percentage of the slope calculated from the luminance-contrast-only model, and averaging the data (weighting to correct for the unequal spacing of the points along the abscissa). For an animal responding only to luminance contrast, one would obtain a figure of 100%; for an animal responding only to chromatic contrast, one would obtain 0%. The result of these calculations for the data of Fig. 3 is that the average slope for the carotenoid-deprived birds is 67% and for the normal birds is 26%.

These figures support the conclusion that the carotenoid-deprived birds are intermediate between normal birds and what would be expected for completely color-blind birds. Before considering other explanations, the involvement of the rods was assessed.

Although the luminance levels of the apparatus were within the human photopic range, there is abundant evidence of rod function at light levels generally considered photopic. This evidence comes from large-field spectral sensitivity measurements (Yager, 1970) and low-frequency flicker studies (Walters, 1971). Furthermore, there is substantial evidence for the participation of rods in color vision. Blackwell and Blackwell (1961) have explicitly shown some wavelength discrimination in a cone monochromat, and Weale (1953), in an earlier study of a cone monochromat, indicated that the subject lacked wavelength discrimination only with foveal targets. In addition, dichromats can show trichomatic color vision if the stimuli are not confined to the fovea (Smith and Pokorny, 1977). In normal subjects, rod activity apparently affects large-field color matches (Trezona, 1970).

To test the possibility of rod involvement, the experiment was repeated at a lower luminance level with a carotenoid-deprived bird that was dark-adapted. These circumstances should enhance the contribution of the rods. Figure 4 shows the results for a dark-adapted bird at a luminance 2 log units below that of Fig. 3. The curves seem

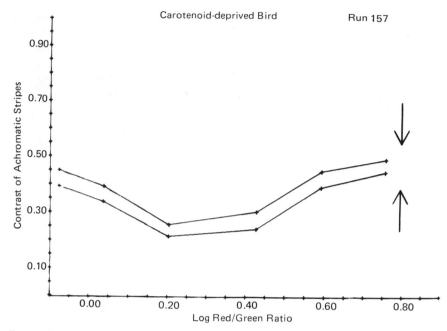

Fig. 4. Results of optomotor response experiment. Carotenoid-deprived bird. Mesopic conditions.

more like those of the normal birds. The average slope was 50% of the luminance-contrast-only model (compared to the average slope of 67% in Fig. 3b and the 26% slope for the normal birds in Fig. 3a).

Lowering the luminance seems to make the color vision of the carotenoid-deprived birds more normal. This is a somewhat surprising result because, in normal pigeons, increased luminance results in steeper wavelength-generalization curves, an indication of better wavelength discrimination (Blough, 1972). The present results suggest that, in the carotenoid-deprived birds, the rod can contribute to color vision.

There is other evidence for rod/cone interactions in birds. Blough (1958) discovered a peculiarity of dark adaptation in the pigeon which can best be understood as the result of the rods inhibiting the cones. I have found similar evidence of rods inhibiting cones in electroretinogram (ERG) experiments. The flicker ERG to a 40-Hz stimulus (presumably stimulating only the cones) is inhibited by dark adaptation. This effect has a time course roughly similar to that of the increase in rod sensitivity. Conceivably, rod/cone interactions are especially pronounced in birds.

EFFECT OF EXOGENOUS CAROTENOIDS ON THE OIL DROPLETS AND COLOR VISION OF CAROTENOID-DEPRIVED BIRDS

A pilot study was undertaken to see whether it is possible, by feeding carotenoids, to reverse the effects of carotenoid deprivation on the oil droplets and on color vision. If exogenous carotenoids are incorporated into the oil droplets of adult birds raised on the carotenoid-deficient diet, and if, as a result, a reasonably normal pattern of oil droplet pigmentation is produced, assessment of the color vision of these birds would confirm the results of the original deprivation study. Furthermore, one could feed carotenoids not normally available to carotenoid-deprived birds and thereby perhaps obtain birds with particular color-vision abnormalities.

Methods

One adult male quail, which had been raised from hatching on a carotenoid-deficient diet, as had its parents, was tested on two occasions in the optomotor apparatus, yielding two complete runs. The quail was then maintained on a diet containing 2.67 g/kg of carotenoid activity in the form of a stabilized carotenoid preparation fed at the level of 66.7 g/kg of diet. This is approximately 70 times the amount of carotenoid fed to laying hens as a supplement to produce eggs with yolks of moderate pigmentation. (The carotenoid preparation consisted of equal parts—by carotenoid activity—of Pigmentene Yellow-Gold, which is principally lutein, and Pigmentene Red, which is principally capsanthin. Both are manufactured by Special Nutrients, Inc., Bay Harbor Island, Florida.)

After 7 weeks on the carotenoid-supplemental diet, the bird was retested on 2 separate days in the optomotor apparatus and then sacrificed, and its retina was compared with that of a normal bird. Photographs of both retinas were made under the same conditions and on the same roll of film.

Results and Discussion

The result of the carotenoid supplementation was to produce a retina clearly containing three types of oil droplets. Their colors appeared similar to those of the normal bird, but were less intense. There seemed to be greater variation across the retina in the oil droplet colors of the experimental bird, but this was not explored systematically.

The results of the behavioral tests are shown in Fig. 5. Compared to the bird's earlier tests and to those of other carotenoid-deprived

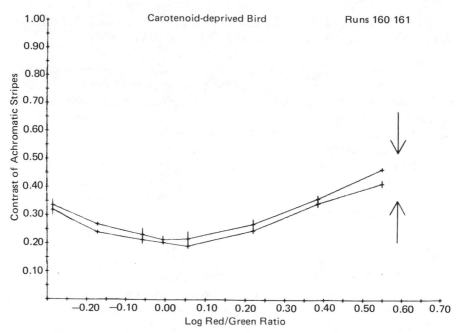

Fig. 5. Results of optomotor response experiment. Carotenoid-deprived bird after maintenance on diet with high carotenoid concentration.

birds, this bird was less luminance dependent. The average slope was
32% of the luminance model curve, compared to 67% for the carotenoid-deprived birds and 26% for the normals. Therefore, the deficiencies
in color vision produced by carotenoid deprivation can be at least
partially reversed by administration of carotenoids.

GENERAL DISCUSSION

The first experiment reported here shows that birds whose oil
droplets are all identical respond to a red/green grating principally on
the basis of the luminance information of the grating, whereas normal
birds respond principally to wavelength information. This difference
constitutes evidence that the oil droplets play a role in color vision in
the Japanese quail.

Since Bowmaker and Knowles (1977) have measured the absorption
spectra both of the cone visual pigments and of the oil droplets associated with measured cones in the chicken (a rather close relative of

the Japanese quail), we have an opportunity to estimate the effect of carotenoid deprivation on the receptor mechanisms present. Bowmaker and Knowles found six different combinations of oil droplet and visual pigment present in the chicken retina, and calculated the spectral sensitivity curves that each of these receptor types would have. Four were very similar: broadband curves, all having a maximum at 569 nm (the λ_{max} of the associated visual pigment). The curves differed only in the short-wavelength region, with large differences only below 500 nm. The effect of carotenoid deprivation would be to make these four receptor types identical to the receptor with the broadest curve, the one with the clear oil droplet.

The remaining two receptor types have much narrower curves, one peaking in the green (533 nm), the other in the red (606 nm), with very little overlap. Coincidentally, the dominant wavelengths of the stimuli used in the present experiments are almost exactly the peak wavelengths of these two receptors. In fact, the green used even had the same shape and bandwidth as the green receptor. This no doubt accounts for the fact that the normal birds' performance depended almost entirely on chromatic rather than luminance differences. In the carotenoid-deprived birds, the "red" receptor would become identical with the broadband receptors described above, while the "green" receptor would shift over to 497 nm. The result would be that the "red" receptor would now be more sensitive to my green stimulus than to my red stimulus, and the "green" receptor's sensitivity to the green stimulus would diminish more than would its sensitivity to the red stimulus. These results are consistent with the finding that the carotenoid-deprived birds rely much more on luminance than chromatic difference, even though the two stimuli do not appear identical.

Recently, there have been two other studies published on the color vision of quail raised on a diet similar to, but developed independently of, the one reported here (diet of Meyer, 1971, and Meyer et al., 1971). Kovach et al. (1976) investigated color preference in two genetically selected lines, one selected for preference of red over blue, the other selected for the reverse preference. In both lines, there was a modest increase in red preference. Dücker and Schulze (1977) found that carotenoid-deprived birds could easily distinguish narrowband light from white light of any intensity, but there were differences in their color preferences compared to that of normals. The normals preferred, in decreasing order, green, yellow, blue, red; the carotenoid-deprived birds preferred green, blue, yellow, red. The authors suggest that this represents a shift in preference toward short wavelengths, but in view of the careful studies of Kovach et al., with different results, it seems possible that, in the absence of the "red" narrowband receptor, the yellow and red stimuli might appear similar and thus acquire similar preference values.

In conclusion, the results reported here show that pigmented oil droplets are not essential for color vision in the Japanese quail, but, if they are removed, color vision deteriorates, and if they are replaced, color vision improves. Rod/cone interactions may be partly responsible for the remaining color vision, but the most likely explanation is that the two or three receptor types remaining after carotenoid depletion permit substantial color vision. Nevertheless, these results show that the oil droplets do play a role in avian color vision.

ACKNOWLEDGMENTS. I am grateful to Paul K. Brown, who introduced me to the mysteries of the retina, and to Ann M. Graybiel, who intially collaborated on this project. The design of the appartus and the carrying out of the experiments benefited from the generous assistance of Hildur V. Colot and Martha M. Constantine-Paton. Dr. Bernard Wentworth, then of the University of Massachusetts, donated the birds that formed the breeding stock. I would also like to thank my advisors in graduate school, Drs. Roger S. Payne, Charles Walcott, and Benjamin Dane for encouragement and assistance, and Dr. Kenneth D. Roeder for inspiration and advice.

REFERENCES

Blackwell, H. R., and Blackwell, O. M.: Rod and cone receptor mechanisms in typical and atypical congenital achromatopsia. *Vision Res.* **1**:62–107 (1961).

Bloch, S., and Martinoya, C: Are colour oil droplets the basis of the pigeon's chromatic space? *Vision Res. Suppl.* **3**:411–418 (1971).

Bloch, S., and Maturana, H.: Oil droplet distribution and color discrimination in the pigeon. *Nature (London) New Biol.* **234**:284–285 (1971).

Blough, D. S.: Rise in the pigeon's threshold with a red test stimulus during dark adaptation. *J. Opt. Soc. Am.* **48**:274 (1958).

Blough, P. M.: Wavelength generalization and discrimination in the pigeon. *Percept. Psychophys.* **12**:342–348 (1972).

Bowmaker, J. K., and Knowles, A.: The visual pigments and oil droplets of the chicken retina. *Vision Res.* **17**:755–764 (1977).

Bridges, C. D. B.: Visual pigments of the pigeon (*Columba livia*). *Vision Res.* **2**:125–137 (1962).

Brush, A. H.: Pigments in hybrid, variant and melanic tanagers (birds). *Comp. Biochem. Physiol.* **36**:785–793 (1970).

Crescitelli, R., Wilson, B. W., and Lilyblade, A. L.: The visual pigments of birds. I. The turkey. *Vision Res.* **4**:275–280 (1964).

Delius, J. D., Thompson, G., Allen, K. L., and Emmerton, J.: Colour mixing and colour preferences in neonate gulls. *Experientia* **28**:1244–1246 (1972).

Detwiler, S. R.: *Vertebrate Photoreceptors.* Macmillan, New York (1943).

Donner, K. O.: On the effect of the coloured oil droplets on the spectral sensitivity of the avian retina. In *Proc. XIIth Int. Ornithol. Congr., Helsinki* (1960). Pp. 167–172.

Dücker, G.: Untersuchungen über die hormonale Beeinflussbarkeit der Farbbevorzugung von Feuerwebern (*Euplectes orix franciscanus*). *J. Ornithol.* **111**:19–29 (1970).

Dücker, G., and Schulze, I.: Color vision and color preference in Japanese quail (*Coturnix coturnix japonica*) with colorless oil droplets. *J. Comp. Physiol. Psychol.* **91**:1110–1117 (1977).

Fox, M. R. S., and Briggs, B. M.: Salt mixtures for purified-type diets. III. An improved salt mixture for chicks. *J. Nutr.* **72**:243–250 (1960).

Fox, M. R. S., and Harrison, B. N.: Use of Japanese quail for the study of zinc deficiency. *Proc. Soc. Exp. Biol. Med.* **116**:256–259 (1964).

Fujimoto, K., Yanase, T., and Hanaoka, T.: Spectral transmittance of retinal colored oil globules re-examined with microspectrophotometer. *Jpn. J. Physiol.* **7**:339–346 (1957).

Ganguly, J., Mehl, J. W., and Deuel, H. J.: Studies on carotenoid metabolism. XII. The effect of dietary carotenoids on the carotenoid distribution in the tissues of chickens. *J. Nutr.* **50**:59–72 (1953).

Gough, B. J., Shellenberger, T. E., and Escuriex, L. A.: Response of Japanese quail fed purified diets. *Quail Q.* **5**:2–6 (1968).

Govardovskii, V. I.: Color vision mechanism in birds: Visual pigments in pigeons and chicks. *Dokl. Transl. Biol. Sci.* **228**:257–259 (1976).

Govardovskii, V. I., and Zueva, L. V.: Visual pigments of chicken and pigeon. *Vision Res.* **17**:537–543 (1977).

Graf, V., and Norren, D. V.: A blue sensitive mechanism in the pigeon retina: λ_{max} 400 nm. *Vision Res.* **14**:1203–1209 (1974).

Hailman, J. P.: Coding of the colour preference of the gull chick. *Nature (London)* **204**:710 (1964).

Hailman, J. P.: Mirror-image color-preferences for background and stimulus-object in the gull chick (*Larus atricilla*). *Experientia* **22**:257–258 (1966).

Hailman, J. P.: The ontogeny of an instinct. The pecking response in chicks of the laughing gull (*Larus atricilla* L.) and related species. *Behaviour Suppl.* **15**:1–159 (1967).

Hamilton, W. F., and Coleman, T. B.: Trichromatic vision in the pigeon as illustrated by the spectral hue discrimination curve. *J. Comp. Psychol.* **15**:183–191 (1933).

Impekoven, M.: Motivationally controlled stimulus preferences in chicks of the black-headed gull (*Larus ridibundus* L). *Anim. Behav.* **17**:252–270 (1969).

Jitsumori, M: Anomaloscope experiment for a study of color mixture in the pigeon. *Jpn. Psychol. Res.* **18**:126–135 (1976).

Kear, J.: Colour preference in young Anatidae. *Ibis* **106**:361–369 (1964).

King-Smith, P. E.: Absorption spectra and function of the colored oil drops in the pigeon retina. *Vision Res.* **9**:1391–99 (1969).

Konishi, T.: Developmental studies on the retinal oil globules in Japanese quail, *Coturnix coturnix japonica. Zool. Mag.* **74**:119–131 (1965).

Kovach, J. K., Wilson, G., and O'Connor, T.: On the retinal mediation of genetic influences in the color preferences of Japanese quail. *J. Comp. Physiol. Psychol.* **90**:1144–1151 (1976).

Lashley, K. S.: The color vision of birds. I. The spectrum of the domestic fowl. *J. Anim. Behav.* **6**:1–26 (1916).

LeGrand, Y.: Colorimetrie du poulet théorique. *Vision Res.* **2**:81–83 (1962).

Liebman, P. A.: Microspectrophotometry of photo-receptors. In Dartnall, H. J. A. (ed.): *Handbook of Sensory Physiology VII/1.* Springer-Verlag, Berlin (1972).

Liebman, P. A., and Granda, A. M.: Super-dense carotenoids in cone oil droplets. *Nature (London)* **253**:370 (1975).

Mayr, I.: Über die Ölkugelverteilung in der Retina männlicher und weiblicher Feuer-
weber (*Euplectes orix franciscanus*). *J. Ornithol.* **111**:30–37 (1970).

Mayr, I.: Verteilung, Lokalisation und Absorption der Zapfenölkugeln bei Vögeln (Plo-
ceidae). *Vision Res.* **12**:1477–1484 (1972).

Meyer, D. B.: The effect of dietary carotenoid deprivation on avian retinal oil droplets.
Ophthalmic. Res. **2**:104–109 (1971).

Meyer, D. B., Stuckey, S. R., and Hudson, R. A.: Oil droplet carotenoids of avian cones.
I. Dietary exclusion: Models for biochemical and physiological studies. *Comp.
Biochem. Physiol.* **40B**:61–70 (1971).

Muntz, W. R. A.: Inert absorbing and reflecting pigments. In Dartnall, H. J. A. (ed.):
Handbook of Sensory Physiology VII/1. Springer-Verlag, Berlin (1972).

Norren, D. V.: Two short wavelength sensitive cone systems in pigeon, chicken and
daw. *Vision Res.* **15**:1164–1166 (1975).

Nyström, M.: The development of stimulus preferences in the pecking behaviour of
young herring gulls (*Larus argentatus*). I. Methods for the quantification of neonatal
responses. *Psychol. Res. Bull.* **9(8)**:1–17 (1969a).

Nyström, M.: The development of stimulus preferences in the pecking behaviour of
young herring gulls (*Larus argentatus*). III. A replica of Tinbergen and Perdeck's
classical investigation with an alternative interpretation. *Psychol. Res. Bull.* **9(10)**:1–
10 (1969b).

Oppenheimer, R. W.: Color preferences in the pecking response of newly hatched ducks
(*Anas platyrhynchos*). *J. Comp. Physiol. Psychol. Monogr. Suppl.* **66**:1–17 (1968).

Orlov, O. Y., and Maksimova, E. M.: The role of intracone light filters (Mechanism of
color vision of lizard and tortoise). *Dokl. Biophys.* **154**:11–14 (translation of *Dokl.
Akad Nauk SSR* **154**:463–466, 1964).

Pedler, C., and Boyle, M.: Multiple oil droplets in the photoreceptors of the pigeon.
Vision Res. **9**:525–528 (1969).

Peiponen, V. A.: Experimentelle Untersuchungen über das Rotkehlchen, *Erithacus rubecula* (L.). *Ann. Zool. Soc. Vanamo* **24(8)**:1–49 (1963).

Peiponen, V. A.: Zur Bedeutung der Ölkugeln im Farbensehen der Sauropsiden. *Ann.
Zool. Fenn.* **1**:281–302 (1964).

Riggs, L. A., Blough, P. M., and Shafer, K. L.: Electrical responses of the pigeon eye to
changes in wavelength of the stimulating light. *Vision Res.* **12**:981–991 (1972).

Roaf, H. E.: The absorption of light by the coloured globules in the retina of the domestic
hen. *Proc. R. Soc. London Ser. B* **105**:371–374 (1929).

Roaf, H. E.: Colour vision. *Physiol. Rev.* **13**:43–79 (1933).

Romeskie, M., and Yager, D.: Psychophysical studies of pigeon color vision. I. Photopic
spectral sensitivity. *Vision Res.* **16**:501–506 (1976a).

Romeskie, M., and Yager, D.: Psychophysical studies of pigeon color vision. II. The
spectral photochromatic interval function. *Vision Res.* **16**:507–512 (1976b).

Schneider, B.: Multidimensional scaling of color differences in the pigeon. *Percept.
Psychophys.* **12**:373–378 (1972).

Sillman, A. J.: The visual pigments of several species of birds. *Vision Res.* **9**:1063–1077
(1969).

Smith, V. C., and Pokorny, J.: Large-field trichromacy in protanopes and deuteranopes.
J. Opt. Soc. Am. **67**:213–220 (1977).

Strother, G. K.: Absorption spectra of retinal oil globules in turkey, turtle and pigeon.
Exp. Cell Res. **29**:349–355 (1963).

Taylor A., Sluckin, W., and Hewitt, R.: Changing colour preferences of chicks. *Anim.
Behav.* **17**:3–8 (1969).

Trezona, P. W.: Rod participation in the "blue" mechanism and its effect on colour
matching. *Vision Res.* **10**:317–332 (1970).

Wald, G., and Zussman, H.: Carotenoids of the chicken retina. *J. Biol. Chem.* **122**:446–460 (1938).

Wald, G., Brown, P. K., and Smith, P. H.: Iodopsin. *J. Gen. Physiol.* **38**:623–681 (1955).

Wallman, J.: The role of the retinal oil droplets in color vision of Japanese quail. *Am. Zool.* **10**:506–507 (1970).

Wallman, J.: The role of the retinal oil droplets in the color vision of the Japanese quail. Ph.D. dissertation, Tufts University (1972).

Wallman, J.: A simple technique using an optomotor response for visual psychophysical measurements in animals. *Vision Res.* **15**:3–8 (1975).

Walls, G. L., and Judd, H. D.: The intra-ocular colour-filters of vertebrates. *Br. J. Ophthalmol.* **17**:641–675, 705–725 (1933).

Walters, J. W.: Scotopic vision at photopic levels. *Vision Res.* **11**:787–798 (1971).

Weale, R. A.: Cone-monochromatism. *J. Physiol.* *(London)* **121**:548–569 (1953).

Wolbarsht, M. L.: The function of intraocular color filters. *Fed. Proc.* **35**:44–50 (1976).

Wright, A. A.: Psychometric and psychophysical hue discrimination functions for the pigeon. *Vision Res.* **12**:1447–1464 (1972a).

Wright, A. A.: The influence of ultraviolet radiation on the pigeon's color discrimination. *J. Exp. Anal. Behav.* **17**:325–339 (1972b).

Wright, A. A., and Cumming, W. W.: Color-naming functions for the pigeon. *J. Exp. Anal. Behav.* **15**:7–17 (1971).

Yager, D.: Spectral sensitivity with the freely moving eye. *Vision Res.* **10**:521–523 (1970).

Yazulla, S., and Granda, A. M.: Opponent-color units in the thalamus of the pigeon. *Vision Res.* **13**:1555–1563 (1973).

19

Synaptic Layers of the Retina: A Comparative Analysis with [125I]-α-Bungarotoxin

STEPHEN YAZULLA

INTRODUCTION

Substantial amounts of acetylcholine (AcCh) have been found in all vertebrate retinas so far investigated, suggesting a role for this compound as a retinal neurotransmitter (see Graham, 1974, for review). In support of this idea, both the synthesizing enzyme choline acetyltransferase (CAT) (Ross and McDougal, 1976) and the hydrolytic enzyme acetylcholinesterase (AcChE) (Francis, 1953; Nichols and Koelle, 1968) also are located in retinal cells, with the greatest concentration in amacrine cells and their processes. Experiments with perfused retinas consistently show effects of AcCh, cholinergic mimics, and antagonists on the light-evoked discharge of ganglion cells (Straschill, 1968; Ames and Pollen, 1969; Masland and Ames, 1976). All of this evidence has led to the hypothesis that there is a class of amacrine cells which uses AcCh as a neurotransmitter, with ganglion cells as the likely target.

The issue is by no means settled, for in some species the outer plexiform layer (OPL) may be involved in cholinergic transmission. In the newt, AcChE is found in horizontal cell processes (Dickson et al., 1971); in the frog, the ERG b wave is depressed by atropine, a mus-

STEPHEN YAZULLA • Department of Biology, State University of New York, Stony Brook, New York 11794. This work was supported by NIH Grant RO1 EYO1682.

carinic antagonist; in carp, perfusion with AcCh enhances the light response of horizontal cells (Kaneko and Shimazaki, 1976); in the turtle, atropine depresses horizontal cell activity (Gerschenfeld and Piccolino, 1977).

One solution for the problem of identifying cholinergic cells is the use of a labeled probe specific for AcCh receptors. Such a probe exists for the neuroeffector junctions of skeletal muscle and electric organ. α-Bungarotoxin (αBgt), the principal component of the venom from the banded krait (*Bungarus multicinctus*), binds specifically and irreversibly to nicotinic-AcCh receptors in the peripheral somatic nervous system (Bourgeois et al., 1972; Changeux, 1975; Fertuck and Salpeter, 1974).

α-Bungarotoxin has been used to search for AcCh receptors in the central nervous system as well (Salvaterra and Moore, 1973; Eterović and Bennett, 1975; Polz-Tejera et al., 1975; Hunt and Schmidt, 1978). Similarly, in the retinas of rabbit and chick (Vogel and Nirenberg, 1976) and goldfish, turtle, and pigeon (Yazulla and Schmidt, 1976, 1977) αBgt binds specifically and with high affinity to receptor sites in both the OPL and IPL. The question which naturally arises is whether or not the toxin receptors in the retina represent AcCh receptors, as is the case for the peripheral somatic nervous system.

METHODS

Subjects were goldfish (*Carassius auratus*), turtles (*Pseudemys scripta*), chicks (*Gallus domestica*), and homing pigeons (*Columba livia*). After decapitation, the eye was excised and the retina was dissected free of the pigment epithelium under ordinary room-light conditions. At this stage, the retina was weighed and prepared for either biochemical assay or histology.

Biochemistry

Preparation of Homogenates. The freshly dissected retina was homogenized in 20–50 volumes of 0.2 M sodium phosphate, pH 7.2 (unless stated otherwise), using a small glass tissue grinder. Approximately 100 strokes sufficed to produce a fine dispersion of tissue fragments. The homogenate was used immediately for binding studies.

Radiotoxin. [^{125}I]-αBgt was prepared as described previously (Lowy et al., 1976). Specific activity was approximately 10^6 Ci/mole or lower, depending on the age of the preparation. Biological activity, defined as the ability to bind to AcCh receptors from *Torpedo californica*, was retained over several iodine-125 half-lives.

In Vitro Binding Assay. Samples of retinal homogenates were incubated with [^{125}I]-αBgt in 1.5-ml microfuge tubes; the amount of toxin was measured in the particular fraction, obtained by centrifuging for 2 min in a model 3200 Eppendorf bench-top centrifuge. For radioactivity measurements, the top of the plastic centrifuge tube was sliced off and the tube was inserted into a transparent polystyrene counting tube and counted in an Isodyne model 1185 automatic gamma counter. Specific details are provided in the appropriate figure legends.

Autoradiography

After dissection, retinas were treated under a variety of conditions prior to incubation in [^{125}I]-αBgt. All substances, unless otherwise noted, were dissolved in Sorensen's 200 mM sodium phosphate buffer (pH 7.2), which is the same buffer used for the biochemical assays. All incubations were conducted at room temperature (21°C). Prior treatment with various cholinergic drugs lasted for 30 min, after which [^{125}I]-αBgt was added, resulting in a final toxin concentration of 5 × 10^{-9} M. Prior treatment consisted of incubation for 30 min in any one of the following:

1. 200 mM sodium phosphate buffer—control.
2. 30 μM eserine sulfate—10 min, after which 1 mM AcCh in 30 μM eserine sulfate was added for 20 min.
3. 30μM eserine sulfate—10 min, after which 1 mM butyrylcholine chloride (BuCh) in 30 μM eserine sulfate was added for 20 min.
4. Nicotine—10 μM, 100 μM, 1000 μM.
5. *d*-Tubocurarine—10 μM, 1000 μM.
6. 1 μM native αBgt.

After 30 min incubation in [^{125}I]-αBgt, the tissue was subjected to six 5-min rinses in phosphate buffer, which reduced the amount of free toxin remaining to about 15% of the bound toxin. The tissue was fixed overnight at 4°C in 2% glutaraldehyde and for 1 hr in 1% OsO$_4$; it was then dehydrated and embedded in Epon 812. For light microscopy, 4-μm sections were taken on a Sorvall JB-4 microtome and placed on acid-cleaned subbed slides. The slides were dipped in Kodak NTB-2 nuclear track emulsion (diluted 1:1 with Dreft water) at 40°C, dried in a humid chamber for 2 hr, exposed at 4°C for 1–4 weeks, developed at 18°C in undiluted D-19, and stained for 5 sec in methylene blue–sodium borate (0.1%). For electron microscopy, gold sections were collected on 300-mesh grids and coated with a monolayer of Ilford L4 emulsion by the loop technique. After exposures ranging from 4 to 16 weeks, sections were developed in D-19, fixed in a nonhardening fixer, and double stained in uranyl acetate and lead citrate. Specimens were viewed on a Jelco 100B electron microscope at ×1600–×14,000.

RESULTS

Toxin Binding in Vitro

Results of biochemical assays show that the retinas of goldfish, turtle, and pigeon bind $[^{125}I]$-αBgt with high affinity and great specificity. These results are summarized in Table 1. The half-saturation constants (K_d) are quite similar for the three species, ranging from 8 × 10^{-11} M for goldfish to 3 × 10^{-10} M for turtle and pigeon, values which are fairly close to the dissociation constant of 5.6 × 10^{-11} M determined for the binding of $[^{125}I]$-αBgt to rat brain extracts (Lowy et al., 1976). The total toxin binding per retina shown in the second column is much higher in pigeon than in turtle or goldfish. This is entirely due to the difference in size of the respective eyes. If the values per retina are adjusted for retinal diameter and retinal thickness (excluding the outer segments), the values/mg retina in the third column are obtained. These values, clustered around 26 fM/mg, are remarkably similar for the three species. The outer segments were discounted in the previous calculations for two reasons. First, all retinal isolations were performed in the light, resulting in most outer segments becoming detached. Outer segments, therefore, were not included in the original weight from which total binding was calculated. Second, outer segments do not occupy the same proportion of retinal space in the three species. In goldfish, in particular, the photoreceptors occupy nearly two-thirds of the retinal thickness, with outer segments occupying one-third of the total. In pigeon and turtle, outer segments and photoreceptors take up a much smaller percentage of retinal thickness. It should be pointed out that the absolute value of αBgt binding will decrease with increases in the ionic strength of the incubating medium (Yazulla and Schmidt, 1977). The values just cited were obtained in 10 mM phosphate buffer. In the

Table 1. In Vitro Binding of αBgt in the Retina

	K_d (M)	$[^{125}I]$-αBgt/ (fM) retina	$[^{125}I]$-αBgt/ (fM) mg retina
Goldfish	8 × 10^{-11}	330	26.8
Turtle	3 × 10^{-10}	550	27.4
Pigeon	3 × 10^{-10}	1800	24.4

following figures where an attempt is made to compare biochemical and histological data, 200 mM buffers were used in all experiments.

Toxin-Binding Localization

Initially, we (Yazulla and Schmidt, 1976) wished to determine where toxin binding occurs in the retinas of goldfish and turtle and whether such binding could be blocked by the cholinergic ligand, nicotine. As seen in the autoradiographs of Figs. 1 and 2, under control conditions toxin binding is largely restricted to the two plexiform layers. In both species, the heavier, more dense label is found in the outer plexiform layer (OPL). When the retina is simultaneously treated in 10^{-5} M nicotine, toxin binding is greatly reduced, and there is little evidence of specific binding in the plexiform layers. The high affinity and specificity of this toxin binding, plus its sensitivity to blockage by low concentrations of nicotine, led to the suggestion that these toxin-

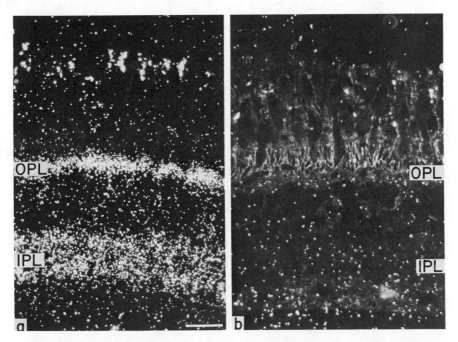

Fig. 1. Dark-field autoradiographs of goldfish retina incubated in 5×10^{-9} M $[^{125}I]$-αBgt under control conditions (a) and in the presence of 10^{-5} M nicotine (b). Abbreviations for all micrographs: OPL, outer plexiform layer; IPL, inner plexiform layer; PE, pigment epithelium. Calibration marker for Figs. 1–5, 25 μm.

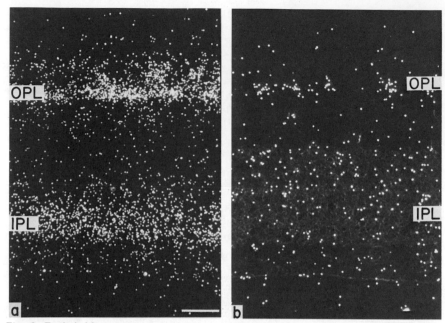

Fig. 2. Dark-field autoradiograph of turtle retina incubated in 5×10^{-9} M [^{125}I]-αBgt under control conditions (a) and in the presence of 10^{-5} M nicotine (b).

binding sites represented acetylcholine receptors (Yazulla and Schmidt, 1976).

Further experiments on chick and pigeon retinas were not so easily interpreted. Under control conditions, pigeon retina displayed the same qualitative pattern of toxin binding in both plexiform layers as was seen in goldfish and turtle (Fig. 3a). However, the effect of nicotine was quite different in that toxin binding in the OPL appeared to be unaffected by nicotine at concentrations as high as 10^{-3} M (Fig. 3b), even though binding in the IPL was significantly reduced at 10^{-5} M and approached background levels at 10^{-3} M. This was a very surprising result, because αBgt, a specific probe for nicotinic-cholinergic receptors, was completely unaffected by nicotine in the pigeon OPL. Further comparative tests were performed on turtle and pigeon to determine if similar differences could be found with other cholinergic ligands. Native (i.e., nonradioactive) αBgt (10^{-6} M) completely abolished toxin binding in the retinas of both species, once again demonstrating the specificity of this binding. This was especially important for the pigeon OPL, where nonspecific binding was a possible explanation for its insensitivity to nicotine. Atropine, a muscarinic ligand

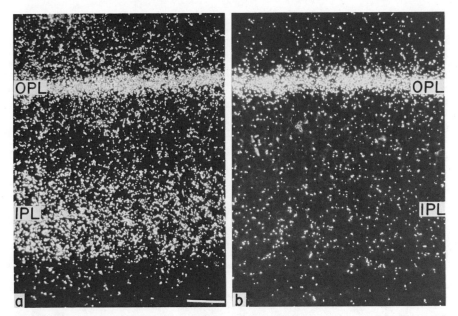

Fig. 3.Dark-field autoradiograph of pigeon retina incubated in 5×10^{-9} M [^{125}I]-αBgt under control conditions (a) and in the presence of 10^{-3} M nicotine (b). From Yazulla and Schmidt (1977).

at 10^{-3} M, had little inhibitory effect on toxin binding in either species (Figs. 4a and 5a), while the nicotinic ligand d-tubocurarine effectively inhibited toxin binding in both plexiform layers in both species at concentrations from 10^{-5} to 10^{-3} M (10^{-3} M shown, Figs. 4b and 5b). In addition, acetylcholine (10^{-3} M) and butyrylcholine (10^{-3} M) inhibited toxin binding in both plexiform layers in the eserinized (10^{-5} M) pigeon retina (Yazulla and Schmidt, 1977). The results show that toxin binding in the synaptic layers of pigeon and turtle is similarly affected by all cholinergic ligands tested except nicotine.

This apparent insensitivity to nicotine in the pigeon OPL was investigated in more detail by Yazulla and Schmidt (1977). It seemed possible that nicotine was prevented from acting at the OPL by some localized uptake mechanism or enzymatic degradation. These possibilities may be tested using a biochemical drug-competition assay in which the amount of toxin bound is plotted against the concentration of the competing drug. The concentration at which binding is reduced to 50% of the control is called the inhibition constant. A homogeneous receptor population will result in a simple inhibition curve, whereas the presence of multiple receptor types will give rise to a more complex function. Effects due to local enzyme action will be eliminated, since

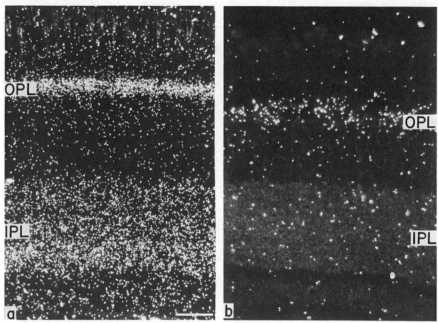

Fig. 4. Dark-field autoradiograph of pigeon retina incubated in 5×10^{-9} M [^{125}]-αBgt in the presence of 10^{-3} M atropine sulfate (a) and 10^{-3} M d-tubocurarine chloide (b). Figure b from Yazulla and Schmidt (1977).

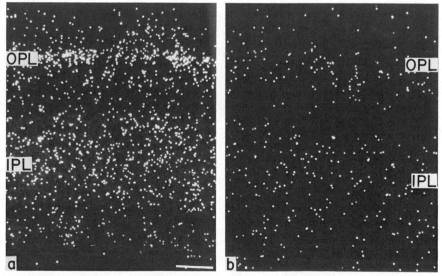

Fig. 5. Dark-field autoradiograph of turtle retina incubated in 5×10^{-9} M [^{125}I]-αBgt in the presence of 10^{-3} M atropine sulfate (a) and 10^{-3} M d-tubocurarine chloride (b).

homogenization of the tissue would evenly distribute any such enzymes throughout the preparation. The net result would be an overall reduction in the sensitivity of the binding sites to nicotine.

Figure 6 shows the results of this experiment. Curare, as expected, shows a simple curve, with an inhibition constant of 10^{-6} M. Nicotine, on the other hand, displays a two-component function: the first one, which is very sensitive to nicotine, with an inhibition constant of 5×10^{-7} M, and a second, less sensitive component with an inhibition constant at about 3×10^{-3} M. This experiment shows that the resistance to inhibition by nicotine is probably a property of the receptor itself.

In order to conclusively link the nicotine-resistant shoulder shown in Fig. 6 with toxin receptors in the outer plexiform layer, it is necessary to selectively block toxin binding in one plexiform layer, and by a drug competition study show a concomitant change in the inhibition function for nicotine. If the pigment epithelium is left attached to the retina, αBgt does not bind in the OPL within an incubation period of 30 min. Figure 7 shows a autoradiograph of a piece of pigeon retina in which the pigment epithelium is attached and detached over adjacent portions of the retina. Binding in the IPL shows little change across the section, while binding in the OPL decreases rapidly as the area with an intact pigment epithelium is entered. It is clear that diffusion from both retinal surfaces is necessary for adequate labeling of the retina.

The protective effect of the pigment epithelium can be utilized for a biochemical analysis in the following manner. In an eyecup preparation, with the pigment epithelium adhering to the retina, toxin receptors in the IPL are selectively blocked by adding native αBgt to the bathing medium. After excess toxin has been washed out, the retina is isolated and homogenized, and the affinity of the remaining unblocked toxin receptors for nicotine is measured using the toxin competition assay. Figure 8 shows that such treatment results in the elimination of the nicotine-sensitive component, thereby isolating the insensitive plateau. This experiment confirms that it is the toxin receptor residing in the OPL and protected by the pigment epithelium that is relatively insensitive to nicotine.

The question which immediately comes to mind is whether the toxin receptor in the outer plexiform layer has anything to do with synapses. We tried to get at this question by EM autoradiography. This is not the ideal method, because of the poor resolution. Localization of the radioactive source is a statistical problem with a fair amount of uncertainty, half-distance 800 A (Fertuck and Salpeter, 1974). Yet the synaptic arrangement at photoreceptor terminals is extensive, with many invaginating processes. If photoreceptors or horizontal cells were cholinergic, interactions which take place within the pedicle would be

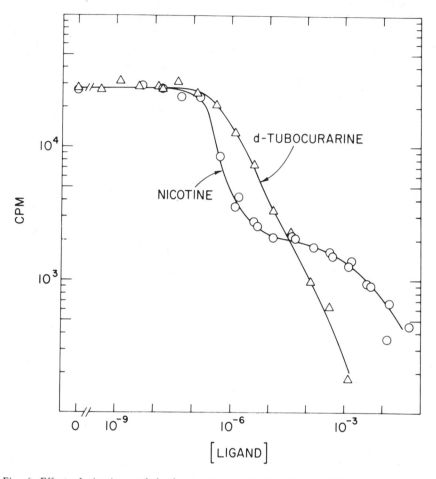

Fig. 6. Effect of nicotine and d-tubocurarine on the binding of $[^{125}I]$-αBgt. Retina homogenates, representing 3.8 mg of fresh tissue, are incubated with the indicated concentrations of cholinergic ligand in 0.3–0.4 ml of 0.2 M sodium phosphate, pH 7.2. After 30 min at room temperature, 0.02 ml of 6.3×10^{-8} M $[^{125}I]$-αBgt is added, and the toxin-binding reaction is allowed to proceed for 30 min to approximately 90% of completion (as determined by long-term incubation under the same conditions in the absence of the drug). The incubation is terminated by addition of 1.0 ml of 0.2 M sodium chloride immediately followed by centrifugation. The supernatant fluid is removed by aspiration, and the pellet is washed by resuspension in 1.4 ml of 0.2 M sodium chloride and centrifugation; this wash procedure is repeated once whereupon the particulate fraction is counted. Data are corrected for nonspecific binding. From Yazulla and Schmidt (1977).

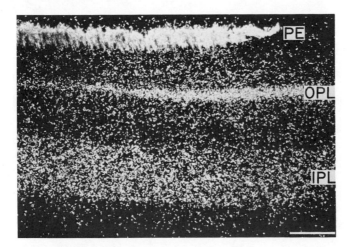

Fig. 7. Dark-field autoradiograph of pigeon retina incubated in 5×10^{-9} M [^{125}I]-αBgt. The pigment epitheleum, indicated by the uppermost bright band, is attached only over the left portion of the section. Calibration marker, 50 μm. From Yazulla and Schmidt (1977).

easily identified. Synaptic interactions outside the pedicle would prove more difficult. The following micrographs were taken from the "red field" of the pigeon retina where the vast majority of receptors are cones.

Figure 9 shows cone pedicles and associated silver grains. Note that the grains are located slightly proximal to the synaptic ribbons, not around them. In each of the remaining micrographs, the same proximal location of silver grains can be observed. Only rarely are silver grains seen over processes associated with a synaptic ribbon (arrow, Fig. 9a). The specific localization of toxin binding is amply demonstrated in Fig. 10a. Here a myriad of neurites of the OPL are bounded distally by two photoreceptor terminals and proximally by a large dendrite. Note that all of the silver grains are located in this plexus of small processes. This can be seen less dramatically in Fig. 9a. The most puzzling feature of these micrographs is that none of the grains is located consistently near an identifiable synaptic structure. It is possible that the silver grains could be associated with unconventional synaptic junctions such as flat contacts or basal or distal junctions. Some of these contacts, indicated by arrows in Fig. 10b, do not have nearby silver grains. However, the grains are so large that any underlying contact would be hidden. The resolution is just not good enough to identify the location of the toxin receptors.

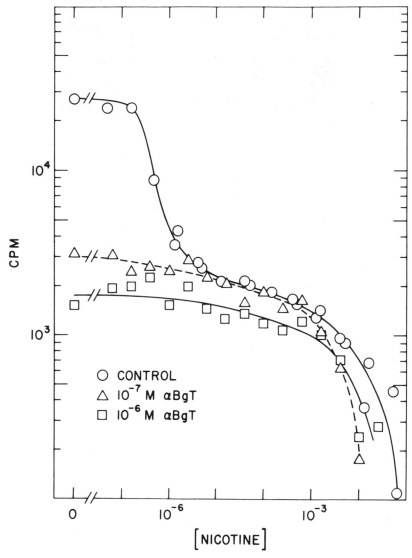

Fig. 8. Effect of pretreatment of intact retina with native αBgt on binding properties. Freshly excised retinas with the pigment epithelium attached are incubated in 200 mM sodium phosphate at the indicated concentrations of native αBgt, washed with six changes of toxin-free buffer, and homogenized. Aliquots of the homogenate representing 3.8 mg of fresh tissue are then incubated at various concentrations of nicotine, and the effect of nicotine on the binding of [^{125}I]-αBgt is measured as described in the caption of Fig. 6. From Yazulla and Schmidt (1977).

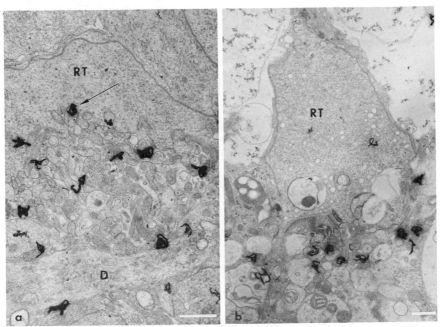

Fig. 9. Electron microscopic autoradiographs of the pigeon OPL, exposure 12 weeks. Calibration marker, 1 μm. See text for details. Abbreviations: RT, receptor terminal; D, dendrite.

DISCUSSION

α-Bungarotoxin binds to the synaptic layers in the retinas of all species so far investigated in this laboratory. These include goldfish, swamp turtle, pigeon, and chick. This binding is specific in that it is saturable and can be blocked by low concentrations of native αBgt, and it occurs with high affinity as judged by the low dissociation constant values, ranging from 8×10^{-11} to 30×10^{-11} M (Yazulla and Schmidt, 1976, 1977). In addition, the binding of αBgt can be inhibited by curare, AcCh, BuCh, and, except at the avian OPL, nicotine. Atropine, a muscarinic antagonist, is a much less effective competitor for αBgt than are the nicotinic agents. The histological results obtained with native αBgt, curare, AcCh, and atropine in this study are further supported by drug-competition studies in chick retina (Vogel and Nirenberg, 1976). Thus, for the most part, αBgt reacts in a similar competitive fashion with retinal receptor sites as it does with AcCh receptors at peripheral neuroeffector junctions of electric organ (Schmidt and Raftery, 1973), as well as with αBgt-binding sites in rat brain (Schmidt,

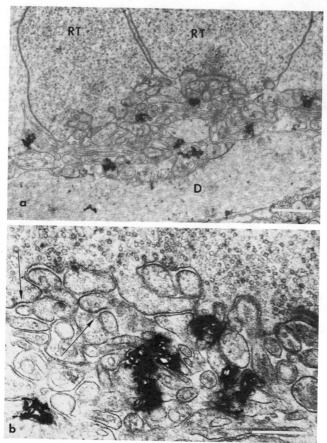

Fig. 10. Electron microscopic autoradiographs of the pigeon OPL, exposure 12 weeks. Abbreviations: RT, receptor terminal; D, dendrite. Calibration markers, 1 μm (a) and 0.5 μm (b). Arrows in (b) indicate specialized junctions not involving synaptic ribbons.

1977) and chick sympathetic ganglia (Greene, 1976). Since there is little doubt that AcCh acts as a neurotransmitter in the retina (see Graham, 1974, for review), is it appropriate at this time to identify toxin-binding sites in the retina with nicotinic-AcCh receptors as in the neuromuscular junction and electric organ? In my opinion, the answer at this time is "not yet." It is true that a strong case can be made for the IPL, with such evidence as the histochemical localization of AcChE and CAT in amacrine cells and their processes (Francis, 1953; Nichols and Koelle, 1968; Ross and McDougal, 1976), the sensitivity of αBgt receptors to nicotinic ligands (Vogel and Nirenberg, 1976; Yazulla and Schmidt, 1976, 1977), the localization of an αBgt-HRP complex postsynaptically to amacrine and bipolar cell synapses (Vogel et al., 1977), the developmental appearance of αBgt receptors relative to synapse formation in chick embryos (Vogel and Nirenberg, 1976), and the light-evoked release of AcCh with its effect on ganglion cell discharges in rabbit retina (Masland and Ames, 1976; Masland and Livingstone, 1976). The case is weaker for the OPL, since neither AcChE nor CAT has been demonstrated in appreciable quantities in this area (Francis, 1953; Nichols and Koelle, 1968; Nichols et al., 1972; Ross and Mc-Dougal, 1976). Thus, if AcCh were a neurotransmitter in the OPL, it would have to be deactivated either by diffusion or, more likely, by a high-affinity uptake mechanism, unusual for a cholinergic system but typical for the amino acids (Snyder et al., 1973). Although precise localization of αBgt binding is not known for the OPL as yet, it is clear from EM autoradiography that the processes associated with cone pedicles in pigeon are not the sites of αBgt binding. The appearance of label among the small processes of the OPL is not peculiar to the pigeon but has been seen in goldfish as well. Label also was seen penetrating high into the photoreceptor terminals, which contained bipolar but not horizontal cell dendrites, suggesting that bipolar dendrites contain αBgt receptors in goldfish retina (Schwartz and Bok, 1979). On the positive side, except for nicotine in the avian OPL, αBgt receptors in the OPL show the same sensitivity to blockage by cholinergic ligands as do their counterparts in the IPL. In spite of all these data, the critical point is that in neither plexiform layer has αBgt been shown to block cholinergically induced neural activity. Until this is done, one should not claim, as have Vogel and Nirenberg (1976), that αBgt receptors in the retina are nicotinic AcCh receptors.

Similar problems in establishing such an identity have been reported for nicotinic synapses in the spinal cord of frog (Miledi and Szczepaniak, 1975) and cat (Duggan et al., 1976), as well as in ganglionic fibers in guinea pig (Bursztajn and Gershon, 1977). In none of these cases did αBgt behave as a nicotinic antagonist on evoked neural activity. In mouse and guinea pig ganglia, no binding of rhodamine-labeled αBgt could be observed (Bursztajn and Gershon, 1977). This is in contrast to membrane fragments of chick sympathetic ganglia in which highly specific αBgt binding could be traced through development (Greene, 1976), and in rat superior cervical ganglion in which αBgt binding could be demonstrated but application of αBgt was without any physiological effect (Brown and Fumagulli, 1977). Binding of αBgt has been amply demonstrated in brain tissue, also (Salvaterra and Moore, 1973; Polz-Tejera et al., 1975; Schmidt, 1977), even to the point of locating $[I^{125}]$-αBgt to synaptic membranes in rat hippocampus by EM autoradiography (Hunt and Schmidt, 1978). Yet the crucial physiological evidence is lacking here as well.

It is obvious that nicotinic receptors in vertebrate nervous systems cannot be considered as a unitary class, and results obtained in the spinal cord cannot be generalized to those in the brain, periphery, or retina. Even in the retinas of chick and pigeon, there are two types of αBgt receptors which differ markedly in their sensitivity to blockage by nicotine. It is possible that differences may be found between αBgt receptors in the OPL and IPL of other species after treatment with other pharmacological agents. αBgt has proven invaluable in the study of the neuromuscular junction. Given the chance, with appropriate caution, αBgt may prove equally valuable in determining the role of AcCh in information transfer in the vertebrate retina.

ACKNOWLEDGMENTS. I would like to acknowledge the collaboration of Dr. Jakob Schmidt in this work as well as the technical assistance of Ging-Kuo Wang, Indhira Handy, and Mark Rosenthal.

REFERENCES

Ames, A., and Pollen, D. A.: Neurotransmission in central nervous tissue: A study of isolated rabbit retina. *J. Neurophysiol.* **32**:424–442 (1969).

Bourgeois, J. P., Ryter, A., Menez, A., Fromageot, P., Boquet, P., and Changeux, J. P.: Localization of the cholinergic receptor protein in electrophorus electroplax by high resolution autoradiography. *FEBS Lett.* **25**:127–133 (1972).

Brown, D. A., and Fumagulli, L.: Dissociation of alpha bungarotoxin binding and receptor block in the rat superior cervical ganglion. *Brain Res.* **129**:165–169 (1977).

Bursztajn, S., and Gershon, M. D.: Discrimination between nicotinic receptors in vertebrate ganglia and skeletal muscle by alpha-bungarotoxin and cobra venoms. *J. Physiol. (London)* **269**:17–31 (1977).

Changeux, J.: The cholinergic receptor protein from fish electric organ. In Iverson, L. U., Iverson, S. D., and Snyder, S. H. (eds.): *Handbook of Psychopharmocology,* Vol. 6: *Biogenic Amine Receptors.* Plenum, New York (1975). Pp. 235–302.

Dickson, D. H., Flumerfelt, B. A., Hollenberg, M. J., and Gwyn, D. G.: Ultrastructural localization of cholinesterase activity in the outer plexiform layer of the newt retina. *Brain Res.* **35**:299–303 (1971).

Duggan, A. W., Hall, J. G., and Lee, C. Y.: Alpha-bungarotoxin, cobra neurotoxin and excitation of Renshaw cells by acetylcholine. *Brain Res.* **107**:166–170 (1976).

Eterović, V. A., and Bennett, E. L.: Nicotinic cholinergic receptor in brain detected by binding of α-[^{3}H] bungarotoxin. *Biochim. Biophys. Acta* **363**:346–355 (1975).

Fertuck, H. C., and Salpeter, M. M.: Localization of acetylcholine receptor by ^{125}I-labeled α-bungarotoxin binding at mouse motor end plates. *Proc. Natl. Acad. Sci. USA* **71**:1376–1378 (1974).

Francis, C. M.: Cholinesterase in the retina. *J. Physiol. (London)* **120**:435–439 (1953).

Gerschenfeld, H. M., and Piccolino, M.: Muscarinic antagonists block cone to horizontal cell transmission in turtle retina. *Nature (London)* **2568**:257–259 (1977).

Graham, L. T.: Comparative aspects of neurotransmitters in the retina. In Davson, H., and Graham, L. T. (eds.): *The Eye,* Vol VI. Academic Press, New York (1974). Pp. 283–342.

Greene, L.: Binding of α-bungarotoxin to chick sympathetic ganglia: Properties of the receptor and its rate of appearance during development. *Brain Res.* **111**:135–145 (1976).

Hunt, S., and Schmidt, J.: The electron microscopic autoradiographic localization of α-bungarotoxin binding sites within the CNS of the rat. *Brain Res.* **142**:152–159 (1978).

Kaneko, A., and Shimazaki, H.: Synaptic transmission from photoreceptors to the second-order neurons in the carp retina. In Zettler, F., and Weiler, R. (eds.): *Neural Principles of Vision.* Springer-Verlag, New York (1976). Pp. 143–157.

Lowy, J., McGregor, J., Rosenstone, J., and Schmidt, J.: Solubilization of an α-bungarotoxin-binding component from rat brain. *Biochemistry* **15**:1522–1527 (1976).

Masland, R. H., and Ames, A.: Responses to acetylcholine of ganglion cells in an isolated mammalian retina. *J. Neurophysiol.* **39**:1220–1235 (1976).

Masland, R. H., and Livingtone, C. J.: Effect of stimulation with light on synthesis and release of acetylcholine by an isolated mammalian retina. *J. Neurophysiol.* **39**:1210–1219 (1976).

Miledi, R., and Szczepaniak, A. C.: Effect of *Dendroaspis* neurotoxin on synaptic transmission in the spinal cord of the frog. *Proc. R. Soc. London Ser B* **190**:267–274 (1975).

Nichols, C. W., and Koelle, G. B.: Comparison of the localization of acetylcholinesterase and non-specific cholinesterase activities in mammalian and avian retinas. *J. Comp. Neurol.* **133**:1–16 (1968).

Nichols, C. W., Hewitt, J., and Laties, A. M.: Localization of acetylcholinesterase in the teleost retina. *J. Histochem. Cytochem.* **20**:130–136 (1972).

Polz-Tejera, G., Schmidt, J., and Karten, H. J.: Autoradiographic localization of α-bungarotoxin binding sites in the central nervous system. *Nature (London)* **258**:349–351 (1975).

Ross, C. D., and McDougal, D. B., Jr.: The distribution of choline acetyltransferase activity in vertebrate retina. *J. Neurochem.* **26**:521–526 (1976).

Salvaterra, P. M., and Moore, W. J.: Binding of [^{125}I]-αBungarotoxin to particulate fractions of rat and guinea pig brain. *Biochem Biophys. Res. Commun.* **55**:1311–1318 (1973).

Schmidt, J.: Drug binding properties of an α-bungarotoxin-binding component from rat brain. *Mol. Pharmacol.* **13**:283–290 (1977).

Schmidt, J., and Raftery, M. A.: A simple assay for the study of solubilized acetylcholine receptors. *Anal. Biochem.* **52**:349–354 (1973).

Schwartz, I. R., and Bok, D.: Electron microscopic localization of ^{125}I-αbungarotoxin binding sites in the outer plexiform layer of the goldfish retina. *J. Neurocytol.* In press (1979).

Snyder, S. H., Young, A. B., Bennett, J. P., and Mulder, A. H.: Synaptic biochemistry of amino acids. *Fed. Proc.* **32**:2039–2047 (1973).

Straschill, M.: Action of drugs on single neurons in the cats retina. *Vision Res.* **8**:35–47 (1968).

Val'tsev, V. B.: Role of cholinergic structures in outer plexiform layer in the electrical activity of frog retina. *Fed. Proc. Trans. Suppl.* **25**:T765–T766 (1966).

Vogel, Z., and Nirenberg, M.: Localization of acetylcholine receptors during synapatogenesis in retina. *Proc. Natl. Acad. Sci. USA* **73**:1806–1810 (1976).

Vogel, Z., Maloney, G. J., Ling, A., and Daniels, M. P.: Electron microscopic identification of nicotinic acetylcholine receptor sites in retinal synapses. *Proc. Natl. Acad. Sci. USA* **74**:3268–3272 (1977).

Yazulla, S., and Schmidt, J.: Radioautographic localization of ^{125}I-αbungarotoxin binding sites in the retinas of goldfish and turtle. *Vision Res.* **16**:878–880 (1976).

Yazulla, S., and Schmidt, J.: Two types of receptors for α-bungarotoxin in the synaptic layers of the pigeon retina. *Brain Res.* **138**:45–47 (1977).

20

Quantitative Morphological Investigations of Retinal Cells in the Pigeon: A Golgi, Light Microscopic Study

MEL LOCKHART

INTRODUCTION

The fovea is a small, pit-shaped depression located on the vitreal surface of the retina. It is produced by the centrifugal displacement of the inner retinal layers from the center of the area centralis, a retinal thickening caused by local increases in cell density (Slonaker, 1897; Polyak, 1941, 1957; Walls, 1942; Duke-Elder, 1958). Two general forms of foveas have been described in vertebrates: shallow, saucer-shaped, or concaviclivate foveas are found in some fish, turtles, and primates, while deep, pit-shaped, or convexiclivate foveas are found in many diurnal lizards and some fish (Walls, 1942; Duke-Elder, 1958). Most avian foveas are centrally located and should probably be classified as convexiclivate, although the foveas of ground-feeding and nocturnal birds are shallower than those of diurnal predators (Slonaker, 1897; Walls, 1942; Oehme, 1961, 1962; Galifret, 1968; Blough, 1971, 1973; Fite and Rosenfield-Wessels, 1975). Many avian predators exhibit two foveas—a central fovea and a temporal fovea—while some bird species have only a

MEL LOCKHART • Department of Psychology, Lafayette College, Easton, Pennsylvania 18042. Present address: Jules Stein Eye Institute, University of California at Los Angeles, Los Angeles, California 90024.

single temporal fovea (Slonaker, 1897; Walls, 1942; Duke-Elder, 1958; Fite and Rosenfield-Wessels, 1975).

In primates, the centrally located fovea appears to mediate static acuity, since foveal lesions produce significant decrements in spatial resolution (Yarczower et al., 1966; Weisenkrantz and Cowey, 1967; Cowey and Ellis, 1967; Rolls and Cowey, 1970). Two anatomical features are thought to contribute to the enhanced spatial resolution associated with foveal vision in primates. First, as noted above, cell densities are typically higher in foveal and parafoveal areas than in more peripheral portions of the retina (Walls, 1942; Polyak, 1957). Anatomically, foveal cells are usually smaller than their peripheral counterparts (e.g., Ramón y Cajal, 1892; Polyak, 1941, 1957). Second, electrophysiological recordings indicate that ganglion cells from the foveal region of primates have very small receptive fields (Hubel and Weisel, 1960; Gouras, 1968; deMonasterio and Gouras, 1975). Taken together, these factors essentially increase the retinal "grain" in the foveal area. Data described by Walls (1942) suggest that resolution in the fovea is further enhanced by direct magnification since differences in the refractive indices of the retina and vitreous produce an enlarged image when light intersects the foveal slope.

The precise function of the avian fovea has been a matter of some debate (Walls, 1937, 1942; Pumphrey, 1948, 1961). Walls (1942) stressed the functional similarities between primate and avian central foveas, arguing that both structures mediate static acuity. He suggested that the deeper foveal clivus characteristic of most birds simply produces a greater magnification of the image falling on foveal receptors. Thus visual acuity should be best in those species which have very deep convexiclivate foveas (Walls, 1942).

Pumphrey (1948, 1961) challenged Walls's analysis of foveal functioning in birds, pointing out that the rapidly changing slope of the convexiclivate fovea would distort as well as enlarge the visual image. Such aberrational effects would be most severe in those species with the deepest foveas and would interfere with spatial resolution, according to Pumphrey. The distorted image produced by deep avian foveas could potentially increase sensitivity to angular movement, however, since an image focused on the foveal pit would become asymmetrical as it moved across the sloped side of the fovea. Pumphrey therefore hypothesized that the avian fovea was specifically designed for aiding the exact alignment and fixation of the eye in tracking moving objects. The accurate fixation of moving contours is critically important for diurnal avian predators, precisely those species which possess the deepest convexiclivate foveas (Slonaker, 1897; Walls, 1942; Duke-Elder, 1958; Oehme, 1961, 1962; Fite and Rosenfield-Wessels, 1975).

Behavioral evidence pertaining to the function of avian foveas is inconclusive. Psychophysical studies indicate that minimum separable acuity in diurnal birds approaches or exceeds that of humans and other primates (Blough, 1971; Fite et al., 1975; Fox et al., 1976; Hodos et al., 1976a). In such visual discrimination tasks, birds are reported to fixate distant targets on the central retina prior to responding (Blough, 1971; Fox et al., 1976), leading some investigators to assume that the centrally located fovea mediates static acuity in birds, as it does in primates. However, lesion studies suggest that the pigeon fovea is not critically involved in the resolution of fine spatial detail, since foveal lesions produce little change in acuity (Yarczower, 1964; Blough, 1973).

Movement detection, or dynamic acuity, has only recently been investigated in avian species. Hodos et al. (1976b) used several procedures to determine the minimum detectable velocity of movement in pigeons. Threshold values obtained by Hodos and his colleagues (4.1–6.01 deg/sec) are substantially higher than those previously reported for humans and other primates (Brown, 1931; Carpenter and Carpenter, 1958). Furthermore, Mulvanny (1978) found that pigeons were less sensitive than humans to changes in velocity. However, target distances in the studies of Hodos et al. (1976b) and Mulvanny (1978) were relatively short (43–62 mm from stimulus field to nodal point); therefore, the targets were probably focused on the dorsotemporal retina rather than on the central fovea (Catania, 1964; Blough, 1973). Earlier studies by Nye (1968, 1973) had evaluated responses to movement in both the frontal and lateral fields in pigeons. Nye's data indicated that pigeons were more responsive to movement in the frontal field than to movement in the lateral field. However, Nye (1973) noted that the reduced sensitivity shown toward moving stimuli in the lateral field (served by the central fovea) may have been an artifact of his testing procedures. Thus the dynamic acuity of the central fovea in birds remains to be evaluated behaviorally.

The structural organization of the avian fovea may provide additional evidence as to its functional significance. Ramón y Cajal (1889, 1892) first reported that cells in the foveas of sparrows and chameleons were smaller than peripheral cells. Polyak (1941) found a similar relationship in the primate retina. The close correspondence in size between the dendritic fields of foveal bipolars and the bases of receptor cells, and between the dendritic fields of small foveal ganglion cells and the axonal terminations of nearby bipolars, led Polyak to hypothesize that these "midget" bipolars and "midget" ganglion cells formed a "private line" for transmitting information from individual foveal receptors to the central nervous system. The foveal midget system is thought to mediate static acuity in primates (Polyak, 1941, 1957; Boycott and Dowling, 1969). Subsequent authors have often assumed that a comparable midget system capable of maintaining a one-to-one relationship between receptors and ganglion cells exists in birds (e.g., Oehme, 1961, 1962). However, that assumption has yet to be confirmed experimentally by a detailed quantitative analysis of individually impregnated cells.

The present morphological investigation examined cells of the central fovea and the red field in the pigeon. The central fovea of the pigeon, located in the yellow field, serves a monocular, lateral field of view, and is thought to mediate responses for distant targets (Blough, 1973). The red field, which serves a binocular, frontal field, seems to be used for near-field vision (Catania, 1964; Galifret, 1968; Blough, 1971, 1973). The central red field contains a circumscribed area of increased cell density, called the area dorsalis (Galifret, 1968; Binggeli and Paule, 1969). Several authors have suggested that the shallow central fovea of the pigeon is homologous to the central foveas of other birds (e.g., Blough, 1971, 1973), and that the area dorsalis corresponds to the temporal foveas found in some avian species (e.g., Binggeli and Paule, 1969).

Light microscopic studies of Golgi-impregnated tissue compared cell dimensions in the fovea, central red field, and periphery of the pigeon retina. In addition, evidence for a midget system, comparable to that found in primates, was evaluated. Cells in the foveal region of the bluejay were also measured in an effort to confirm the suggestion that the central fovea of the pigeon is structurally similar to the deeper central foveas of other birds.

METHODS AND MATERIALS

The retinas of 17 White Carneaux pigeons (*Columba livia*) and 13 northern bluejays (*Cyanocitta cristata*) were studied. The pigeon is reported to possess a shallow, convexiclivate central fovea (Slonaker, 1897, Chard and Gundlach, 1938; Galifret, 1968; Blough, 1971), while the bluejay exhibits a deeper convexiclivate fovea, similar in shape to those of several predatory birds (Slonaker, 1897; Fite and Rosenfield-Wessels, 1975).

Eyes were removed under chloroform anesthesia and opened by removing the cornea and lens. To prepare flat mounts, the retina was dissected from the eye cup, then sandwiched according to the procedure described by Stell and Witkowsky (1973). Tissue was processed using both the Stell (Stell and Witkovsky, 1973) and Colonnier (1964) variations of the Golgi technique. Only tissue processed by the Colonnier method was examined further, since tissue prepared using the Stell method was inadequately impregnated. Nineteen retinas of each species were sufficiently impregnated to permit microscopic examination.

Transverse sections were obtained by processing whole eye cups following the Colonnier (1964) procedure. Impregnated eyes were then embedded in celloidin using the procedure described by Fite (1973) for low-viscosity nitrocellulose (LVN), but substituting celloidin for LVN. Following embedding, sections of 100 μm were cut with a sliding microtome, paying careful attention to the maintenance of retinal orientation and the order of sections.

Foveal cell dimensions were obtained in flat-mounted tissue for receptor bases and basal processes, and for cell bodies and process fields of horizontal, bipolar, amacrine, and ganglion cells. A concentric-ring eyepiece micrometer was centered on the structure in question, then the length of the longest diameter was measured. The length of a second diameter which passed through the midpoint of the first diameter was also recorded. Displacement of bipolar cells was determined in transverse sections by measuring the horizontal distance from dendritic to axonal expansion. All measurements were made through an oil-immersion lens at a magnification of × 1000.

Although the foveal depression was readily discernible in transverse sections, its location in flat-mounted tissue was more difficult to determine. Previous authors had located the foveal area in flat-mounted primate retinas by the absence of blood vessels (Ogden, 1974) or by determining the cone density (Boycott and Kolb, 1973). However, the entire avian retina is avascular (Pumphrey, 1961), and the relative rod/cone densities have not been determined for pigeons or bluejays. As described below, the distinctive arrangement of bipolar cells in the foveal region of these species suggested a procedure which permits the accurate localization of the foveal pit in flat-mounted avian retinas.

For purposes of quantitative analysis, the foveal area was defined as encompassing a circular area of 1.5 mm diameter, the center of which coincided with the center of the foveal pit. Yazulla (1974) estimated the width of the foveal clivus in pigeons to be approximately 0.5 mm, while Fite and Rosenfield-Wessels (1975) reported that the clivus of bluejay was about 0.7 mm in width. Data obtained in the present study indicated that the lateral displacement of the axons of bipolar cells in the foveal region frequently exceeded 0.3 mm. Additional lateral displacement of information derived from foveal receptors which is less easily quantified may occur via horizontal or amacrine cells. Hence ganglion cells located as much as 0.8 mm from the center of the foveal pit may receive input from receptors located within the area of the foveal clivus.

The central red field, which includes the area dorsalis, was located prior to impregnation by the clearly discriminable red hue produced by the large numbers of red and orange oil droplets in that area. The peripheral region was arbitrarily defined as the 2-mm-wide region adjacent to the scleral border of the retina.

In order to permit interspecies comparisons, estimates of the size of the visual field and the length of the retina were obtained for three retinas from each species studied. An estimate of the mean number of micrometers per visual degree was then calculated using the procedure described by Fite and Rosenfield-Wessels (1975).

RESULTS

Examination of transverse horizontal sections of the retinas of pigeons confirmed the existence of a shallow central fovea in that species (Fig. 1). In addition, a very distinctive lateral displacement of bipolar cell processes was observed in the foveal region which was not

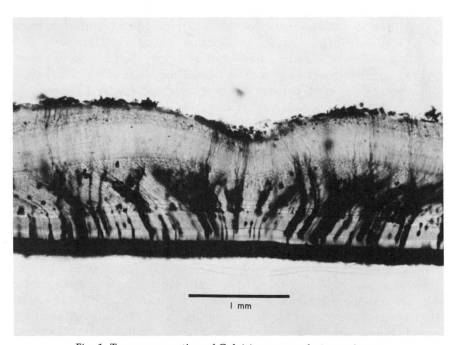

Fig. 1. Transverse section of Golgi-impregnated pigeon fovea.

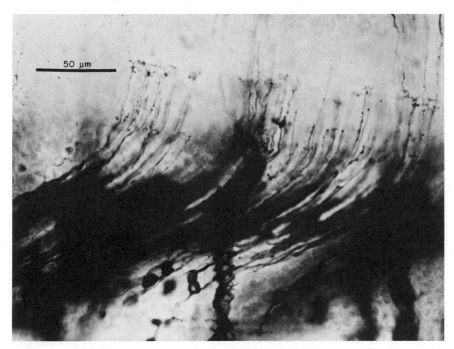

Fig. 2. Enlargement of parafoveal bipolar cells in transverse section. Axonal terminals are displaced from more centrally located dendritic processes.

evident in other retinal areas (Fig. 2). Inner-plexiform-layer terminals of the foveal bipolar cells were displaced by approximately 300 μm from corresponding outer-plexiform processes. This phenomenon permitted the accurate localization of the fovea in flat-mounted retinas, since bipolars appear to radiate symmetrically from the center of the foveal pit (Fig. 3).

Cells occurring in flat-mounted retinas were classified as receptor, horizontal, bipolar, amacrine, ganglion, or glial cells on the basis of location of cell bodies and processes. The five categories of neural cells were further divided into subclasses on the basis of shape and size. Two types of receptor bases, three types of horizontal cells, two types of bipolar cells, two classes of amacrine cells, and one type of ganglion cell were present in sufficient numbers in each retinal area studied to permit meaningful quantitative comparisons. (Various cell types have been designated by initial and number, e.g., bipolar 1 or B1.)

The dimensions of retinal cells were found to vary systematically with retinal locus in the pigeon. The relationship of retinal locus to process-field diameters paralleled that of locus to cell-body dimensions.

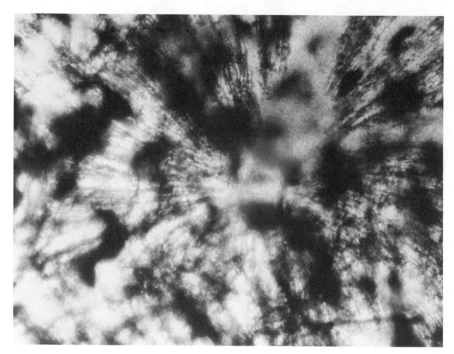

Fig. 3. Golgi-impregnated foveal area of the pigeon retina, flat mounted. Bipolar cells appear to radiate from the center of the foveal pit.

Since the former differences were somewhat larger in magnitude, only the dimensions of process fields will be presented in detail. As shown in Table 1, processes terminating on the outer plexiform layer (receptor basal processes, horizontal and bipolar dendritic fields) exhibited the following relationship: dimensions for foveal cells were very similar to those of cells found in the dorsotemporal red field, and the dimensions of both foveal and red-field cells were smaller than those of their peripheral counterparts.

Bipolar and amacrine terminations occurring within the inner plexiform layer were larger in the dorsotemporal area than in the foveal region (see Table 2). Furthermore, the dimensions of both varieties of dorsotemporal cells approached those of their peripheral counterparts. The dendritic fields of ganglion cells were similar in the fovea and the central red field, and smaller there than in the periphery.

The preceding quantitative data indicate that bipolar and ganglion cells with relatively small dendritic fields exist in both the fovea and the central red field. As seen in Fig. 4, small foveal bipolars extend fingerlike dendritic projections into the region occupied by the bases

Table 1. Mean Dimensions of the Process Fields of
Cells Terminating in the Outer Plexiform Layer of
the Pigeon Retina[a]

Cell type	Location		
	Foveal	Dorsotemporal	Peripheral
Receptor 1	4 × 9	5 × 8	6 × 13
Receptor 2	13 × 19	13 × 18	17 × 24
Receptor 3	14 × 23	15 × 19	14 × 21
Horizontal 1	19 × 23	17 × 21	21 × 32
Horizontal 2	22 × 32	27 × 36	34 × 55
Bipolar 1	7 × 10	8 × 11	12 × 17
Bipolar 2		8 × 12	10 × 14

[a] Dimensions are given in micrometers.

of receptor cells. Foveal bipolars, as noted above, are quite long, with axonal terminations displaced from the dendritic arborization by up to 300 μm. Occasionally, a foveal bipolar cell could be traced for its entire length in transverse sections (see Fig. 5). However, these cells were particularly difficult to follow in flat-mounted tissue, where retinal

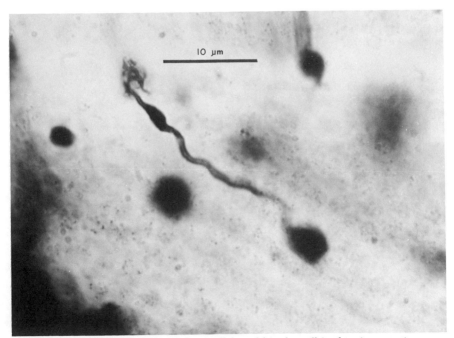

Fig. 4. Dendritic arborization of a small foveal bipolar cell in the pigeon retina.

Table 2. Mean Dimensions of the Process Fields of Cells Terminating in the Inner Plexiform Layer of the Pigeon Retina[a]

Cell type	Location		
	Foveal	Dorsotemporal	Peripheral
Bipolar 1	7 × 11	10 × 15	9 × 14
Bipolar 2	7 × 9	11 × 15	11 × 15
Amacrine 1	48 × 60	125 × 138	150 × 190
Amacrine 2	33 × 45	58 × 105	60 × 98
Amacrine 3	78 × 113	150 × 225	150 × 218
Ganglion 1	25 × 42	30 × 45	35 × 70

[a] Dimensions are given in micrometers.

thickness reduced resolving power for deep structures, particularly in foveal regions. Bipolar cells in the red field showed no such lateral displacement: axonal terminations occurred directly proximal to the dendritic arborization, and it was usually possible to measure both dendritic and axonal dimensions for each bipolar cell.

Small ganglion cells (G1), which were found both in the fovea and in the red field, were typically multidendritic, with fine processes

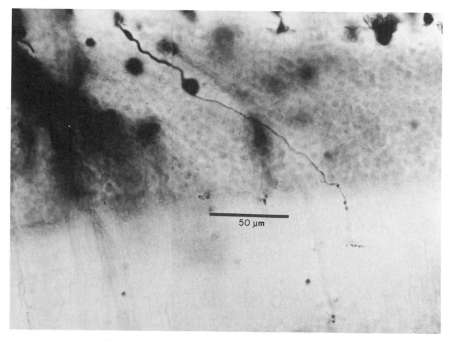

50 µm

Fig. 5. Photomontage of the entire bipolar cell shown in Fig. 4.

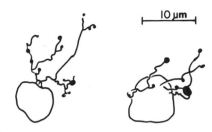

Fig. 6. Tracings of small ganglion cells from the pigeon fovea.

terminating in small bulbous expansions (Fig. 6). Larger, more elaborately branched, and multistratified ganglion cells were found in some portions of the retina, but they were rare in the fovea and were always larger than the G1 cells in other areas.

In order to provide a basis for evaluating a possible "midget system" in the pigeon fovea, a distribution of bipolar dendritic field dimensions was constructed by calculating the approximate area of each dendritic expansion using the formula $A = \frac{1}{4}\pi ab$, where a and b represent diameter measurements. As shown in Fig. 7, the distribution is apparently bimodal, with clusters occurring between 20 and 30 μm^2 and above $50 \mu m^2$. Also shown in the figure is the range of sizes found for the basal process fields of foveal photoreceptors. Note that many of the bipolar cells exhibited dendritic fields which were smaller in size than the process fields of the photoreceptors.

A similar analysis compared the dimension of foveal bipolar axonal terminations with the areal extent of foveal ganglion cells (Fig. 8). Only the smallest ganglion cell fields were comparable in size to the axonal expansions of the bipolar cells. As noted above, retinal thickness and cell density in the foveal area made it impossible to trace bipolars from their dendritic to their axonal expansions in flat-mounted tissue. Consequently, the dendritic diameters of small (less than 32 μm^2) bipolars could not be obtained directly.

In order to estimate the size of the inner-plexiform-layer terminations of the small foveal bipolars, a correlational analysis was performed. The correlation between dendritic and axonal areal extent was obtained for nonfoveal bipolars, since both measurements could be obtained for each cell. The Pearson product-moment correlation coefficients were found to be $r = 0.55$ for B1 cells and $r = 0.56$ for B2 cells. The largest of the small-field bipolar cells had a dendritic area of 32 μm^2. A regression analysis indicated that a B1 cell of that size would have an axonal area greater than 45 μm^2 less than 1% of the time, while a B2 cell of comparable size would have an axonal area greater than 100 μm^2 less than 1% of the time. No ganglion cells with dendritic fields as small as 45 μm^2 were found in any of the

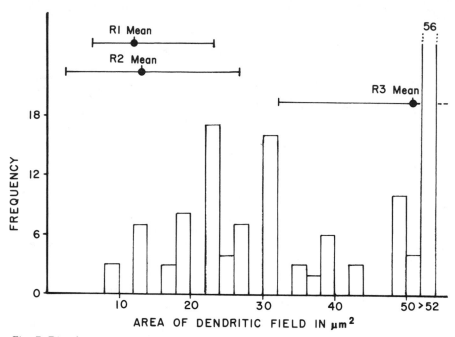

Fig. 7. Distribution of dendritic-field sizes for foveal bipolar cells in the pigeon retina. Brackets (⊢——⊣) above the distribution indicate the range of sizes found for the basal fields of foveal photoreceptors, R1, R2, and R3. Mean size for each cell type is indicated by ●

Table 3. *Summary of the Quantitative Analysis of Potential "Midget" Cells in the Pigeon's Fovea and Red Field* [a]

	Fovea		Red Field	
Cell type	Maximum process area, μm^2	Proportion	Maximum process area, μm^2	Proportion
Receptor	32	—	28	—
"Midget" bipolar				
Dendritic terminal	32*	0.41	28*	0.20
Axonal terminal				
B1	45[b]	—	85	—
B2	100[b]	—	120	—
"Midget" ganglion	45**	0.00	85	0.08
	100**	0.03	120	0.13

[a] Maximal size of bipolar dendritic terminals was limited by the extent of receptor-cell process dimensions (*), and, similarly, maximal size of "midget" ganglion cell fields was determined by the size of "midget" bipolar axonal terminations (**).
[b] Estimates of the areas of "midget" bipolar axonal terminals were obtained using a regression analysis. The values represent the upper end of the 99% confidence interval.

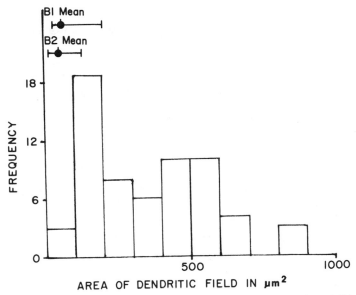

Fig. 8. Distribution of dendritic-field sizes for small (less than 1000 μm) G1 ganglion cells in the pigeon fovea. The range (⊢——⊣) and mean (●) of bipolar axonal areas are shown in the upper left for foveal B1 and B2 cells.

retinas investigated, and only 3% of the impregnated cells were found to have fields smaller than 100 μm^2. It therefore seems highly unlikely that even the smallest ganglion cells could make exclusive contact with a single small-field foveal bipolar cell.

Table 3 summarizes the quantitative analysis of receptor, bipolar, and ganglion cell characteristics. The maximal area observed for the basal processes of foveal receptors was equal to 32 μm^2, and 41% of the foveal bipolar cells impregnated with the method used here exhibited fields of 32 μm^2 or less. The correlational analysis suggested that the maximum value to be expected for the axonal terminals of small-field bipolars would be 45 μm^2 and 100 μm^2 for B1 and B2, respectively. Only 3% of the ganglion cells examined had dendritic areas as small as 100 μm^2. The smallest area observed was 75 μm^2.

Comparisons of field sizes for receptor, bipolar, and ganglion cells found in the red field were based on direct measurement, since both dendritic arborizations and axonal terminals could be observed for individual bipolars there. Data obtained from that analysis are also summarized in Table 3. In the dorsotemporal retina of the pigeon, approximately 20% of the bipolars exhibited dendritic fields smaller than receptor basal-process fields, while 13% of the ganglion cells had dendritic expansions smaller than the axonal arborizations of the small-field bipolars.

The structural and quantitative analysis of foveal cells described in the pigeon was repeated in the bluejay, which is reported to possess a relatively deep, convexiclivate central fovea similar to those observed in other predatory birds (Slonaker, 1897; Fite and Rosenfield-Wessels, 1975). In general, cells found in the retinas of both species were structurally similar. Furthermore, the relationship between eye size and visual field of view was quite similar for the two species. Measurements indicated that the species differed by less than 3% in this characteristic (pigeon, 175 μm/deg; bluejay, 170 μm/deg). Therefore, cellular dimensions were compared directly.

As Table 4 indicates, foveal cells in the bluejay were considerably smaller than their peripheral counterparts, as was the case in pigeon (refer to Tables 1 and 2). The magnitude of the size increase from fovea to periphery was much larger in the bluejay than in the pigeon. Not only were most foveal cells in the bluejay smaller than those found in the pigeon, but also most peripheral cells were larger in the bluejay than in the pigeon. This finding suggests that the pigeon retina is somewhat more homogeneous than the bluejay retina with respect to cell size.

The investigation of a possible midget system in the blue jay was comparable to that completed in pigeons. As shown in Fig. 9, the dendritic fields of many foveal bipolars were quite small in the bluejay. Typically fields were as small as, or smaller than, the fields of surrounding receptor cells. However, foveal G1 ganglion cells in the bluejay were similar in size to their pigeon counterparts. Thus, since the regression analysis indicated that small foveal bipolar cells would be expected to have axonal fields as large as 66 μm^2 less than 0.1% of the time, and

Table 4. Mean Field Dimensions of Retinal Cells in the Bluejay[a]

Outer-plexiform-layer processes			Inner-plexiform-layer processes		
Cell type	Fovea	Periphery	Cell type	Fovea	Periphery
Receptor 1	2.5 × 3	5 × 7	Bipolar 1	6 × 10	10 × 18
Receptor 2	7 × 8	20 × 32	Bipolar 2	6 × 11	12 × 22
Receptor 3	8 × 10	16 × 23	Amacrine 1	70 × 103	280 × 325
Horizontal 1	10 × 12	33 × 67	Amacrine 2	—	85 × 125
Horizontal 2	17 × 19	59 × 85	Amacrine 3	58 × 100	150 × 230
Bipolar 1	4 × 6	12 × 21	Ganglion 1	16 × 35	90 × 100
Bipolar 2		14 × 27			

[a] Diameters are given in micrometers.

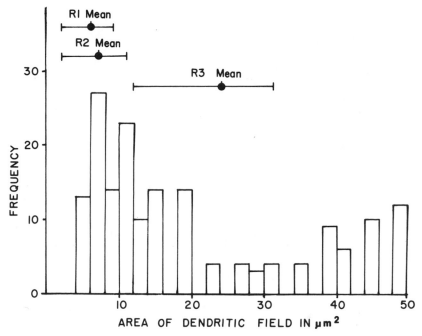

Fig. 9. Distribution of dendritic-field sizes for foveal bipolar cells in the bluejay retina. Range (⊢——⊣) and mean (●) size of photoreceptor basal fields are shown in the upper left.

since the diameter of the smallest ganglion cell observed in the bluejay was 117 μm^2, it was concluded that exclusive contact between foveal bipolars and individual ganglion cells was unlikely. This conclusion receives further verification from the observation that even the largest axonal terminations of foveal bipolars are smaller than the dendritic fields of most foveal ganglion cells, as shown in Fig. 10.

DISCUSSION

The dimensions of the process fields of cells observed in the pigeon and bluejay retinas varied systematically with retinal locus. In both species, foveal cells were smaller than their peripheral counterparts, although the difference observed from fovea to periphery was larger in bluejay than in pigeon. This observation supports the notion that the relatively shallow fovea of the pigeon is homologous to the deeper, clearly convexiclivate central foveas of other avian species (Blough,

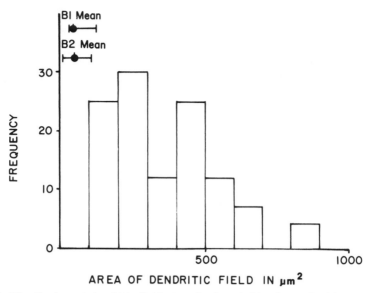

Fig. 10. Distribution of dendritic-field sizes for foveal G1 cells in the bluejay. Range (——) and mean (●) size of bipolar axonal terminations are shown in the upper left.

1971, 1973). Thus the cells of the pigeon retina differ only quantitatively from those of the bluejay retina: the pigeon retina is more homogeneous with respect to cell size than is the bluejay retina.

Cell dimensions were also investigated in the dorsotemporal red field of the pigeon retina. Typically, the dimensions of cells in the red field were similar to those of foveal cells, although bipolar axonal terminations and amacrine cell fields were larger in the red field than in the fovea. The central red field contains an area of increased cell density, the area dorsalis, which may correspond to the temporal fovea found in some predatory birds (Galifret, 1968; Binggeli and Paule, 1969). However, the precise location of the area dorsalis can be determined only on the basis of cell density counts which are difficult to obtain from flat-mounted tissue. Consequently, data reported for the dorsotemporal retina, which were obtained from the entire red field rather than from the area dorsalis, may overestimate the actual dimensions of cells in the latter area. Informal observations suggest that cell dimensions were smaller in the central red field than in surrounding areas.

Potential "midget" cells observed in the pigeon retina can be compared both morphologically and quantitatively with midget cells described in primate retinas by Polyak (1941, 1957) and by Boycott and Dowling (1969). Morphologically, the smallest foveal bipolar and ganglion cells were strikingly different in the primate and pigeon retinas. Two varieties of midget bipolar cell have been observed in the primate retina: invaginating and flat midget bipolars (Boycott and Dowling, 1969; Kolb et al., 1969; Kolb, 1974). The flat bipolar has a small, flat dendritic expansion, while the invaginating midget bipolar is characterized by small but distinct apical processes at the point of dendritic termination. The dendritic arborizations of the small-field bipolars found in the pigeon retina resembled those of the invaginating midget bipolar. No flat midget bipolars were observed in the tissue studied. The extensive lateral displacement of the axonal terminal from the dendritic terminal found in avian foveal bipolars is not observed in primates, although receptor pedicle bases are displaced laterally from the receptor cell body in the primate foveal area (Polyak, 1957).

Neither variety of ganglion cell found in the avian retina investigated was similar structurally to the foveal midget ganglion cells observed in primates. Midget ganglion cells found in primate retinas usually have dendritic expansions which emanate from a single central trunk attached to the cell body (Polyak, 1957; Boycott and Dowling, 1969). As seen in Fig. 6, the smaller of the avian ganglion cells (G1) usually had three or more branches extending from the cell body and ending in small (1 μm) terminal bulbs. The processes of the small G1 cells observed in the foveal region usually terminated in the inner half of the inner plexiform layer, often at more than one level.

In order to compare retinal cells from the pigeon and the rhesus monkey quantitatively, dimensions obtained by Boycott and Dowling (1969) were corrected for species differences in eye size and visual field of view. Fite and Rosenfield-Wessels (1975) reported that 1 visual degree in the rhesus monkey retina subtends an arc of approximately 211 μm in length. Data obtained in the present study using similar methods indicate that 1 visual degree is approximately equal to 175 μm for the pigeon.

Boycott and Dowling (1969) reported that primate midget bipolars have dendritic spreads ranging from 4 to 7 μm (mean 5 μm), while midget ganglion cells have field diameters of less than 10 μm, more commonly 4–5 μm. A pigeon bipolar with a dendritic spread of about 4 μm would correspond in size to an average midget bipolar for rhesus monkey, and a ganglion cell with a 4 μm field would be comparable in size to an average primate midget ganglion cell. The upper limit of size for midget bipolar and ganglion diameters becomes, respectively, 6 and 8 μm. On the basis of the corrected dimensions, the fovea was found to contain many bipolars with dendritic spreads comparable to those of primate cells. Cells with distal field diameters of as little as 4 μm were commonly observed. Foveal ganglion cells were not as small as primate midget ganglion cells: the smallest ganglion cell found in the foveal area of the pigeon had a dendritic field of 10 μm in diameter. Thus, while small foveal bipolars in the pigeon retina are similar in size to primate midget bipolars, the small foveal ganglion cells are much larger than primate ganglion cells.

Clearly, the most critical aspect of the primate midget system is neither the absolute size of the cells nor their anatomical configuration, but rather the relative diameter of (1) bipolar dendritic fields and receptor synaptic bases and (2) ganglion cell dendritic fields and bipolar axonal expansions. A primate bipolar cell is classified as a midget bipolar if its distal field is so small that contact with more than one receptor is unlikely; a ganglion cell is called a midget ganglion cell when its dendritic field is so small that contact with more than one midget bipolar cannot occur. Traditionally, the relationships described have been stated more directly: midget bipolar fields must be as small as or smaller than cone pedicle bases, while ganglion cell dendritic fields must be as small as or smaller than midget bipolar axonal expansions. Frequently, light microscope photographs showing bipolar axons and ganglion cell dendrites which occur in close proximity have been provided to buttress assumptions of nearly exclusive synaptic interaction (e.g., Boycott and Dowling, 1969).

The bimodal distribution of bipolars in the foveal region of the pigeon retina suggests that two distinct classes of bipolars exist in that area, as Ramón y Cajal (1892) reported for other species. Furthermore, a comparison of the size of bipolar fields with the size of receptor synaptic bases indicated that one-to-one contact between receptors and the smaller bipolars could occur. The "one-to-one" contact mediated by the first stage of the midget system refers to the fact that a midget bipolar may contact only one receptor, but does not require that the contacts of any receptor be limited to only one bipolar. (This point has occasionally been misinterpreted, e.g., by Pedler, 1969.) It would appear then, on the basis of these light microscopic observations, that a midget bipolar comparable to the midget bipolar of primates does exist in the pigeon central fovea.

The second relational requirement for a "midget system" is two-fold, involving a comparison of ganglion-cell field dimensions with those of midget bipolar proximal terminations. In order to argue that a given ganglion cell could receive input from only one bipolar, it must be shown that ganglion-cell fields are as small as, or smaller than, bipolar axonal expansions. G1 cells, the smallest ganglion cells and therefore the strongest candidate for midget ganglion cell, were typically larger than surrounding bipolar axonal terminations in the fovea. Further, individual ganglion cells often ended at multiple levels within the inner plexiform layer. The smallest foveal ganglion cells observed did correspond in size to the very largest bipolar axonal expansions. Hence, if the diffuse G1 cells form synaptic contact only at the ends of their dendritic processes, it is possible that the smallest G1 cells *could* contact a single bipolar. However, a statistical analysis indicated that it was extremely unlikely that a *midget* bipolar would exhibit an axonal termination as large as the dendritic field of the small foveal ganglion cells.

Quantitative morphological data detailed above suggest that a functional midget system may exist in the central red field of the pigeon. Approximately 20% of the bipolar cells found in the red field morphologically resemble the invaginating midget bipolar of primates and meet the relational criteria for midget bipolars described above. In addition, 13% of the ganglion cells impregnated had dendritic fields as small as the axonal terminations of the midget bipolar cells, although the ganglion cells were structurally different from primate midget ganglion cells.

Some care must be taken in evaluating the data from this (or any) Golgi study. First, many different Golgi procedures have been developed, and they may each impregnate different types of cells, or different cells in different species. Frequently, studies using different methods have independently confirmed the existence of similar cells in different vertebrate retinas, for example, horizontal cells in turtle (Leeper, personal communication), pigeon (Lockhart, 1976), and cat (Dowling et al., 1966; Fisher and Boycott, 1974). However, while observation of a given type of cell clearly confirms its existence, the absence of a cell type must be interpreted with caution. Furthermore, since the processes by which the various Golgi procedures impregnate cells are largely unknown, one cannot assume that impregnation occurs randomly. Thus, while quantitative data as to cell size are probably reliable, information as to the proportions of cells present in a particular species or in a given retinal area must be considered to be an estimate.

Bearing in mind these limitations, the following statements can be made concerning presumptive midget systems in the pigeon retina. First, a rudimentary midget system, composed of midget bipolar and midget ganglion cells, has been found in the dorsotemporal red field. Second, although many small foveal bipolar cells meet relational criteria for midget bipolars, the "midget" bipolars were up to 300 μm long from dendrite to axon. Furthermore, the small foveal ganglion cells observed differed from primate midget ganglion cells in that they were larger, less numerous and multidendritic, and they exhibited many dendritic varicosities. To date, no ganglion cells morphologically or quantitatively comparable to primate midget ganglion cells have been observed in avian retinas either in Ramón y Cajal's (1892) early work, which used the rapid Golgi procedures, or in the present study, which used the Colonnier (1964) modification of the Golgi method. Each of those methods impregnates numerous midget ganglion cells in the foveal region of primates (Polyak, 1941, 1957; Boycott and Dowling, 1969).

The present study supplements a growing body of data which suggests that the central fovea of birds is organized differently from that of primates. Foveal lesions produce significant decrements in near-field acuity in primates (Yarczower et al., 1966; Weisenkrantz and Cowey, 1967; Cowey and Ellis, 1967; Rolls and Cowey, 1970), but not in pigeons (Yarczower, 1964; Blough, 1973). The central fovea of primates subserves a frontal binocular field of view, while the central foveas of most birds serve a monocular lateral field, because of the lateral placement of the eye in those avian species (Galifret, 1968; Blough, 1973). Finally, synaptic relations seem to be more complex in the inner plexiform layer of the pigeon fovea than in the primate fovea. Although the ratio of conventional synapses to ribbon synapses is lower in the foveal region of the pigeon retina than elsewhere (Yazulla, 1974), as it is in primates (Dubin, 1970), the foveal and parafoveal ratios obtained by Yazulla (1974) for pigeon are significantly higher than those reported for the primate fovea by Dubin (1970).

The observation of a rudimentary midget system in the dorsotemporal retina is most intriguing, since that area is thought to mediate near-field acuity in the pigeon (Catania, 1964; Blough, 1971, 1973; Nye, 1973). Like the primate fovea, the dorsotemporal retina of most birds subserves a frontal, binocular field of view (Galifret, 1968; Blough, 1973). Efforts to establish a possible analogy between the primate central fovea and the dorsotemporal areas or foveas of birds are not without problems, however. For example, Yazulla (1974) reported that the dorsotemporal red field has the highest conventional-to-ribbon-synapse ratio in the pigeon retina, although the primate fovea has the lowest ratio for that retina (Dubin, 1970).

The apparent absence of a completely developed midget system in the pigeon retina may be related to a significant feature of visual processing in that species. A number of investigators have reported that ganglion cells in the pigeon's retina are responsive to relatively

complex characteristics of visual stimuli, such as movement, orientation, and directionality (Maturana, 1962; Maturana and Frenk, 1965;
Holden, 1969; Pearlman and Hughes, 1976). Dowling (1970) has argued
that much complex processing may occur within the inner plexiform
layer of species such as pigeon, while Sjostrand (1976) has recently
suggested that coding of movement or directionality could occur in the
outer plexiform layer of some species. In any event, since processing
of complex stimuli is presumably occurring within the retina of the
pigeon, it may not be necessary to maintain the fine retinal grain
established at the receptor level in the fovea or area dorsalis into the
central nervous system. Clearly, even in primates, the one-to-one relationship between receptors and higher-order neurons cannot be
maintained indefinitely within the central nervous system.

The possibility that the majority of small-field ganglion cells found
in the fovea and red field may act as *functional* midget cells cannot be
ruled out completely by the present study. Cells observed in this study
were classified on the basis of anatomical criteria such as shape and
size, criteria which have traditionally been used to distinguish midget
cells from other varieties. Recently, some authors have demanded that
more stringent criteria, including demonstration of exclusive synaptic
contact between midget ganglion cell and midget bipolar, be met (e.g.,
Bunt, 1976). Such criteria may be overly restrictive, however, since
both Polyak (1957) and Boycott and Dowling (1969) have indicated that
midget ganglion cells in the primate fovea are probably synaptically
related to diffuse bipolars and amacrine cells, in addition to a single
midget bipolar. Electrophysiological recordings from presumed midget
ganglion cells have demonstrated a center-surround organization of the
receptive fields, indicating that synaptic relationships within the primate midget system cannot be exclusively one-to-one-to-one (Hubel
and Weisel, 1960; Gouras, 1968; deMonasterio and Gouras, 1975).

Most of the small ganglion cells found in the pigeon retina were
larger than the terminations of the vast majority of midget bipolars.
Therefore, it is unlikely that numerous instances of exclusive contact
between ganglion cell and individual midget bipolars occur in that
retina. However, while the size of the ganglion cell dendritic fields
suggests that the smaller cells are postsynaptic to more than one cell,
it is possible that the presynaptic complex is made up of a single
midget bipolar and additional diffuse bipolars or amacrine cells. Such
an arrangement is exactly the same as that postulated by Polyak (1957)
and Boycott and Dowling (1969) for midget ganglion cells in the primate
fovea. As yet, the actual synaptic relations of small ganglion cells have
not been determined for either primates or pigeons, although that

could be accomplished using electron microscopic techniques in conjunction with Golgi methods.

REFERENCES

Binggeli, R. L., and Paule, W. J.: The pigeon retina: Quantitative aspects of the optic nerve and ganglion cell layer. *J. Comp. Neurol.* **137**:1–17 (1969).

Blough, P. M.: Visual acuity in the pigeon for distant targets. *J. Exp. Anal. Behav.* **15**:57–69 (1971).

Blough, P. M.: Visual acuity in the pigeon. II. Effect of target distance and retinal lesions. *J. Exp. Anal. Behav.* **20**:333–343 (1973).

Boycott, B. B., and Dowling J. E.: Organization of the primate retina: Light microscopy. *Philos. Trans. R. Soc. London Ser. B* **255**:109–176 (1969).

Boycott, B. B., and Kolb, H.: The horizontal cells of the rhesus monkey retina. *J. Comp. Neurol.* **148**:115–140 (1973).

Brown, J. F.: The thresholds for visual movement. *Psychol. Forsch.* **14**:249–268 (1931).

Bunt, A. H.: Ramification patterns of ganglion cell dendrites in the retina of the albino rat. *Brain Res.* **103**:1–8 (1976).

Carpenter B., and Carpenter, J.T.: The perception of movement by young chimpanzees and human children. *J. Comp. Physiol. Psychol.* **51**:782–784 (1958).

Catania, A. C.: On the visual acuity of the pigeon. *J. Exp. Anal. Behav.* **7**:316–366 (1964).

Chard, R. D., and Gundlach, R. H.: The structure of the eye of the homing pigeon. *J. Comp. Psychol.* **25**:249–272 (1938).

Colonnier, M.: The tangential organization of the visual cortex. *J. Anat.* **98**:327–344 (1964).

Cowey, A., and Ellis, C. M.: Visual acuity of rhesus and squirrel monkeys. *J. Comp. Physiol. Psychol.* **64**:80–84 (1967).

deMonasterio, F. M., and Gouras, P.: Functional properties of ganglion cells of the rhesus monkey retina. *J. Physiol. (London)* **251**:167–195 (1975).

Dowling, J. E.: Organization of vertebrate retinas. *Invest. Ophthalmol.* **9**:655–680 (1970).

Dowling, J. E., Brown, J. E., and Major, D.: Synapses of horizontal cells in rabbit and cat retinae. *Science* **153**:1639–1641 (1966).

Dubin, M. W.: The inner plexiform layer of the vertebrate retina. A quantitative and comparative electron microscope analysis. *J. Comp. Neurol.* **140**:479–506 (1970).

Duke-Elder, S.: *System of Ophthalmology*, Vol. 1: *The Eye in Evolution*. Kimpton, London (1958).

Fisher, S. K., and Boycott, B. B.: Synaptic connexions made by horizontal cells within the outer plexiform layer of the retina of the cat and the rabbit. *Proc. R. Soc. London Ser. B* **186**:317–331 (1974).

Fite, K. V.: Anatomical and behavioral correlates of visual acuity in the great horned owl. *Vision Res.* **13**:219–230 (1973).

Fite, K. V., and Rosenfield-Wessels, S.: A comparative study of deep avian foveas. *Brain Behav. Evol.* **12**:97–115 (1975).

Fite, K. V., Stone, R. J., and Conley, M.: Visual acuity in the northern blue jay: Behavioral and anatomical correlates. Paper presented at Neuroscience Society, New York (1975).

Fox, R., Lehmkehle, S. W., and Westendorf, D. H.: Falcon visual acuity. *Science* **192**:263–265 (1976).

Galifret, Y.: Les diverses aires functionelles de la rétine du pigeon. *Z. Zellforsch. Mikrosk. Anat.* **86**:535–545 (1968).

Gouras, P.: Identification of cone mechanisms in monkey ganglion cells. *J. Physiol.* (*London*) **199:**533–547 (1968).

Hodos, W., Leibowitz, R. W., and Bonbright, J. C.: Near-field visual acuity of pigeons: Effect of head location and stimulus luminance. *J. Exp. Anal. Behav.* **25:**129–141 (1976a).

Hodos, W., Smith, L., and Bonbright, J. C.: Detection of velocity of movement of visual stimuli by pigeons. *J. Exp. Anal. Behav.* **25:**143–156 (1976b).

Holden, A. L.: Receptive properties of retinal and tectal cells in the pigeon. *J. Physiol.* (*London*) **200:**56–57P (1969).

Hubel, D. H., and Weisel, T. N.: Receptive fields of optic nerve fibers in the spider monkey. *J. Physiol.* (*London*) **154:**572–580 (1960).

Kolb, H.: Organization of the outer plexiform layer of the primate retina: Electron microscopy of Golgi-impregnated cells. *J. Comp. Neurol.* **155:**1–14 (1974).

Kolb, H., Boycott, B. B., and Dowling, J. E.: A second type of midget bipolar cell in the primate retina. *Philos. Trans. R. Soc. London Ser. B* **255:**177–184 (1969).

Lockhart, M.: Quantitative analysis of horizontal cells in pigeon and blue jay retinae: Golgi studies. Paper presented at Association for Research in Vision and Ophthalmology Meeting, Sarasota, Fla. (1976).

Maturana, H. R.: Functional organization of the pigeon retina. Proceedings of the International Union of Physiological Science, XXII International Congress. Leiden (1962).

Maturana, H. R., and Frenk, S.: Directional movement and horizontal edge detectors in the pigeon retina. *Science* **150:**359–361 (1965).

Mulvanny, P.: Velocity discrimination by pigeons. *Vision Res.* **18:**531–537 (1978).

Nye, P. W.: The binocular acuity of the pigeon measures in terms of modulation transfer function *Vision Res.* **8:**1041–1053 (1968).

Nye, P. W.: On the functional differences between frontal and lateral visual fields of the pigeon. *Vision Res.* **13:**559–574 (1973).

Oehme, H.: Vergleichend-histologische Untersuchungen an der Retina von Eulen. *Zool. Jahrb. Abt. Anat. Ontog. Tiere* **79:**439–478 (1961).

Oehme, H.: Das Ruge von Mauersegler, Star und Amsel. *J. Ornithol.* **103:**187–212 (1962).

Ogden, T. E.: The morphology of retinal neurons of the owl monkey, *Aotes*. *J. Comp. Neurol.* **153:**399–427 (1974).

Pearlman, A. L., and Hughes, C. P.: Functional role of efferents to the avian retina. I. Analysis of retinal ganglion cell receptive fields. *J. Comp. Neurol.* **166:**111–122 (1976).

Pedler, C.: Rods and cones—A new approach. *Int. Rev. Gen. Exp. Zool.* **4:**219–274 (1969).

Polyak, S. L.: *The Retina.* University of Chicago Press, Chicago (1941).

Polyak, S. L.: *The Vertebrate Visual System.* University of Chicago Press, Chicago (1957).

Pumphrey, R. J.: The theory of the fovea. *J. Exp. Biol.* **25:**299–312 (1948).

Pumphrey, R. J.: Sensory organs: Vision. In Marshall, A. J. (ed.): *Biology and Comparative Physiology of Birds,* Vol. 2. Academic Press, New York (1961). Pp. 22–68.

Ramón y Cajal, S.: Sur la morphologie et les connexions des éléments de la rétine des oiseaux. *Anat. Anz.* **4:**111–121 (1889).

Ramón y Cajal, S.: *The Structure of the Retina* (1892). Translated by S. A. Thorpe and M. Glickstein. Charles C. Thomas, Springfield, Ill. (1972).

Rolls, E. T., and Cowey, A.: Topography of the retina and striate cortex and its relationship to visual acuity in rhesus and squirrel monkeys. *Exp. Brain Res.* **16:**1–14 (1970).

Sjostrand, F. S.: The outer plexiform layer of the rabbit retina, an important data processing center. *Vision Res.* **16:**1–14 (1976).

Slonaker, J. R.: A comparative study of the area of acute vision in vertebrates. *J. Morphol.* **13:**445–494 (1897).

Stell, W. K., and Witkovsky, P.: Retinal structure in the smooth dogfish, *Mustelus canis:*

General description and light microscopy of giant ganglion cells. *J. Comp. Neurol.* **148:**1–32 (1973).

Walls, G. L.: The significance of the foveal depression. *Arch. Ophthalmol.* **18:**912–917 (1937).

Walls, G. L.: *The Vertebrate Eye and Its Adaptive Radiations.* Cranbrook Press, Bloomfield Hills, Mich. (1942).

Weisenkrantz, L., and Cowey, A.: Comparison of the effects of striate cortex and retinal lesions on visual acuity in monkeys. *Science* **155:**104–106 (1967).

Yarczower, M.: The development of a behavioral system to evaluate visual performance in animals. Report for the Institute of Behavioral Research (August 1964).

Yarczower, M., Wolbarst, M. L., Galloway, W. D., Fligsten, K. E., and Malcolm, R.: Visual acuity in the stumptail macaque. *Science* **152:**1392–1393 (1966).

Yazulla, S.: Intraretinal differentiation in the synaptic organization of the inner plexiform layer of the pigeon retina. *J. Comp. Neurol.* **153:**309–324 (1974).

21

Optokinetic Nystagmus and the Pigeon Visual System

KATHERINE V. FITE

INTRODUCTION

Optomotor or optokinetic nystagmus (OKN) is among the most uni-versal of visually elicited behaviors that can be induced in both ver-tebrates and invertebrates alike. Exposure to a continuously moving pattern of black and white stripes or almost any array of regular or irregular contours will typically elicit a well-defined sequence of pur-suit–saccadic eye and/or head movements. The pursuit or tracking phase (which occurs in the same direction as pattern motion) has traditionally been regarded as an involuntary response to maintain relative stabilization of the moving image(s) on the retina, while the saccadic or return phase enables the fixation of contours just entering the field of view. Bárány (1921) introduced the use of a rotating drum covered with alternating black and white stripes to objectively study visual functions. Subsequent investigators have utilized this technique and OKN to study a wide variety of visual abilities including visual acuity, color vision, motion perception, dark adaptation, binocular rivalry, monocular dominance, and even visual imagery (Smith and Bojar, 1938; Enoksson, 1963, 1968; Fox et al., 1975; Graham, 1970). OKN has also been used extensively in the clinical analysis and diagnosis of neurological impairment and brain damage which are frequently ac-

KATHERINE V. FITE • Department of Psychology, University of Massachusetts, Am-herst, Massachusetts 01002.

companied by disorders of oculomotor function (Reinecke, 1961; Baloh et al., 1977). However, relatively little is known about the neural substrates of OKN, despite numerous studies on a wide variety of species.

Several investigators have suggested that a dichotomy of OKN response types and mechanisms may exist; these have been variously referred to as Look ("Schau") and Stare ("Stier") nystagmus (Ter Braak, 1936, 1962; Fite, 1968) or "active" and "passive" nystagmus (Scala and Spiegel, 1938; Ter Braak et al., 1971), "cortical" and "subcortical" nystagmus (Rademaker and Ter Braak, 1948; Pasik et al., 1959; Ter Braak and Van Vliet, 1963), and "foveal" and "peripheral" OKN (Hood, 1967). Ter Braak (1936, 1962) has described Look or active nystagmus as occurring only in animals with a specialized retinal area or macula and requiring visual attention. Stare or passive nystagmus, on the other hand, presumably occurs in its purest form in animals with no macular vision and serves to counteract the displacement of the entire retinal image. Since OKN can be observed in vertebrates with only rudimentary telencephalic development and in decerebrate mammals and pigeons, several authors have proposed that this subcortically mediated nystagmus may correspond to Stare or passive nystagmus and represent a primitive retinocollicular field-holding reflex (Ter Braak, 1936, 1962; Scala and Spiegel, 1938; Rademaker and Ter Braak, 1948; Walls, 1962, Ter Braak et al., 1971).

OKN can be elicited by stimulation of almost any portion of the retina (Smith and Bojar, 1938); for example, Dodge and Fox (1928) reported a clinical case in which foveal vision was eliminated by a central scotoma, yet OKN could still be induced with peripheral retinal stimulation. More recently, evidence has been presented that suggests two distinct and separate mechanisms mediating the fast phase of OKN in humans, one involving foveal vision and the other being mediated by peripheral vision. Elaborating on an earlier proposal by Bárány and others, Hood (1967) has suggested that foveal nystagmus is controlled by frontal cortical areas controlling voluntary gaze, while peripheral OKN, which is more reflexive in nature, is mediated by occipital cortical visual areas. Dix and Hood (1971) have provided some evidence for this duality of cortical mechanisms from clinical studies. Simultaneous presentation of conflicting central and peripheral OKN stimuli (i.e., movement in opposite directions) leads to different perceptual experiences. Exocentric motion perception (illusion of self-motion) depends on peripheral stimulation when the central field of stimulation is 30 deg or less in diameter, while egocentric motion perception (remaining stationary in a moving surround) and suppression of the perception of self-motion occur when the central stimulus is increased to a diameter of 100 deg (Brandt et al., 1973). Occlusion of foveal vision subtending 5 deg or less produces no observable change in OKN, but further increase in the size of the occlusion leads to a decrease in OKN frequency and amplitude and to its eventual loss with a 30-deg occlusion (Cheng and Outerbridge, 1972). Thus foveal or macular vision does not appear essential for the maintenance of a typical nystagmus in humans.

Relatively few quantitative studies of OKN have been reported for nonmammals, and most of the research has been concerned primarily with the directional asymmetry which occurs with monocular stimulation. Mowrer (1936) first described in pigeons that temporal-to-nasal pattern movement elicited nystagmus, whereas movement in the opposite direction (nasal-to-temporal) produced little or no response. Mowrer believed that this monocular asymmetry was due to the complete decussation of the optic tracts in pigeons, an explanation which now appears to be incorrect, since S. P. Hunt (personal communication) has recently demonstrated that several areas, including the dorsal thalamus, the pretectal complex, and the accessory optic nuclei of pigeons, receive a small number of ipsilateral retinal afferents. Tauber and Atkin (1968) have suggested that the asymmetrical or "unidirectional" OKN occurs in animals that do not have a fovea, while bidirectional or symmetrical OKN occurs only in foveate species. Unfortunately, they erroneously classified the pigeon as afoveate. There are, in fact, two specialized retinal areas in pigeons, a somewhat shallow fovea centralis and a second area dorsalis located in the red field (Galifret, 1968), which are used for lateral and frontal fields of view, respectively.

Since the domestic pigeon has become one of the most frequently studied nonmammalian vertebrates with respect to vision, studies of OKN should be of considerable comparative value in further understanding the complexities and neural mechanisms of this remarkably common, visually guided behavior.

STUDIES OF OKN IN PIGEON

Optomotor Response Types

Two types of optomotor response in the domestic pigeon were described in a study which utilized two rather different methods of stimulus presentation (Fite, 1968), after earlier observations had revealed an apparent mixture of response types. Measurement of the average frequency of saccadic head movements as pattern velocity was gradually increased from low to higher velocities (3–60 deg/sec) revealed a highly regular response whose frequency and amplitude increased as velocity was increased and which ceased abruptly at higher velocities (Fig. 1A). The total number of density of contours in the pattern was varied from 6 to 44 stripes, but no change was observed in the OKN frequency/velocity function. This response thus appeared to be related to the velocity of a single stripe, and was named "Look" nystagmus, in keeping with terminology first introduced by Ter Braak (1936). A second type of optomotor response was observed with discrete, pseudorandom changes in pattern velocity. The topography of this response was irregular, with conspicuous and seemingly random variations in amplitude at any given velocity (Fig. 1B). Although some slight change in the average frequency of head movement occurred at lower velocities (3–24 deg/sec), an asymptotic response frequency was observed beyond approximately 24 deg/sec. However, a marked in-

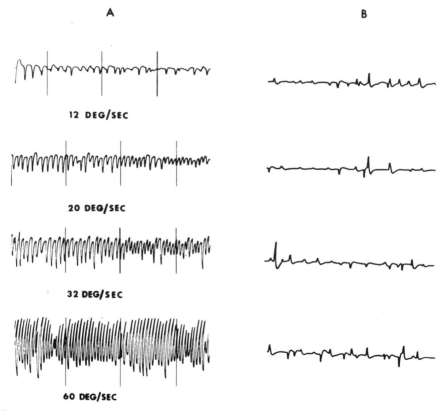

A

B

12 DEG/SEC

20 DEG/SEC

32 DEG/SEC

60 DEG/SEC

Fig. 1. Sample polygraph records of head movements in response to a black-and-white striped pattern moving at velocities of 12, 20, 32, and 60 deg/sec. A: Look nystagmus. B: Stare nystagmus.

crease in the average response frequency was observed with increases in pattern density. When OKN frequency at any given velocity was plotted as a function of the number of stripes (log axis), a linear function was obtained. Thus this second type of optomotor response varied not with pattern velocity but rather with the total number of contours moving in the field of view. This response type was termed "Stare" nystagmus, since it appeared to be based on visual information derived from a large portion of the visual field. Look nystagmus appears to be a genuine pursuit, tracking response, unlike Stare nystagmus, which perhaps should not be labeled "nystagmus" at all, since it is highly irregular in character. However, the quantitative relationships obtained as pattern density was varied raise some new and important questions concerning the ability of pigeons to respond to the number of contours moving in the visual field—a capacity which may be of significance in the context of flight or detection of predators anywhere in the field of view.

Effects of Foveal Lesions

The pigeon retina contains a distinct although somewhat shallow fovea located near the central retina which is used for lateral viewing of distant objects. [Pigeons are hypermetropic for this portion of the visual field (Catania, 1964; Millodot and Blough, 1971; Nye, 1973).] A series of studies was carried out to assess what role, if any, the pigeon fovea plays in Look nystagmus and whether or not the degree of directional asymmetry which occurs with monocular stimulation could be modified following selective destruction of the foveal photoreceptors (Conley, 1975). Both binocular and monocular Look nystagmus response functions were obtained over a stimulus velocity range of 1.5–70 deg/sec. With monocular stimulation, OKN response functions were obtained for both temporal-to-nasal and nasal-to-temporal directions of pattern movement. Discrete foveal lesions were produced under anesthesia with an ophthalmic ruby laser photocoagulator. A barely noticeable change in the appearance of the fundus following a laser pulse indicated a lesion restricted primarily to the photoreceptor layer.

Postlesion measures of Look nystagmus obtained with binocular stimulation revealed little change in the OKN frequency/velocity functions except at the higher pattern velocities. Foveally centered lesions in two birds were correlated with an increase in the range of effective velocities; that is, OKN could be obtained at higher velocity levels than prelesion by some 25–30 deg/sec (Figs. 2 and 3). A similar although less pronounced effect was observed in a third pigeon which received a large foveal lesion in one eye and a parafoveal lesion in the other eye.

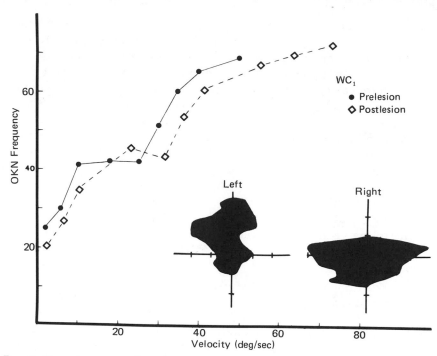

Fig. 2. Binocular pre- and postlesion measures of Look nystagmus: OKN frequency (average number of head movements/min) vs. pattern velocity (deg/sec) for subject WC_1. Insert shows the extent of photoreceptor damage in the foveal center of each eye (1 division = approximately 120 μm).

Using monocular stimulation, three of four subjects showed a more limited range of effective velocities for nasal-to-temporal stimulation but no major differences in OKN frequency when compared with temporal-to-nasal stimulation for the same velocity range. When tested after lesion, foveal lesions in monocularly tested eyes correlated either with no change or with an *increase* in the range of effective velocities for nasal-to-temporal stimulation; thus there was a loss of asymmetry with respect to the effective range of stimulus velocities. This observation is also consistent with the effects obtained using binocular stimulation and foveal lesions in both eyes.

Thus a loss of foveal vision may result in a slight facilitation of nystagmus with respect to the range of effective velocities. If Look nystagmus does reflect a tendency to foveate moving contours, the loss of foveal vision may produce an "open loop," with reduced feedback from this high-acuity retinal area. Far from being adversely affected, Look nystagmus remained quite robust, raising the question of the

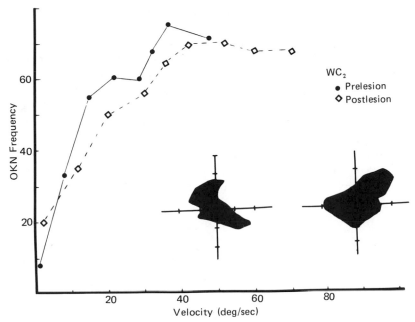

Fig. 3. Similar measurements obtained for subject WC₂ (see Fig. 2 caption).

retinal locus of origin for OKN. Both the large parafoveal area (approximately 10 deg in diameter) and the area dorsalis remain candidates in
this regard. Alternatively, any portion of the retina may mediate Look
nystagmus, with an "equipotentiality" of OKN function. These possibilities can be tested experimentally with lesions in a wide variety of
retinal areas. However, in keeping with observations on humans, foveal stimulation in pigeons is neither necessary nor essential for OKN.

Neural Correlates of OKN

Relatively few studies have examined the neural bases of OKN in
nonmammalian vertebrates despite the advantage of reduced complexity in their nervous systems and visually guided behaviors. Visser and
Rademaker (1934) reported that a decerebrate pigeon showed OKN that
was little different from normal, with the exception that it was somewhat more regular in its occurrence. Similar observations have been
reported following forebrain ablation in frog (Birukow, 1937) and turtle
(Hertzler and Hayes, 1969), visual cortex ablation in cat (Baden et al.,
1965; Spear and Braun, 1969; Wood et al., 1973), and massive cortical
ablations in monkey (Pasik and Pasik, 1964). Furthermore, the optic

tectum does not appear to be essential for OKN in turtles (Hertzler and Hayes, 1969), frogs (Lazar, 1973), or mammals (Proctor, 1962; Collewijn, 1971), including primates (Pasik and Pasik, 1964; Pasik et al., 1966). However, Lazar (1973) has reported that destruction of the nucleus of the basal optic root (nBOR), a major component of the accessory optic system, or section of the basal optic tract completely abolished OKN in frogs. Destruction of the pretectal region also produced some deficits, indicating that both regions play a significant role in mediating OKN in frogs.

Lazar's conclusions are of particular interest, since Karten et al. (1977) have recently demonstrated in pigeons that a unique and little-understood class of retinal neurons—the displaced ganglion cell—pro-

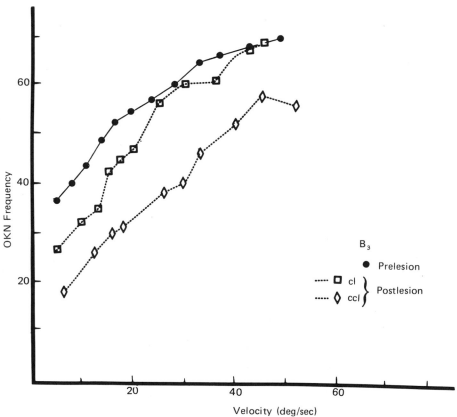

Fig. 4. Binocular OKN response functions obtained before and after bilateral lesions of nBOR in subject B_3. Clockwise and counterclockwise directions of pattern movement are shown separately for postlesion response measures.

ject specifically to nBOR, which is the major component of the accessory optic nuclei in pigeons as well. nBOR, in turn, projects directly to the vestibulocerebellum as mossy fibers terminating within the granule cell layer of folia IXc, IXd, and paraflocculus (uvula). nBOR also projects to the oculomotor complex (Brecha et al., 1977). Both of these projections suggest that this system may play an important role in oculomotor reflexes. Indeed, the size of the displaced ganglion cells (20 × 30 μm) and their extensive dendritic spread indicate that they probably receive information from large retinal areas.

Binocular and monocular Look nystagmus functions were obtained on five pigeons, each of which received bilateral, stereotaxically placed electrolytic lesions in nBOR. Extensive postlesion testing was followed by injections of approximately 100 μCi of [³H]proline into each eye 24–

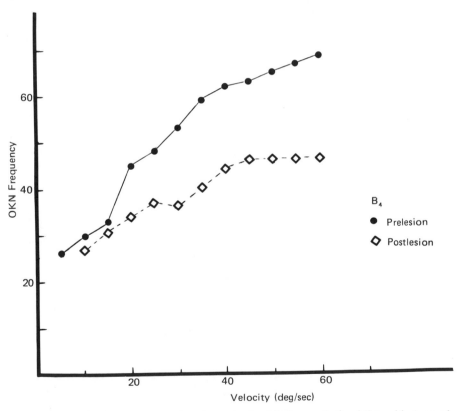

Fig. 5. Binocular OKN response functions obtained before and after bilateral lesions of nBOR in subject B_4.

48 hr prior to sacrifice to enable a precise evaluation of retinal input to each nBOR. In one subject, lesions infringed on nBOR but were incomplete, leaving both nuclei largely undamaged. Postlesion testing in this animal revealed Look nystagmus response functions that were identical to those obtained prelesion. However, in three other birds with substantial or complete bilateral damage to nBOR and no remaining retinal input, the frequency of Look nystagmus was reduced over much of the effective velocity range, particularly at higher velocities (Figs. 4, 5, and 6). The only instance in which OKN could not be obtained after lesion occurred with subject B_3 when tested monocularly with the right eye. As can be seen from Fig. 4, a dissociation of OKN functions was also observed binocularly for clockwise (temporal-to-nasal for the left eye) and counterclockwise (temporal-to-nasal for the right eye) directions of pattern rotation. For subject B_5 (Fig. 6), postlesion testing showed a decrease in OKN frequency above 50 deg/sec, but the response continued up to a velocity of 120 deg/sec.

Thus it appears that the accessory optic system and displaced ganglion cells mediate at least some portion of Look nystagmus in the pigeon, although OKN was not abolished with complete loss of retinal

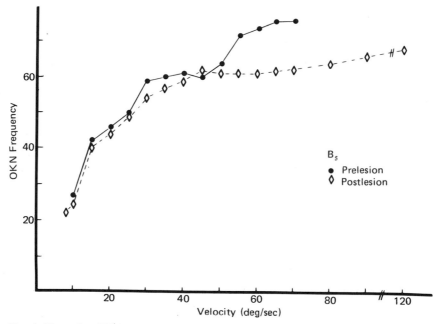

Fig. 6. Binocular OKN response functions obtained before and after bilateral lesions of nBOR in subject B_5.

input to nBOR. The pretectal complex may mediate a substantial portion of this optomotor behavior as well. Many investigators have previously concluded that OKN is not mediated by a single neural structure or "center," and it seems likely that OKN is multiply mediated and distributed throughout the vertebrate visual system. Further studies of OKN in pigeons should be of great value in the future development of a model neural network underlying OKN which may be applicable to a wide variety of vertebrates.

REFERENCES

Baden, J. P., Urbaitis, J. C., and Meikle, T. H.: Effects of serial bilateral neocortical ablations on a visual discrimination by cats. *Exp. Neurol.* **13**:233-251 (1965).

Baloh, R. W., Honrubia, V., and Sills, A.: Eye tracking and optokinetic nystagmus. Results of quantitative testing in patients with well-defined nervous system lesion. *Ann. Otol. Rhinol. Laryngol.* **86**:1-7 (1977).

Bárány, R.: Zur Klinik und Theorie des Eisenbahn-Nystagmus. *Arch. Augenheilk.* **88**:139-142 (1921).

Birukow, G.: Untersuchungen über den optischen Drehnystagmus und über die Sehscharfe des Grasfrosches (*Rana temporaria*). *Z. Vergl. Physiol.* **25**:92-122 (1937).

Brandt, T., Dichgans, J., and Koenig, E.: Differential effects of central vs. peripheral vision on egocentric and exocentric motion perception. *Exp. Brain Res.* **16**:476-491 (1973).

Brecha, N., Karten, H. J., and Hunt, S. P.: A visual quickie: A bisynaptic retinal pathway to the vestibulocerebellum and oculomotor nuclear complex. *Neurosci. Abstr.* 1977.

Catania, A. C.: On the visual acuity in the pigeon. *J. Exp. Anal. Behav.* **7**:361-366 (1964).

Cheng, M., and Outerbridge, J. S.: Optokinetic nystagmus during selective retinal stimulation. *Exp. Brain Res.* **23**:129-139 (1972).

Collewijn, H.: The optokinetic system of the rabbit. *Doc. Ophthalmol.* **30**:227-236 (1971).

Conley, M.: The effects of foveal lesions on optokinetic nystagmus in the domestic pigeon. Unpublished honors thesis, University of Massachusetts (1975).

Dix, M. R., and Hood, J. D.: Further observations upon the neurological mechanism of optokinetic nystagmus. *Acta Otolaryngol.* **71**:217-226 (1971).

Dodge, R., and Fox, J. C.: Optic nystagmus. *Arch. Neurol. Psychiatr.* **20**:812-823 (1928).

Enoksson, P.: Binocular rivalry and monocular dominance studies with optokinetic nystagmus. *Acta Ophthalmol.* **41**:544-563 (1963).

Enoksson, P.: Studies in optokinetic binocular rivalry with a new device. *Acta Ophthalmol.* **46**:71-74 (1968).

Fite, K. V.: Two types of optomotor response in the domestic pigeon. *J. Comp. Physiol. Psychol.* **66**:308-314 (1968).

Fox, R., Todd, S., and Bettinger, L. A.: Optokinetic nystagmus as an objective indicator of binocular rivalry. *Vision Res.* **15**:849-853 (1975).

Galifret, Y.: Les diverses aires fonctionelles de la rétine du pigeon. *Z. Zellforsch. Mikrosk. Anat.* **86**:535-545 (1968).

Graham, K. R.: Optokinetic nystagmus as a criterion of visual imagery. *J. Nerv. Ment. Dis.* **151**:411-414 (1970).

Hertzler, D. R., and Hayes, W. N.: Effects of monocular vision and midbrain transection on movement detection in the turtle. *J. Comp. Physiol. Psychol.* **67**:473–478 (1969).

Hood, J. D.: Observations upon the neurological mechanism of optokinetic nystagmus with especial reference to the contribution of peripheral vision. *Acta Otolaryngol.* **63**:208–215 (1967).

Karten, H. J., Fite, K. V., and Brecha, N.: Specific projection of displaced retinal ganglion cells upon the accessory optic system in the pigeon (*Columba livia*). *Proc. Natl. Acad. Sci. USA* **74**:1753–1756 (1977).

Lazar, G.: Role of the accessory optic system in the optokinetic nystagmus of the frog. *Brain Behav. Evol.* **5**:443–460 (1973).

Millodot, M., and Blough, P.: The refractive state of the pigeon eye. *Vision Res.* **11**:1019–1022 (1971).

Mowrer, O. H.: A comparison of the reaction mechanisms mediating optokinetic nystagmus in human beings and pigeons. *Psychol. Monogr.* **47**:2 Whole No. 212 (1936).

Nye, P.: On the functional differences between frontal and lateral visual fields of the pigeon. *Vision Res.* **13**:559–574 (1973).

Pasik, T., and Pasik, P.: Optokinetic nystagmus: An unlearned response altered by section of chiasma and corpus callosum in monkeys. *Nature (London)* **203**:609–611 (1964).

Pasik, T., Pasik, P., and Krieger, H. P.: Effect of cerebral lesions upon optokinetic nystagmus in monkeys. *J. Neurophysiol.* **22**:297–304 (1959).

Pasik, T., Pasik, P., and Bender, M. B.: The superior colliculi and eye movements. *AMA Arch. Neurol.* **15**:420–436 (1966).

Proctor, L. R.: Experimental observations on postural nystagmus. III. Lesions of the colliculi. *Ann. Otol. Rhinol.* **71**:891–912 (1962).

Rademaker, G. G. J., and Ter Braak, J. W. G.: On the central mechanisms of some optic reactions. *Brain* **71**:48–76 (1948).

Reinecke, R. D.: Review of optokinetic nystagmus from 1974–1960. *Arch. Ophthalmol.* **65**:609–615 (1961).

Scala, N. P., and Spiegel, E. A.: The mechanism of optokinetic nystagmus. *Trans. Am. Acad. Ophthalmol.* **43**:277–299 (1938).

Spear, P. D., and Braun, J. J.: Pattern discrimination following removal of visual neocortex in the cat. *Exp. Neurol.* **25**:331–348 (1969).

Smith, K. U., and Bojar, S.: The nature of optokinetic reactions in mammals and their significance in the experimental analysis of the neural mechanisms of visual functions. *Psychol. Bull.* **21**:309–376 (1938).

Tauber, E. S., and Atkin, A.: Optomotor responses to monocular stimulation: Relation to visual system organization. *Science* **160**:1365–1367 (1968).

Ter Braak, J. W. G.: Untersuchungen über optokinetischen Nystagmus. *Arch. Neerl. Physiol.* **21**:309–376 (1936).

Ter Braak, J. W. G.: Optokinetic control of eye movement, in particular optokinetic nystagmus. In *Optic and Vestibular Factors in Motor Coordination.* International Physiological Congress, Leyden (1962).

Ter Braak, J. W. G., and Van Vliet, A. G. M.: Subcortical optokinetic nystagmus in the monkey. *Psychiat. Neurol. Neurochirug.* **66**:277–283 (1963).

Ter Braak, J. W. G., Schenk, V. W. D., and Van Vliet, A. G. M.: Visual reactions in a case of long-lasting cortical blindness. *J. Neurol. Neurosurg. Psychiat.* **34**:140–147 (1971).

Visser, J. A., and Rademaker, G. G. J.: Die optischen Reactionene grosshirnloser Tauben. *Arch. Neerl. Physiol.* **19**:482–501 (1934).

Walls, G. L.: The evolutionary history of eye movements. *Vision Res.* **2:**69–80 (1962).

Wood, C. C., Spear, P. D., and Braun, J. J.: Direction-specific deficits in horizontal optokinetic nystagmus following removal of visual cortex in the cat. *Brain Res.* **60:**231–237 (1973).

22

Visual Lemniscal Pathways in Birds

HARVEY J. KARTEN

INTRODUCTION

The visual capabilities of birds are more highly developed than those of any other class of vertebrates. Yet until the past decade our understanding of central visual pathways in birds was extremely limited, and even the very components of the visual system were unknown. This chapter is a brief résumé of some of our work of the past decade on the organization of central visual pathways in birds. These studies have not only resulted in a major revision of our concepts of vision in birds and other vertebrates but also markedly altered most of our earlier notions concerning the evolutionary origins of neocortex.

This chapter will deal with only a few limited features of the avian visual system. However, these should provide the reader with an overview and indicate the striking similarities that exist in the organization of the visual system of all vertebrates. I will specifically describe (1) the tectofugal system, (2) the thalamofugal system, and (3) the accessory optic system.

Although several components of the avian visual system were extensively described by Ariens Kappers et al. (1936), the major deficiency of this monumental work was the seeming lack of a concept of

HARVEY J. KARTEN • Departments of Psychiatry and Behavioral Science and Anatomical Sciences, Health Sciences Center–School of Medicine, State University of New York, Stony Brook, New York 11794.

the lemniscal nature of the visual and other sensory systems extending to the telencephalon. The optic tectum was considered to be the single dominant structure in the visual system and was often treated as the "highest visual center" of the avian brain—an apparent condensation of the mammalian tectum-colliculus/geniculostriate system—despite the recognized existence of substantial ascending tectofugal paths to the thalamus. This was perhaps due to three notable problems: (1) the notion that the pronounced laminar development of the optic tectum in birds, combined with the lack of an obvious telencephalic region similar to mammalian striate cortex, meant that the tectum was a functional–morphological equivalent (i.e., analogous, not homologous) of the highly laminated mammalian visual striate cortex; (2) the mistaken belief that the prominent nucleus rotundus thalami received a diversity of inputs in addition to that derived from the optic tectum and hence could not be considered to be a specific visual lemniscal channel; and (3) the failure to recognize the existence of a major ascending visual tectal projection to the thalamus in mammals. This last point is particularly intriguing in any history of our understanding of both avian and mammalian visual systems, for it resulted in the belief of several simultaneously opposing ideas: (1) that mammals lack a tectothalamic system; (2) that mammals are capable of conscious visual abstractions and imagery consequent to the development of the telencephalic elaboration of neocortex, particularly the geniculostriate system; (3) that birds lack a neocortex (a point we know now to be false); (4) that if birds have an ascending tectothalamic system it further bespeaks the unusual nature of the organization of the visual system of this class of vertebrates; (5) that the ascending system in birds does none of the things which are done by the neocortex in mammals. Virtually all these postulates now appear to be erroneous.

There were still further variations on this theme, including the notion that in mammals the degree of development of the striate cortex and that of the tectum were inversely related, i.e., the larger the striate cortex, the smaller the tectum. This was given an evolutionary framework suggesting that functions of the optic tectum were gradually taken over by the striate cortex with an associated diminution in the extent of the tectum. This concept of "encephalization" of vision may have some validity, but is likely to be the consequence of the elaboration of stereopsis with a different manner of processing information probably reflecting major differences in the development and organization of the retina itself. The evidence for this last point, however, still remains largely speculative.

Recent experimental studies in birds, reptiles, and mammals have revealed the fallacious nature of virtually all the original postulates.

These recent studies have shown that (1) birds, reptiles, and mammals all possess distinct ascending tectothalamic projections; (2) lesions of this ascending tectal system in birds, reptiles, and mammals produce strikingly similar deficits; (3) birds, reptiles, and mammals all possess a distinctive thalamofugal system (the extent of development of the thalamofugal system in some birds rivals and exceeds that of some mammals); (4) there is no simple relationship in the relative sizes of the tectofugal and thalamofugal systems.

Indeed, the formulation of the visual system that now emerges is of an amazingly consistent organizational pattern of the visual pathways in all amniotes. Although the pattern of cell assemblies may differ in birds and mammals (e.g., clonal vs. laminar), the identities, sequence of development, and functions of homologous neurons do not appear to differ in any major way.

The modern era of investigation of the pigeon visual system began with the experimental study of retinal projections using the degenerating axon and terminal methods (Cowan et al., 1961). The study was notable in several major regards, foremost being the effective application to a nonmammalian vertebrate of a modified Nauta and Gygax (1954) method for degenerating axons. This study confirmed the pattern of retinal termination within the optic tectum described by Ramón y Cajal (1891,1909) on the basis of his study of Golgi-stained material, projections to the ventral nucleus of the lateral geniculate nucleus, accessory optic nucleus, and various pretectal nuclei, as well as a small but distinct projection directly on the dorsal thalamus. This study also demonstrated the presence of retrograde degeneration in the nucleus isthmoopticus, confirming a much earlier suggestion by Wallenberg (1892) that the nucleus is the source of centrifugal fibers projecting on the retina. The subsequent elegant and extensive investigation on the part of Cowan and his students and co-workers of the centrifugal system and its connections, development, and differentiation during embryogenesis is well known and has recently been summarized by Cowan and Clarke (1976). Excellent and somewhat more detailed studies of the pattern of retinal projections, particularly on the optic tectum, are those of Repérant (1973). Hirschberger (1971), Hunt and Webster (1972), Karten et al. (1973), and Karten and Nauta (1968) also reported the presence of a somewhat more extensive retinal projection on the dorsal thalamus.

TECTOFUGAL SYSTEMS

Karten and Revzin (1966), Revzin and Karten (1966/1967), and Karten and Hodos (1970) demonstrated that the stratum griseum centrale

(SGC) of the optic tectum gives rise to an ascending projection on the ipsilateral nucleus rotundus thalami. Karten, Hodos, and Revzin pursued a series of experiments that appear to justify the conclusion that the nucleus rotundus is a specific visual relay nucleus, which projects in turn on the ectostriatum of the telencephalon. Studies by Hunt (1973) and Hunt and Kunzle (1976a,b) using autoradiography further revealed that the optic tectum also projects on the contralateral nucleus rotundus, a finding further substantiated by Benowitz and Karten (1976) using retrograde transport of horseradish peroxidase (HRP) (see Fig. 1).

Benowitz and Karten (1976) further demonstrated the complex organization of this pathway. The SGC of the optic tectum was found to contain at least four sublaminae, each projecting on cytoarchitectonically distinct portions of the nucleus rotundus. Furthermore, a separate portion of the nucleus rotundus was found to receive an input from the nucleus subpretectalis (SP) (see Fig. 2). Karten and Hodos (1970) reported that the nucleus rotundus projects in a seemingly topograpic fashion on the ectostriatal core (E) but apparently does not directly enter or terminate within the surrounding smaller-celled periectostriatal belt (Ep). Benowitz and Karten (1976) discovered that the topography of the rotundoectostriatal system consists of at least five parallel subsets, with each subnucleus of rotundus projecting on a separate subnucleus of the ectostriatal core (Fig. 2). More recently, Cohen and his collaborators investigated the subsequent projections of the ectostriatal core, using a variety of anatomical and physiological methods. Ritchie and Cohen (1977) suggested that the core region projects on the Ep, and Ep projects on a variety of targets, including the neostriatum intermedium laterale (NIL) and a sharply restricted portion of the archistriatum intermedium (Ai) (Fig. 3). Zeier and Karten (1971) reported that the portion of the archistriatum involved in this system is the source of a series of descending connections to the brainstem and optic tectum, and more recently Brecha et al. (1976) have demonstrated that the region of Ai receiving the Ep projection projects predominantly on laminae 11, 12, and 13 of the ipsilateral tectum. The pattern of projections is similar to that known to arise from various lateral cortical areas, including the extrastriate cortices and the inferotemporal cortex of mammals. Karten (1969) and Nauta and Karten (1970) further suggested that parts of the archistriatum specifically and selectively resemble layers V and VI of the mammalian neocortex. Indeed, the findings of Karten and co-workers and the recent findings of Ritchie and Cohen (1977) of serial and reciprocal connections of E, Ep, NIL, and Ai are reminiscent of the intrinsic connections of neocortex, particularly regions such as areas 18, 19, 20, and 22 and the inferotemporal cortex of mammals. We may even speculate that the various subdivisions of the

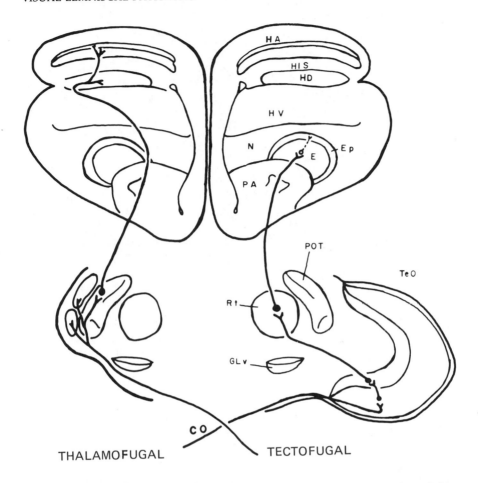

THALAMOFUGAL   TECTOFUGAL

Fig. 1. General schematic of the two major ascending visual lemnisci to the telencephalon. On the right is a tectofugal pathway from retina to tectum (TeO) to rotundus (Rt) to the core nucleus of the ectostriatum (E). The core nucleus projects on the periectostriatal belt (Ep). On the left is the thalamofugal system. This channel appears directly comparable to the geniculostriate system of mammals, with the notable exception of a totally crossed optic nerve projection on the laminated nucleus of the dorsal thalamus (POT). This nucleus projects in turn on a highly laminated portion of the telencephalon, the Wulst, consisting of arrangements of sharply defined laminae, histologically comparable to the mammalian striate cortex. The dorsal thalamus also projects to the contralateral Wulst via the dorsal supraoptic commissure (not shown in this schematic).

ectostriatum represent the avian equivalent of the specific thalamore-cipient neurons of different extrastriate cortical areas of mammals.

   In the mid-1960s, the justification for such a conclusion on the part of Hodos and Karten (1966) was tenuous at best. There was scant evidence at that time in support of the presence of an ascending tec-

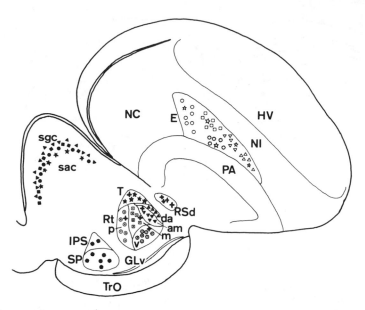

Fig. 2. Topography within the tectofugal system. Ascending projections from the tectum arise from separate sublaminae of the SGC, with each lamina projecting on discrete subdivisions of the nucleus rotundus (Rt). Each of these divisions in turn projects on a discrete domain of the ectostriatal core (E). The topography of this system is indicated by distinct symbols for each sublaminar of tectum on each subdivision of rotundus and of ectostriatum.

tofugal pathway in mammals. The subsequent work of Hall and Diamond (Hall and Ebner, 1970; Diamond, 1973), however, demonstrated that the optic tectum of many mammals projects directly on the nucleus lateralis posterior-inferior pulvinar of the thalamus. The LP-IP complex in turn projects on a variety of extrastriate and middle temporal cortices. These more recent studies now appear to fully justify the original suggestions of Karten, Hodos, and Revzin (Karten and Revzin, 1966; Revzin and Karten, 1966/1967; Karten and Hodos, 1970) concerning the striking similarity of the ascending tectofugal systems of birds and mammals. Hall and Ebner (1970) were further able to demonstrate the presence of this system in turtles and other reptiles.

Behavioral studies on the part of Hodos and Karten (1966, 1970) demonstrated that lesions of this system resulted in severe deficits in visual discrimination. These deficits were again virtually identical to deficits produced by lesions of the corresponding mammalian tectofugal lemniscus described by Diamond (1973), in a variety of mammals, and still more recently by Sprague et al. (1977) in the cat.

Electrophysiological studies of the tectal efferent system by Revzin

(1970), however, resulted in several rather confusing findings. Although clear evidence of a retinotopic projection was found in the superficial layers of the tectum, recordings from the SGC, rotundus, or ectostriatum yielded responses with receptive fields of extremely large dimension (up to 90 deg and occasionally even larger). These findings were most puzzling, as traditional descriptions of the receptive fields of the visual system have always emphasized receptive fields of 0.25–1 deg, with occasional fields of up to 10 deg. Revzin (this volume) has presented evidence of the existence of subsets within the rotundus that correspond to the cytoarchitectonic subfields recently described by Benowitz and Karten (1976) with receptive fields of extraordinarily complex nature, yet distinct and characteristic of each subset. Recordings from the mammalian LP-IP complex are exceedingly rare and do not yet permit detailed comparisons to results in birds.

    Needless to say, we are still far from any reasonable understanding of the mode of operation of the optic tectum or the nature of the transform of narrow receptive fields to virtually global receptive fields found in SGC, rotundus, and ectostriatum (Revzin, 1970). The very

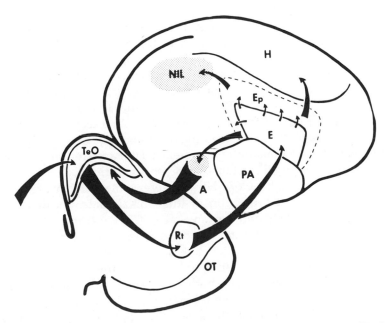

Fig. 3. Subsequent projections of the ectostriatal core based on the studies of Ritchie and Cohen (1977). This figure demonstrates the sequential projections of E on Ep and thence on both neostriatum (NIL) and a distinct portion of the archistriatum (A). The region of A indicated projects back on the optic tectum in a manner similar to that of the projections of mammalian extrastriate visual cortex on the optic tectum.

antiquity of the system and its elaborate development not only in birds but also in reptiles and mammals stress its probable importance in visual processing. Indeed, rather than justifying the concept that the striate cortex of mammals "takes over" functions of the optic tectum, we must now further seek to understand the operations of the optic tectum if we hope to gain further insight into the functions of those extrastriate areas now known to play so important a role in visual performance. For a detailed statement of this concept, the reader is referred to the recent review by Hodos (1976).

THALAMOFUGAL SYSTEM

The thalamofugal system is also known in mammals as the geniculostriate system. Until the past decade, the prevailing notion of the visual system was that the geniculostriate system in mammals evolved to a point of dominance whereupon the tectal system was consigned to relatively mechanical visuomotor operations. It was also suggested that the striate cortical system (area 17) is a uniquely mammalian possession, without significant precedent in nonmammalian vertebrates. Thus by 1966 this led to the seemingly paradoxical conclusion that birds and presumably reptiles had a tectofugal system but no thalamofugal system, whereas mammals had a thalamofugal system but no tectofugal (i.e., tectothalamic) system. By the late 1960s, Diamond and co-workers had effectively demonstrated that mammals possess a very substantial tectofugal system functionally similar to that of birds. While these findings indicated the ubiquity of ascending tectal systems in all vertebrates, they also emphasized the differences between mammalian and nonmammalian thalamofugal systems. This apparent disparity implied that thalamofugal systems were an evolutionary development unique to mammals. In 1967, Hirschberger noted the presence of a massive direct retinal projection on the dorsal thalamus of the owl. Karten and Nauta (1968) and Karten et al. (1973) confirmed this finding in the burrowing owl (*Speotyto cunicularia*) and further noted that the thalamic terminal field contained five or more subnuclei, possibly resembling the various subdivisions or laminae of the mammalian dorsal nucleus of the lateral geniculate body. In keeping with most studies of avian retinal pathways, however, Karten et al. (1973) found the system to be almost totally crossed at the level of the optic chiasm. Employing degeneration methods, Karten and Nauta (1968), Hunt and Webster (1972), and Karten et al. (1973) traced the efferent connections of the dorsal thalamic complex (designated as the OPT or nuclei opticus principalis thalami) in pigeon and owl. They found that each OPT projected *bilaterally* on the telencephalon, bypassing the previously described ectostriatum and entering and terminating in a laminated structure on the dorsal hemisphere, the so-called Wulst (German for "bump" or "elevation"). The Wulst posterior, the specific region of termination, was found to consist of nominally six layers, with a prominent bilaminate granule cell layer (HIS ext and HIS int) forming the third layer from the bottom. This laminar appearance was most apparent in the well-developed owl Wulst. In both histological appearance and pattern of termination, the posterior Wulst bore a striking resemblance to the striate cortex (area 17) of mammals.

Furthermore, the *efferent* connections of the posterior Wulst were amazingly reminiscent of the connections of the mammalian striate cortex, with projections on the dorsal thalamus (OPT) and ventral nuclei or the lateral geniculate, pretectal nuclei, and the superficial layers of the optic tectum. Of particular note was the presence of a projection from the posterior Wulst on the Ep of the tectofugal channel.

The peculiar arrangement of a totally crossed retinal projection but with a bilateral projection from the OPT on the Wulst also seemed to indicate that birds, despite the totally crossed retinal path, should also be capable of stereopsis, but by recrossing of thalamic axons rather than by partial crossing of primary retinal fibers. These findings were confirmed in the pigeon, although the OPT and the Wulst were substantially smaller than in the bifrontal-eyed owl.

These results provided an anatomical explanation of Revzin's (1970) earlier observations of the existence of a discrete retinotopic projection on the Wulst in the pigeon. Of note in this later report was the fact that the receptive fields in the Wulst were small (0.25-2 deg) with only rare receptive fields of up to 10 deg, and clearly different from the fields found in the rotundoectostriatal system. Pettigrew and Konishi (1976) have recorded visual responses from the posterior Wulst of barn owls and confirmed Revzin's report of a clear-cut retinotopic map in the owl Wulst and of the presence of laminarly disposed simple, complex, and hypercomplex cells in various layers of the Wulst, with simple cells predominantly found in the granule cell layer (IHA). Pettigrew and Konishi were further able to demonstrate that the preponderance of units were binocularly responsive, with many "disparity detectors" similar to those reported in mammalian striate cortex. No significant differences were found in the Wulst of owls and the striate cortex of cats.

Pettigrew (personal communication) subsequently extended his earlier studies on barn owls to hawks, kites, and ducks, as well as other species of owls. He suggested that the relative size of the visual Wulst is directly proportional to the degree of binocular overlap and, therefore, presumbly to the degree of development of stereopsis in different birds. These findings might even lead the unwary or enthusiastic reader to conclude that perhaps the striate cortex is not related to "mammal likeness" but rather to the simpler parameter of ocular overlap and stereopsis. I must confess to a certain simple-minded bias on my part in favor of that hypothesis. The argument is certainly not impaired by the recently reported confirmation from several laboratories that lesions in mammals, when confined to the striate cortex without involvement of areas 18, 19, 20, or 22, appear to cause little deficit in visual discrimination (Sprague et al., 1977). Perhaps the role of the striate cortex in visual discrimination has been somewhat overstated.

Hodos and Karten (1974) found that lesions in pigeon OPT and visual Wulst produced meager deficits in visual discrimination performance. The extent of this system in pigeons, however, is much smaller than in the owl, and when such lesions in pigeons were combined with lesions of the tectofugal system, the resultant deficits were far more drastic than with either system alone. Perhaps a fruitful area for further research may be in the study of the details of the interaction between those two systems.

ACCESSORY OPTIC SYSTEM (AOS)

More recently our interests have turned to another major target of the retina and its subsequent projections, the accessory optic system (AOS) and the accessory optic nuclei (AON) (Ariens Kappers et al., 1936; Giolli, 1961, 1963, 1965; Hayhow, 1959, 1966; Tigges, 1966; and Tigges and Tigges, 1969). Their very names suggest the scant attention they have received over the past hundred years. The preponderance of interest in the geniculostriate system (thalamofugal) in mammals, and the emphasis on the optic tectal system in nonmammalian forms, reflected an attempt to conceptualize a functioning visual system centered around a single major structure with other components of progressively lesser importance.

First discovered in mammals by von Gudden in 1881, the largest component of the AOS, the medial terminal nucleus, was subsequently found to occur in virtually all major classes of sighted vertebrates (Ariens Kappers et al., 1936). One of the most striking of its features in many vertebrates is the large size of retinal axons entering this nucleus (Herrick, 1948) and the distinctiveness of a separate tract from the retina to the AON. The tract is called the basal optic root (BOR) in pigeons (Gillilan, 1941; Cowan et al., 1961). The terminal nucleus of the BOR in birds has been called a variety of names, including the nucleus of the basal optic root (nBOR), the nucleus ectomammilaris (nEM), the medial terminal nucleus (MTN), and the nucleus opticus tegmenti. The second-order connections and functions of the accessory optic nuclei were unkown in all vertebrates,although a variety of speculations as to their functions and connections have been advanced over the years, most notably in amphibians and mammals. Thus Herrick (1948) proposed that the BOR of amphibia provided a very-high-speed channel input to nBOR, which projected in turn on the oculomotor complex, resulting in a rapidly responding orienting response to a peripheral stimulus. The primary data supporting a connection with the oculomotor complex, however, were not very persuasive despite the generally high esteem in which Herrick's researches were held. A quite different suggestion emerged from the work of Moore et al. (1967). These authors suggested that in rats the MTN mediated photic stimulation of the pineal and the control of melatonin and estrus. Yet there was little morphological, physiological, or behavioral evidence to support any decisive conclusion concerning its function in any class of vertebrates.

Most recently we have been able to define the afferent and efferent connections of the nBOR in the pigeon, and have substantial evidence to support Herrick's original proposal both in pigeons and in a variety of other classes of vertebrates (Fig. 4).

The initial finding of note was the discovery by Brauth and Karten (1975, 1977), Reiner and Karten (1978), and Finger and Karten (1978), using the retrograde transport of horseradish peroxidase (HRP), that the nBOR projects directly on the vestibulo-cerebellum. Following injections of HRP into the uvula and paraflocculus, Brauth and Karten noted heavy bilateral retrograde labeling of cells of the nBOR. The axons of the nBOR were found to project on the cerebellum via a descending tract, the brachium conjunctivum cerebellopetale (BCP). Following disruption of the BCP unilaterally, there was extensive retrograde cell loss in the *ipsilateral* nBOR (Brauth and Karten, 1977). More recently, Reiner and Karten (unpublished observations) observed massive ipsilateral labeling of nBOR following HRP injections into the BCP. In order to further explore and confirm this projection, Brecha et al. (1977) injected tritiated proline into the nBOR unilaterally. The resultant autoradiographs (ARG) not only confirmed the initial findings of Brauth and Karten revealing the precise projections into the cerebellum but also demonstrated the pathway on the oculomotor complex proposed by Herrick (1948). The efferent axons of nBOR neurons enter the BCP and descend ipsilaterally to the cerebellum. The axons course caudally within the cerebellum to enter the uvula and paraflocculus. The axons of the nBOR were distributed bilaterally within folia

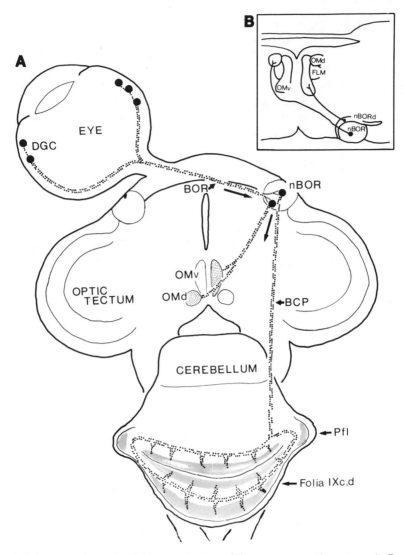

Fig. 4. Summary schematic of the organization of the accessory optic system. A: Projection of peripherally located displaced ganglion cells on the nBOR, which in turn projects directly on both oculomotor nuclei and the vestibulocerebellum. B: Differential projection of the nBOR on the various subdivisions of the oculomotor complex.

IXc and IXd and paraflocculus, and ended within the granule cell layer as mossy fiber terminals (Brecha et al., 1977; Brecha and Karten, 1979).

Perhaps of even greater note was the discovery of a direct projection from the nBOR on the oculomotor complex (Brecha et al., 1977; Brecha and Karten, 1979). More specifically, a projection was found on the ipsilateral ventromedial components of the oculomotor complex and a separate projection on the contralateral dorsolateral nucleus. In order to confirm this projection, we also performed three additional studies: (1) lesions were placed in the nBOR and the brains stained for degeneration, (2) a large dose of tritiated proline was placed in the eye and the oculomotor complex examined for evidence of transynaptic transport, and (3) HRP was placed in the oculomotor complex. While the degeneration study confirmed the presence of a projection from the region of the nBOR on the same divisions of the oculomotor nuclei following large doses of isotope in the contralateral eye, the multiplicity of retinal targets and the presence of transported label to second-, third-, and perhaps even fourth-order structures did not permit the conclusion that the oculomotor projection necessarily arose from the nBOR. The final line of evidence, one we believe to be most convincing, was the demonstration of retrograde transport of HRP from the oculomotor complex to the nBOR. The nBOR complex was seen to consist of three separate components: the nBOR proper, the nBOR pars dorsalis (nBORd), and the nBOR pars lateralis (nBORl). Following unilateral injections of HRP into the oculomotor complex, labeled cells were consistently found in the ipsilateral nBORd and in the contralateral nBOR proper (Brecha et al., 1977; Brecha and Karten, 1979).

These findings were most extraordinary, as they seemed to fully confirm Herrick's original suggestion based on his study of the amphibian visual system using nonexperimental methods. Perhaps equally astounding was the realization that what was found to be the case for birds and amphibians is also likely to be true for virtually all other major classes of vertebrates. In pursuit of this possible generality, Finger and Karten (1978) recently demonstrated the existence of the accessory optic nucleus in catfish and goldfish and its projection on the cerebellum. Observations by Reiner in my laboratory demonstrated the existence of a similar system in turtles (Reiner and Karten, 1978). Studies on the possible presence of a projection on the oculomotor complex in teleosts and reptiles are still in progress.

As mentioned above, however, one of the most striking features of nuclei of the AOS is the prominence of the retinal fiber tract and the large size of its axons in many vertebrates. This well-established observation prompted us to further examine the BOR tract itself, count the number of axons, and determine a fiber spectrum of these axons. Brecha, Karten, Hunt, and Laverack (unpublished data) found that the BOR contained approximately 4500 axons, ranging in size from 2 to 11 μm in diameter. All the axons were heavily myelinated. A precise count, comparable to those obtainable on peripheral nerves, was not possible as the BOR only forms a separate and distinct tract caudal to the optic chiasm. Furthermore, it lies on the lateral margin of the hypothalamus and precise delineation of its dorsal margin proved difficult. Following enucleation of the contralateral eye, fibers of all diameters were found in various stages of degeneration. Binggeli and Paule (1969) reported that the optic nerve of the pigeon contained 1.8 million myelinated axons and 0.6 million unmyelinated axons. Thus the BOR constituted approximately 0.15% of the optic nerve. A fiber spectrum of the BOR and adjacent optic tract indicates a bimodal distribution of axon diameters, with BOR forming a larger and distinct population of axons when compared to the optic tract directed towards the optic tectum.

These observations led to the hopeful anticipation that we might be dealing with a distinctive class of retinal ganglion cells specifically directed to the nBOR. The large size of these axons prompted us to believe that we might be able to selectively label the nBOR with HRP and identify the cells of origin of the BOR. Following injections of HRP confined to the nBOR, Karten et al. (1977a) found labeling in a distinctive and most unusual population of ganglion cells, the displaced ganglion cell of Dogiel (1891) (DGC) (Fig. 5). The DGC is characterized by its presence in the inner nuclear layer at the margin of the inner plexiform layer. The cells are very large (up to 20 by 30 μm), with a prominent axon and with large dendrites confined to layer 1 of the IPL. The morphology of the labeled cells was identical to that shown by Ramón y Cajal in his description of the DGCs of Dogiel. DGCs were never labeled following tectal injections.

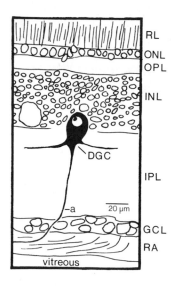

Fig. 5. Camera lucida drawing of a typical displaced ganglion cell found to project on the nBOR.

Although we encountered some variation in our ability to completely label the nBOR stereotaxically, in several cases with complete injections of the nBOR we counted the total number of labeled cells in the contralateral retina. The number of labeled DGCs was between 3800 and 4800, depending on the individual case. This was a most satisfying correspondence with the fiber count of the BOR (approximately 4500) (Karten et al., 1977a).

These findings suggested that the DGCs constitute a distinctive class of cells rather than an anomaly due to failure of migration of ganglion cells during development. Furthermore, they appear to represent a functional grouping specifically directed to only a single target, the nBOR, and they presumably mediate specific functions, i.e., eye movements in response to peripherally moving stimuli. In a broad sense, seen from the perspective of the projection of the nBOR on the cerebellum, the nBOR might be compared to the column of Clarke. The DGCs might then be compared to dorsal root ganglion cells innervating, e.g., muscle spindles, and provide information on the rate of movement of a visual stimulus (or in the case of muscle spindles the rate of contraction of a muscle with the corresponding implication for the rate of movement of a joint).

This led to the question of distribution of the DGCs within the retina and their dendritic morphology. Although we are still in the process of gathering this information, we have sufficient data to report the following: (1) DGCs are large cells with dendrites confined to layer 1 of the IPL; (2) DGCs characteristically have three primary dendrites disposed at approximately 120 deg angles to each other, forming an equilateral triangle; (3) DGCs are most dense at the periphery of the retina and decrease in number toward more central portions of the retina; (4) DGCs are generally most frequent in the inferior temporal retina; (5) In the periphery, the spacing between cells is approximately 140 μm; (6) DGCs, especially in the periphery, form approximations of hexagonal arrays. All of these features are consistent with Herrick's original hypothesis that the nBOR system is a rapidly responding system sensitive to peripheral movements and resulting in orienting movements of eyes and neck to the source of the stimulus.

Physiological data on this system unfortunately are still sparse. Recordings from the nBOR in rabbits (Marg, 1964; Walley, 1967) indicate that the cells of nBOR respond over very large receptive fields, prefer moving stimuli, and show some degree of directional selectivity. Preliminary observations in the pigeon (Revzin, personal communication) also indicate receptive fields that are greater than 30 deg, are movement sensitive and directionally selective, with little response from the region of the area centralis. This last observation is consistent with the study of Galifret (1966). Galifret noted that foveal lesions produced little evidence of axonal degeneration to the nBOR. Fite et al. (unpublished data) found little evidence of labeled DGCs in the region of the fovea.

Our current formulation as to the operation of this system suggests that the nBOR receives its exclusive input from DGCs and that DGCs do not project to any other targets. The DGCs are arrayed mainly in the peripheral retina in a highly ordered fashion, probably in adjacent contiguous fields. They have wide receptive fields sensitive to motion and direction. We presume that they react to moving stimuli and signal the nBOR as to the relative size, speed, and direction of movements of objects as they first appear in the periphery of the visual field. The nBOR directly effectuates an oculomotor response and provides a mossy fiber input to the vestibulo cerebellum. This portion of the cerebellum also receives an input from the vestibular receptors and from the vestibular nuclei, and has an output both to the deep cerebellar nuclei and on the vestibular complex. This latter circuit may provide further compensatory adjustments in both neck and oculomotor neurons. The overall function of this circuit may be to bring the central portion of the retina onto the peripheral stimulus, i.e., the DGCs may trigger a foveopetal movement. The same circuit may operate to keep rapidly moving objects on the fovea. Since the density of DGCs decreases markedly in the region of both the fovea and the red field, the system would again come into action if the object had a tracking speed either higher or lower than the tracking speed of the eye. Thus, as the object drifted off from regions of high acuity, it would again turn on the DGCs and reactivate the circuit. In view of the abovementioned characteristics of the DGCs, we do not believe that they are involved in any form of fine discrimination or fine tracking. This interpretation is also consistent with Lazar's (1972) observation of the participation of the nBOR in optokinetic nystagmus (OKN). OKN consists of both a fast and a slow phase response to vertical stripes moving across the visual field (e.g., railroad nystagmus). OKN may be considered to be a rapid sweep to a peripheral stimulus, fixation on an object, then fine tracking of the object until it passes out of the visual field. At that point another rapid sweep occurs until the eye again fixes on an object, fine tracking, etc. I suggest that lesions of the nBOR may particularly disrupt the rapid sweep phase of OKN.

Further research is necessary to clarify the nature of DGC response, the location of the receptive fields of DGCs, the effect of DGC activation on intracellular responses of the nBOR, the nature of synaptic transmitters, the morphology and physiology of nBOR projections on the oculomotor complex, the precise innervation of the specific muscles by the dorsolateral and ventromedial oculomotor complex, the effect of mossy fibers of the nBOR on cerebellar output in relationship to vestibular inputs, as well as the ontogeny of the system. In regard to this last point, we can already state that on the basis of available data the nBOR not only receives the largest retinal axons but also is among the first of the central visual structures to develop (Karten, unpublished observations) as well as one of the first to receive retinal innervation (Crossland, personal communication). These findings are also consistent with the suggestion of Herrick that this is an early, high-speed system of great survival value to the animal. To the degree that we may suppose that systems arising early in ontogeny reflect phylogenetic antiquity as well as function essential to the survival of the animal, the DGC-nBOR system may well be a candidate for one of the primal mechanisms of visual function. The subsequent sequence of development reveals that the tectofugal system is next to develop and the thalamofugal last to develop among these three lemniscal channels of the visual system in birds. We anticipate that a similar sequence may be characteristic of many other classes of vertebrates as well.

CONCLUSION

In conclusion, we can point to two major consequences of this line of research. The broadest implications are that the avian and mammalian visual systems, indeed the brain itself, follow a fundamentally similar pattern of organization in both of these major classes of vertebrates. One of the major goals of comparative neuroanatomy is to determine the possible existence of universal patterns of neural organization of vertebrate brains. Classical vertebrate neuroanatomy had earlier shown this to be the case for the majority of brain stem structures. This work has extended the validity of this generalization to the thalamus and telencephalon as well. Subsequent work by students of the reptilian brain has demonstrated striking similarities in the organization of the visual system of this major class of vertebrates, permitting us to conclude that there exists a consistent pattern of organization of visual and other systems common to all amniotes, and probably to all vertebrates. The success of this project reflects the validity of the underlying logic of the concept of the comparative approach. The comparative approach claims that the neural circuitry underlying functions common to closely related vertebrate forms is likely to be mediated by homologous neuronal structures. The conclusion, however, reflects to some degree the principle of uncertainty and may at times prove dangerously tautological. The demonstration that common structures mediate common functions also has been relied on to reinforce the postulated proximity of relationships of different vertebrates.

The second major consequence of this research pertains more directly to the issue of the visual system of pigeons, and of birds in general. Both birds and mammals are outstanding among vertebrates for their diversity of behavior and their flexible responses to novel situations. Comparative behaviorists have long noted that birds are truly competitive with the most "intelligent" of mammals in their performance on visual and other discriminative tasks. Until only 10 years ago, the prevailing notion was that the sophistication of avian visual performance was mainly a consequence of the functions of the optic tectum. This implied that birds could do feats with their optic tectum that, in mammals, required the operations of the geniculostriate and extrastriate cortical systems. This earlier concept treated the avian forebrain as a neurological structure concerned with elaborating fixed action patterns as a result of cognitive decision-making on the part of the optic tectum and other brainstem structures. This concept must now be completely revised. The avian thalamus and telencephalon seem to participate in information processing and transformation in a manner still indistinguishable from that performed by the mammalian thalamus and cortex. Indeed, the next major step in our work must be an attempt to understand the differences, not the similarities, in anatomy and function of the avian and mammalian visual forebrain structures. Although a superficial examination of the avian brain may indicate that it lacks the large formal structure of the neocortex, we do not know whether that, in fact, accounts for the functional differences that may occur in processing ability of these two classes of vertebrates. Indeed, we do not even know if there are such differences. The work of Hodos and his colleagues [see Hodos, (1976) for review] has demonstrated that under conditions of careful study many of the purported differences in the functional role of homologous structures prove evanescent. Thus study of the avian visual system actually promises to reveal not only the operations of the visual system of birds but even novel insight into the operational functions of the mammalian neocortex.

In retrospect, when our work first began, Hodos and I had the terribly simple-minded idea that the avian brain provided a simpler nervous system for the analysis of the vertebrate brain. Fortunately for us, we didn't know any better at that time. In truth, we have learned as much about the mammalian visual system as we have about the avian visual system and brain. That should be sufficient justification in an age that has increasingly restricted its research support to projects of "obvious applicability" and "sound research design on problems of urgent merit." Students of the Talmud have long been trained to believe in studying for the pure sense of learning. The exhilaration of novel insights in itself is sufficient motivation to carry on.

ACKNOWLEDGMENT. The author acknowledges the support of National Institutes of Health grants NS 12078 and EY 02146 in pursuit of this research.

REFERENCES

Angaut, P., and Réperant, J.: Fine structure of the optic fiber termination layers in the pigeon optic tectum: A Golgi and electron microscope study. *Neuroscience* **1**:93 (1976).

Ariens Kappers, C. U., Huber, G. C., and Crosby, E. C.: *The Comparative Anatomy of the Nervous System of Vertebrates, Including Man.* Macmillan, New York (1936).

Benowitz, L. I., and Karten, H. J.: Organization of the tectofugal visual pathway in the pigeon: A retrograde transport study. *J. Comp. Neurol.* **167**:503–520 (1976).

Binggeli, R. L., and Paule, W. J.: The pigeon retina: Quantitative aspects of the optic nerve and ganglion cell layer. *J. Comp. Neurol.* **137**:1–18 (1969).

Brauth, S. E., and Karten, H. J.: Direct accessory optic projections to the vestibulocerebellum: A possible channel for oculomotor control systems. *Exp. Brain Res.* **27**:73–84 (1977).

Brauth, S. E., and Karten, H. J.: Accessory optic nuclear projections to the flocculonodular lobe of the cerebellum: A possible channel for eye-neck control systems. *Neurosci. Abstr.* **1**:217 (1975).

Brecha, N., Karten, H. J., and Hunt, S. P.: A visual quickie: A bisynaptic retinal pathway to the vestibulocerebellum and oculomotor nuclear complex. *Soc. Neurosci. Abstr.* **3**:554 (1977).

Brecha, N., and Karten, H. J.: Accessory optic projections upon oculomotor nuclei and the vestibulocerebellum. *Science.* In press. (1979).

Brecha, N., and Karten, H. J.: A visual climbing fiber input to the vestibulocerebellum: An accessory optic-inferior olivary-vestibulocellar projection system. *Soc. Neurosci. Abstr.* **4** (1978a).

Brecha, N., and Karten, H. J.: Projections of the accessory optic nuclei and vestibular nuclei upon the oculomotor nuclear complex in pigeon. *Anat. Rec.* **190**:605–606 (1978b).

Brecha, N., Hunt, S. P., and Karten, H. J.: Relations between the optic tectum and basal ganglia in the pigeon. *Neurosci. Abstr.* **1**:95 (1976).

Cowan, W. M., and Clarke, P. G. H.: The development of the isthmo-optic nucleus. *Brain Behav. Evol.* **13**:345–375 (1976).

Cowan, W. M., Adamson, L., and Powell, T. P. S.: An experimental study of the avian visual system. *J. Anat. (London)* **95**:545–563 (1961).

Diamond, I. T.: The evolution of the tectal-pulvinar system in mammals: Structural and behavioral studies of the visual system. *Symp. Zool. Soc. London* (1973).

Dogiel, A. S.: Uber die nervösen Elemente in der Retine des Menschen. *Arch. Mikro. Anat.* **38**:317–344 (1891).

Finger, T., and Karten, H. J.: The accessory optic system in teleosts. *Brain Res.* **153**:144–149 (1978).

Galifret, Y.: Le système visuel du pigeon: Anatomie et physiologie—Correlations psychophysiologiques. Thèses présentées à la faculté des Sciences de l'Université de Paris (1966). P. 167.

Galifret, Y. : Les diverses aires fonctionelles de la rétine du pigeon. Z. Zellforsch. Mikrosk. Anat. 86:535-545 (1968).

Gillilan, L. A.: The connections of the basal optic root (posterior accessory optic tract) and its nucleus in various mammals. J. Comp. Neurol. 74:367-408 (1941).

Giolli, R. A.: An experimental study of the accessory optic tracts (transpeduncular tracts and anterior accessory optic tracts) in the rabbit. J. Comp. Neurol. 117:77-95 (1961).

Giolli, R. A.: An experimental study of the accessory optic system in the cynomolgus monkey. J. Comp. Neurol. 121:89-108 (1963).

Giolli, R. A.: An experimental study of the accessory optic system and of other optic fibers in the oppossum (Didelphis virginiana). J. Comp. Neurol. 124:229-242 (1965).

Hall, W. C., and Ebner, F.F.: Thalamo-telencephalic projections in the turtle (Pseudemys scripta). J. Comp. Neurol. 140:101-122 (1970).

Harting, J. K.: Descending pathways from the superior colliculus: An autoradiographic analysis in the rhesus monkey (Macaca mulatta). J. Comp. Neurol. 173:583 (1977).

Harting, J. K., Hall, W. C., Diamond, I.T., and Martin, G. F.: Anterograde degeneration study of the superior colliculus in Tupaia glis: Evidence for a subdivision between superficial and deep layers. J. Comp Neurol. 148:361 (1973).

Hayes, B. P., and Webster, K.E.: An electron microscopic study of the retino-receptive layers of the pigeon optic tectum. J. Comp. Neurol. 162:447 (1975).

Hayhow, W. R.: An experimental study of the accessory optic fiber system in the cat. J. Comp. Neurol. 113:281-313 (1959).

Hayhow, W. R.: The accessory optic system in the marsupial phalanger (Trichosurus vulpecula): An experimental degeneration study. J. Comp. Neurol. 126:653-673 (1966).

Hayhow, W. R., Webb, C., and Jervie, A.: The accessory optic fiber system in the rat. J. Comp. Neurol. 115:187-215 (1960).

Herrick, C. J.: The Brain of the Tiger Salamander, Ambystoma tigrinum. Univ. of Chicago Press, Chicago (1948).

Hirschberger, W.: Histologische Untersuchungen an den primaren visuellen Zentren des Eulengehirnes und der retinal Repräsentation in ihnen. J. Ornithol. 108:187-202 (1967).

Hirschberger, W.: Vergleichend experimentell-histologische Untersuchungen zur retinalen Repräsentation in den primaren visuellen Zentren einiger Vogelarten. Unpublished thesis, Frankfurt am Main (1971).

Hodos, W.: Vision and the visual system: A bird's eye-view. In Sprague, J. M., and Epstein, A. M. (eds.): Progress in Psychobiology and Physiological Psychology, Vol. 6 Academic Press, New York (1976). Pp. 29-62.

Hodos, W., and Karten, H. J.: Brightness and pattern discrimination deficits in the pigeon after lesions of nucleus rotundus. Exp. Brain Res. 2:151-167 (1966).

Hodos, W., and Karten, H. J.: Visual intensity and pattern discrimination deficits after lesions of ectostriatum in pigeons. J. Comp. Neurol. 140:53-68 (1970).

Hodos, W. and Karten, H. J.: Visual intensity and pattern discrimination deficits after lesions of the optic lobe in pigeons. Brain Behav. Evol. 9:165-194 (1974).

Hodos, W., Bonbright, J. C., Jr., and Karten, H. J.: Visual intensity and pattern discrimination after lesions of the thalamofugal visual pathway in pigeons. J. Comp. Neurol. 148:447-467 (1973).

Hunt, S. P.: A study of forebrain visual areas in the pigeon. Ph.D. thesis, University College, London (1973).

Hunt, S. P., and Kunzle, H.: Observations on the projections and intrinsic organization of the pigeon optic tectum: An autoradiographic study based on anterograde and retrograde axonal and dendritic flow. *J. Comp. Neurol.* **170**:153 (1976a).

Hunt, S. P., and Kunzle, H.: Selective uptake and transport of label within three identified neuronal systems after injections of ³H-GABA into the pigeon optic tectum: An autoradiographic and Golgi study. *J. Comp. Neurol.* **170**:173 (1976b).

Hunt, S. P., and Webster, K. E.: Thalamo-hyperstriate interrelations in the pigeon. *Brain Res.* **44**:647–651 (1972).

Hunt, S. P., and Webster, K. E.: The projection of the retina upon the optic tectum of the pigeon. *J. Comp. Neurol.* **162**:433 (1975).

Jassik-Gerschenfeld, D., and Guichard, J.: Visual receptive fields of single cells in the pigeon's optic tectum. *Brain Res.* **40**:303 (1972).

Jassik-Gerschenfeld, D., Minois, F., and Conde-Courtine, F.: Receptive field properties of directionally selective units in the pigeon's optic tectum. *Brain Res.* **24**:407 (1970).

Jassik-Gerschenfeld, D., Guichard, J., and Tessier, Y.: Localization of directionally selective and movement sensitive cells in the optic tectum of the pigeon. *Vision Res.* **15**:637 (1975).

Karten, H. J.: The organization of the avian telencephalon and some speculations on the phylogeny of the amniote teleucephalon. In Noback, C., and Petros, J. (eds.): *Comparative and Evolutionary Aspects of the Vertebrate Central Nervous System. Ann. N.Y. Acad. Sci.* **167**:146–179 (1969).

Karten, H. J.: Projections of the optic tectum of the pigeon (*Columba livia*). *Anat. Rec.* **151**:369 (1965).

Karten, H. J.: Efferent projections of the wulst of the owl. *Anat. Rec.* **169**:353 (1971).

Karten, H. J., and Hodos, W.: Telencephalic projections of the nucleus rotundus in the pigeon (*Columba livia*). *J. Comp. Neurol.* **140**:35–52 (1970).

Karten, H. J., and Nauta, W. J. H.: Organization of retino-thalamic projections in the pigeon and owl. *Anat. Rec.* **160**:373 (1968).

Karten, H. J., and Revzin, A. M.: The afferent connections in the nucleus rotundus in the pigeon. *Brain Res.* **2**:368–377 (1966).

Karten, H. J., Hodos, W., Nauta, W. J. H., and Revzin, A. M.: Neural connections of the "visual wulst" of the avian telencephalon. Experimental studies in the pigeon (*Columba livia*) and owl (*Speotyto cunicularia*). *J. Comp. Neurol.* **150**:253–277 (1973).

Karten, H. J., Fite, K., and Brecha, N.: Specific projection of displaced retinal ganglion cells upon the accessory optic system in the pigeon (*Columba livia*). *Proc. Natl. Acad. Sci. USA* **74**(4):1753–1756 (1977).

Karten, H. J., Fite, K., Brecha, N., and Hunt, S. P.: Projections of displaced cells in the pigeon (*Columba livia*). *Invest. Opthalmol. Visual Science* (Abstr.) **16**(4):87 (1977).

Lazar, G. : Role of the accessory optic system in the optokinetic nystagmus of the frog. *Brain Behav. Evol.* **5**:443–460 (1972).

Marg, E.: The accessory optic system. *Ann. Acad. Sci.* **117**:35–52 (1964).

Moore, R. Y., Heller, A., Wurtman, R. J., and Axelrod, J.: Visual pathway mediating pineal response to environmental light source. *Science* **155**:220–223 (1967).

Munzer, E., and Wiener, H.: Beitrage zur Anatomie und Physiologie des Central-Nerven-Systems der Taube. *Monatschr. Psychiat.* **3**:379 (1898).

Nauta, W. J. H., and Gygax, P. A.: Silver impregnation of degenerating axon terminals in the central nervous system: A modified technique. *Stain Tech.* **29**:91–93 (1954).

Nauta, W. J. H., and Karten, H. J.: A general profile of the vertebrate brain with sidelights on the ancestry of cerebral cortex. In Schmitt, F. O. (ed.): *The Neurosciences: Second Study Program.* Rockefeller Press, New York (1970). Pp. 7–26.

O'Flaherty, J. J.: A Golgi analysis of the optic tectum of the mallard duck. *J. Hirnforsch.* **12**:389 (1970).

Pettigrew, J. D., and Konishi, M.: Neurons selective for orientation and binocular disparity in the visual wulst of the barn owl (*Tyto alba*). *Science* **193**:657–678 (1976).

Ramón y Cajal, S.: Sur la fine structure du lobe optique des oiseaux et sur l'origine réele des nerfs optiques. *Int Monatschr. Anat. Physiol.* **8**:337 (1891).

Ramón y Cajal, S.: *Histologie du Système Nerveux des Hommes et des Vertebrés.* Maloine, Paris (1911).

Reiner, A., and Karten, H. J.: A bisynaptic retinocerebellar pathway in the turtle. *Brain Res.* **151**:163–169 (1978).

Repérant, J.: Nouvelles données sur les projections visuelles chez le pigeon (*Columba livia*). *J. Hirnforsch.* **14**:151 (1973).

Repérant, J.: The orthograde transport of horseradish peroxidase in the visual system. *Brain Res.* **85**:307–312 (1975).

Repérant, J., and Angaut, P.: The retinotectal projections in the pigeon: An experimental optical and electron microscope study. *Neuroscience* **2**:119 (1977).

Revzin, A. M.: Some characteristics of wide-field units in the brain of the pigeon. *Brain Behav. Evol.* **3**:195 (1970).

Revzin, A. M., and Karten, H.J.: Rostral projections of the optic tectum and the nucleus rotundus in the pigeon. *Brain Res.* **3**:264–276 (1966/1967).

Ritchie, T. C., and Cohen, D. H.: The avian tectofugal visual pathway: Projections of its telencephalon target ectostriatal complex. *Neurosci. Abstr.* **3**:94 (1977).

Rodieck, R. W.: *The Vertebrate Retina: Principles of Structure and Function.* Freeman, San Francisco (1973).

Shanklin, W. M.: The comparative neurology of the nucleus opticus tegmenti with special reference to *Chameleon vulgaris. Acta Zool.* **14**:163–184 (1933).

Sprague, J. M., Levy, J., DiBernardino, A., and Berlucchi, G.: Visual cortical areas mediating form discrimination in the cat. *J. Comp. Neurol.* **172**:441–488 (1977).

Tigges, J.: Ein experimentellen Beitrag zum subkortikalen optischen System von *Tupaia glis. Folia Primatol.* **4**:103–123 (1966).

Tigges, J., and Tigges, M.: The accessory optic system in *Erinaccus* (Insectivora) and *Galago* (Primates). *J. Comp. Neurol.* **137**:59–70 (1969).

von Gudden, B.: Ueber den Tractus peduncularis transversus. *Arch. Psych.* **11**:415–423 (1881).

Wallenberg, A.: Das mediale Opticusbundel der Taube. *Neurol. Centralbl.* **17**:S.532 (1892).

Walley, R. E.: Receptive fields in the accessory optic system of the rabbit. *Exp. Neurol.* **17**:27–43 (1967).

Zeier, H., and Karten, H. J.: The archistriatum of the pigeon: Organization of afferent and efferent connections. *Brain Res.* **31**:313–326 (1971).

Index